The
ESSENTIAL
MASSAGE COMPANION

The
ESSENTIAL
MASSAGE COMPANION

Everything You Need to Know
to Navigate Safely Through Today's Drugs and Diseases

Dr. Bryan A. Born

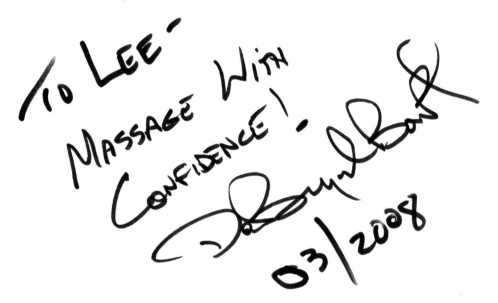

To Lee —
Massage with
Confidence!

03/2008

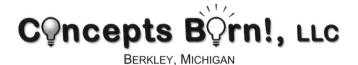

Concepts Born!, LLC

BERKLEY, MICHIGAN

The Essential Massage Companion
Everything You Need to Know to Navigate Safely Through Today's Drugs and Diseases
Bryan A. Born, B.S., D.C.

Published by:
Concepts Born, llc
PO Box 721335
Berkley, MI 48072-0335 USA

Order@ConceptsBorn.com
www.ConceptsBorn.com

FIRST EDITION

10 9 8 7 6 5 4 3 2

ISBN, print edition   0-9749258-0-2

Library of Congress Control Number: 2004096623

Cover Design by Cathi Stevenson, www.BookCoverExpress.com
Graphics by Michael Born

Printed in the United States of America

The publishers have made every effort to trace the copyright holders for borrowed material. If they have inadvertently overlooked any, they will be pleased to make the necessary arrangements at the first opportunity.

We have done our best to make an accurate book. If you discover errors or omissions, please email your findings to comments@ConceptsBorn.com and corrections will be made.

Visit us on the Web:
www.theEssentialMassageCompanion.com

Acknowledgements

Many people have contributed to this monumental endeavor, and my apologies first and foremost to those whom I neglect to mention.

Most importantly, this book would never exist without the strength, love and commitment of my wife, Dr. Carol Born. Her insight, wisdom and support have been critical in my life and the success of this book.

I am indebted to my parents Dr. Bruce Born and Dr. Mary Born, for whom I owe my health, my intelligence, and my fortitude.

I am grateful to have worked with four outstanding principal editors:

Mary Born, ND	Eric Crytzer, JD
Sandi Lynch, ACE	Denise Mussio, CTM

Other colleagues who have provided text review and critical guidance include:

Garry Adkins, NCTMB	Carol Bell, NCTMB	Phil Cutrell, NCTMB
Randy Fillion, NCTMB	Irene Gauthier, CTM	Kathy Gauthier, MSA
Kirk Kelly, DC	Michele Ladiski, BS	Kathy Peltier, MT
Michael Rice, NCTMB	Jeanette Roach, NCTMB	Janet Schrock, NCTMB

Technical supporters included Jonathon Kramer and R. W. Schuck, BSBA.

Graphics and artwork are the genius of Michael Born: Designer, illustrator, brother and treasured friend.

---

*This book is dedicated to the unheralded
therapist, nurturing their passion
to help and heal others.
May you now be free to touch those
in need without fear or uncertainty.*

About the Author

Dr. Bryan Born was persuasively recruited to create a class about pathology for an emerging massage therapy school in southeast Michigan in 1993. He began collecting materials for a series of class handouts. During this period his wife, Dr. Carol Born, was directing the Physical Therapy department at a local hospital. She commented one evening that she'd hired two massage therapists to provide massage room-by-room, but there was no massage reference guide for them to look up the conditions the clients were being treated for. That began the journey that has culminated in the book you now hold.

A second generation Chiropractic Physician, Dr. Born has guided therapists through the complex interactions between massage and disease for over a decade, and his love for teaching shines in his lectures as well as in this book. His energy-filled, passionate teaching style continues to make his pathology program the favorite for many students at Irene's Myomassology Institute in Southeast Michigan. He thrives in clinical practice with his wife, mother and father (all doctors), and continues being taught the wonders of vibrant health by his thriving children, Jessica and Sarah.

Table of Contents

Disclaimer

This book is designed to provide information about the subject matter covered. It is sold with the understanding that the publisher and author are not engaged in rendering legal, medical, or other professional services. If legal, medical, or other expert assistance is required, the services of a physician or another competent professional should be sought.

It is not the purpose of this book to reprint all the information currently known and available to therapists and health care professionals but to crystallize the most practical aspects of that knowledge.

Every effort has been made to make this book as complete and accurate as possible. However, there may be mistakes both typographical and in content. The rapid increase of health information almost makes this a given. Therefore, this text should be used only as a general reference and not as the ultimate source of information. It is not intended in any way to treat any illness.

Medication names, symptoms, effects and side effects are limited to those pertaining to the practice of massage and are an incomplete list. Refer to the documentation that was presented with the medication for a complete reference.

The authors, Concepts Born, L.L.C. and the publishers shall have neither liability nor responsibility to any person or entity with respect to any loss or damage caused or alleged to be caused directly or indirectly by the information contained in this book.

If you do not wish to be bound by the above, you may return this book to the publisher for a full refund.

Introduction

In his book entitled *"Influence, Science and Practice,"* Dr. Robert Cialdini stated that 85 percent of everything we know today *did not exist before 1965.* In my clinical practice every technique and nutritional model has been fundamentally upgraded in the last decade, and I see this trend throughout all of healthcare. Technology has given us remarkable insight into the human condition, and the rate at which new insights are revealed. The sheer volume of information is a heavy load for any professional to keep pace with.

There are undoubtedly more comprehensive texts teaching massage technique and pathophysiology, and this author holds those texts in great esteem. Many of them have been referenced in the making of this quick-reference guide. Those tomes, however, are missing two key ingredients, which are the backbone of *The Essential Massage Companion.* This is the first comprehensive indexed guide covering over 3,000 brand name and generic drugs, specifically focused on the precautions for massage therapy. There is no other published text today in which a massage professional can quickly reference any drug name and read exactly what they must be concerned with concerning their massage techniques.

The Essential Massage Companion also debuts the TILE method of categorizing massage techniques. Over 130 specific massage techniques are grouped in four intensity gradients: TOLERANCE, INCREMENTAL, LIGHT, and ENERGY. Until now there has been no industry-wide standard for understanding massage restrictions within the framework of each style. A bewildering variety of treatment styles refer to "gentle" and "non-invasive," yet there is no objective standard for those words. I think you'll find the TILE system uniquely objective and easy to understand. It accurately guides the therapist to the safest techniques for each condition while giving the greatest amount of professional discretion.

I maintained the "need-to-know" philosophy throughout the text. Life-threatening drug reactions and symptoms are listed at the top of each category. All symptoms pertaining to the practice and effects of massage in all its forms are included. It is a refreshingly direct approach for the time-conscious therapist looking for guidance about the client in their office.

Ten years in the making, you can be reassured that you are holding the most up-to-date information on diseases and drugs, in a format that will maximize your knowledge yet allow you to stay focused on the client's needs. You'll find it the essential companion for your professional security and success.

Bryan A. Born, B.S., D.C.

How To Use This Book

About This Book

I designed *The Essential Massage Companion* to make your life easier as you work with your clients. You don't have to read this book cover to cover and memorize it. Instead, each condition, medical term, abbreviation and drug is listed in the index for easy reference.

Need to know about a condition your client has? Jump right in, and in seconds you have specific information to make your massage safe and effective. And don't worry about keeping precautions in your head for their next visit. The next time you need to recall the precautions, just go back and in seconds you'll have everything you need. There is extra space in the margin of each page to write notes, and feel free to dog-ear the pages too! The more you make the book uniquely yours, the more you'll get out of it.

What This Book is Not About

All drug and disease descriptions have been edited for reading by a healthcare professional for the sole purpose of making educated decisions about their course of action.

This book is not intended as medical advice for the treatment of any disease. It is not an endorsement of any medicine, and self-medicating is strongly discouraged. Consult the proper health care authority for treatment or medication concerns. For a complete listing of the side effects and warnings for any medication, please refer to the insert that came with the prescription.

Conventions Used in This Book

Keeping things consistent makes them easier to understand and will speed up your ability to quickly find what you need. I have made every attempt to define *new terms* (shown in italics) on the same page. Even so, there are over 1,500 terms in the glossary. Odds are good that you'll never need a medical dictionary with *The Essential Massage Companion* at your side!

Every drug class and condition begins with a brief description. Your time is short, so this book focuses on concise, useful facts rather than lengthy explanations. The chemical name (also called the *generic* name) is underlined, and the brand names follow each in parentheses. Example: cyclobenzaprine (Cycloflex, Flexeril).

The TILE System

The TILE system is the most comprehensive tool available for the massage therapist to accurately determine what can and cannot be performed with the client based upon their condition. The four columns signify the four massage technique classifications: TOLERANCE, INCREMENTAL, LIGHT, and ENERGY. Each is explained in greater detail below. The height of the blocks in each column signifies the relative intensity of the technique, with TOLERANCE techniques having the greatest pressure intensity, and ENERGY techniques having the least intensity. Over 130 massage techniques have been researched and categorized based upon the technique's goals and pressure intensity.

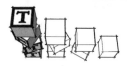 **Tolerance Massage Techniques**

This group consists of massage techniques that routinely use an intense pressure. This pressure is typically beyond the client's "comfort zone" (assuming their senses are not dulled by medications or disease). These techniques have the greatest effect on the circulatory system and may include a local inflammatory reaction to the pressure.

TOLERANCE techniques typically are goal-oriented, striving for greater function or mobility. They typically instigate an active healing response by the body. For example, if the therapist determines that adhesions have formed between a tendon and adjacent tissues, s/he may consider using a deep friction massage across the tendon to break up the adhesions. This forces the body to clean up the remnants and patch up torn tissue. The end result is an improvement in flexibility and function, but it relies heavily upon a properly functioning body to finish the repairs.

Because TOLERANCE techniques are the most taxing to the body and may also be emotionally strenuous, this class of techniques are the first to be eliminated whenever the client's healing strength or resilience is in question.

Massage techniques in the TOLERANCE category include: Ashiatsu Oriental Bar Therapy, Canadian Deep Muscle Massage, Cross-Fiber Massage, Deep Tissue Massage, Endermologie, Hellerwork, Korean Martial Therapy, Lypposage, Myofascial Release, Myoskeletal Alignment Technique, Pfrimmer Deep Muscle Therapy, Postural Integration, Rebalancing, Rolfing, Soft Tissue Release, Soma Neuromuscular Integration, and Structural Integration.

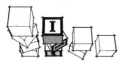 **Incremental Massage Techniques**

There is a wide range of different techniques in the INCREMENTAL group. They typically begin with a relatively light pressure and become more intense as the session progresses. The therapist strives to stay within the client's "comfort zone" with these techniques. This is the common theme linking these techniques together in the INCREMENTAL group. All stretching techniques fall under this classification.

INCREMENTAL techniques also actively stimulate an improvement in the lymph and circulatory systems. The benefits of this stimulation are well established. However, for the same reason that they are powerful stimulators of the healing response, they can have a dramatic effect if the body is unable to handle these effects.

The INCREMENTAL massage techniques may be prohibited for a number of reasons. The body may be overwhelmed by the dramatic circulatory changes that these techniques can create, as explained above. The client may be under the influence of medication that prevents the body from properly reacting to this level of stimulation, such as anti-inflammatory or heart medications. In some instances, the client's immune system may be too fragile from a current or recent condition to handle INCREMENTAL techniques. You may interpret the effects of your techniques differently than this guide; be sure to fully research the client's condition and how it reacts to massage, as well as the medications taken for this condition before disregarding this precaution. Many of the techniques listed here may be considered TOLERANCE techniques if the pressure intensity is high, or LIGHT techniques if the pressure intensity is low. The more knowledgeable you are about your techniques and their effects, as well as your client's conditions, the safer and more effective you will be.

Massage techniques in the INCREMENTAL category include: Acupressure, AcroSage (Inversion Therapy), Amma, Applied Kinesiology, Aston-Patterning, Ayurvedic Massage, Balinese Massage, Berrywork, Bindegewebmassage, Bioenergetics, Biosync, Body Rolling, Bowen Technique, Chair Massage, Champissage, Chi Nei Tsang, Connective Tissue Massage, Conscious Bodywork, Foot Zone Therapy, Gua Sha, Hakomi, HEMME, Hoshino Therapy, Hot Stone Massage, Jamu Massage, Jin Shin Do, Kripalu Bodywork, Kriya Massage, Lastone Therapy, Lomilomi, Lonsdale Method, Looyen Work, Massotherapy, Medical Massage, Movement Therapy, Muscle Energy Technique, Muscle Release Technique, Myomassology, Myotherapy, Naprapathy, Neuro-Structural Bodywork, Neuromuscular Therapy, Nikkon (Okazaki) Restorative Massage, Nuad Bo Rarn, Nuat Thai, Onsen Technique, Orthopedic Massage, Oshiatsu, Prenatal/Pregnancy Massage,

Reflective Healing, Reflexognosy, Reflexology, Reichian Release, Reposturing Dynamics, Restoration Therapy, Russian Massage, Shiatsu, Spinal Release, Sports Massage, St. John's Neuromuscular Therapy, Strain/Counterstrain, Swedish Massage, Taikyo Shiatsu, Tantsu Tantric Shiatsu, Thai Massage, Touch For Health, Trigger Point Myotherapy, Tui Na, Vibrational Healing Massage Therapy, Visceral Manipulation, Watsu, Yogassage, Zen Shiatsu, and Zero Balancing.

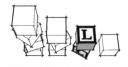 ## Light Massage Techniques

LIGHT massage techniques all include touching the client's body with some application of pressure. My personal definition of light pressure is significantly different than other therapists; indeed, sometimes their "light" techniques go way beyond my comfort zone! After considerable research into the effects of light pressure massage and the techniques listed below, I have come to the conclusion that any discussion of light pressure should include the effects on the body as well as the client's perception. With the vast array of medications available to the client to boost their emotional and physical pain threshold, it falls upon the therapist to determine how much is too much. Obviously, if it is painful to the client, then it falls outside the realm of LIGHT pressure.

This class of technique includes goals for mental relaxation and relief. Physical goals include increasing circulation and reducing tension through nervous system relaxation rather than more intense physical pressure. LIGHT techniques are less likely to be considered "muscle massage" techniques, even though certain mobility techniques would fall into this category. Any stretching is limited to fingertip pressure.

The upper limit of light pressure can be demonstrated as follows: Place your hand palm down on a hard surface. Slowly begin applying pressure with the pad of your middle finger, stopping when you see a whitening of the nail bed by the distal (outer) edge. That pressure or less can be considered light massage pressure.

Massage techniques in the LIGHT category include: Alexander Technique, Bindi, Body-Mind Centering, Breema Bodywork, Esalen Massage, Feldenkrais, Huna Kane, Ingham Method, Insight Bodywork, Integrative Massage, Lymph Drainage Therapy, M Technique, Manual Lymph Drainage, Ortho-Bionomy, Rubenfeld Synergy Method, Trager Approach, Trauma Erase, and UNTIE.

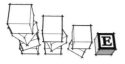 **Energy Massage Techniques**

These techniques may or may not have the therapist make physical contact with the client. Any touch is without pressure and incidental to the technique. This is the only classification in which there is no direct, localized increase in circulation. As a result, almost all conditions can benefit from these techniques. There are notable exceptions listed in the guide, however, so it is still recommended that the therapist reference each condition and not assume that the client is always safe with these techniques. The goals are focused on improving the client's energy, vitality and sense of well-being.

<u>Massage techniques in the ENERGY category include</u>: Attunement Therapy, Barbara Brennan Healing Science, Bioenergy, Biofeedback, Bio-Magnetic Touch Healing, Body-talk, Christopher Method, Craniosacral Therapy, Earth Energy Healing, EMF Balancing Technique, Energy Flow Balancing, Haelan technique, Healing Touch, Holographic Memory Release, Jin Shin Jyutsu, Kundalini Energization, Lenair Technique, Mariel Technique, Polarity Therapy, Pranic Healing, Qigong, Quantum Energetics, Quantum-Touch, Reiki, Ro-Hun Transformation Therapy, Rosen Method Bodywork, Shen Therapy, Shinkiko, Syntropy Insight Bodywork, Therapeutic Touch, Tibetan Point Holding, Trauma Touch Therapy, Tuina Chinese Medical Massage, Turaya Touch System, and Vortex Healing Energetic Therapy.

Individual Interpretation

It must be understood that there is considerable variance within each massage technique. Each therapist also adds a unique quality to his or her techniques. For instance, one therapist's application of Myomassology techniques (listed in the INCREMENTAL class) may be up to the limit of the client's tolerance, in which case it might be more appropriate for that therapist to classify their "normal" massage higher than what is listed in this guide. Likewise, it is entirely possible to perform reflexology techniques (also listed in the INCREMENTAL class) using no pressure whatsoever, thereby enabling this technique to be acceptable for those conditions in which ENERGY techniques are recommended. This guide draws upon the unique skills and knowledge of the therapist to accurately determine the correct classification for their techniques.

Each client will present with a unique set of conditions. It is especially important to note the precautions for every condition the client presents with. For example, the client may have osteoporosis, requiring one set of precautions, and diabetes, which has another set. All precautions should be adhered to.

In this increasingly litigious society it is critical that the therapist has an accurate method of documenting the pressure and scope of each massage session. Applying the TILE method to daily sessions and notes will give the therapist the secure knowledge that s/he is providing the most accurate and appropriate precautions known for client safety.

Icons Used in This Book

Here are all the TILE icons as they will appear with each condition. When you see the caution symbol replacing the letter, it signifies that this class of technique is prohibited. Remember, TILE is an acronym for the four technique classes, and the icons represent the relative intensity from the most intense (TOLERANCE) to the least (ENERGY).

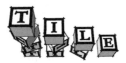

This TILE icon is completely full, which indicates that your full range of massage techniques are encouraged without restriction.

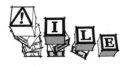

This icon has the TOLERANCE class removed and replaced with a caution symbol. When you see this icon it indicates that the INCREMENTAL, LIGHT and ENERGY techniques are encouraged, but TOLERANCE techniques should be avoided.

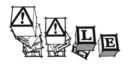

This icon has both the TOLERANCE and INCREMENTAL class of techniques removed and replaced with caution symbols. LIGHT and ENERGY techniques are encouraged.

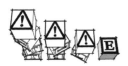

When you see this icon, no circulatory massage should be performed. All pressure techniques should be avoided. ENERGY techniques are encouraged.

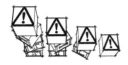

There are certain situations or conditions that are life threatening, and any intervention by a therapist may prove disastrous. If you see this icon, avoid all techniques until the client has stabilized and their physician has given approval.

There are four additional icons following the TILE icon and general precautions:

 This icon alerts you to symptoms that may constitute a medical emergency, or other circumstances that may prohibit general massage. If discussion with the client's physician is necessary, it is explained here.

 This icon tunes you into warnings about specific precautions. Look for these icons to find out what body parts or techniques to avoid in your massage session.

 This icon is used to explain the drug classes that may be prescribed for the current disease. It is also used to list the generic and brand name drugs in the medication sections.

 Because our clients rely on us for hope and inspiration, discussion about every disease ends on a positive note. I use this icon for positive practice tips and hope-inspiring thoughts.

Where To Go From Here

Chapter 1 leads you through stress and the healing response, and Chapter 2 takes an in-depth look at cancer through the eyes of a massage therapist. Feel free to read through those chapters to refresh your knowledge about disease in general. Chapters 3 through 11 discuss conditions and diseases system by system. Jump to any part that interests you, and don't feel as though you're missing something. Every condition is packaged with the information you need, and it will specifically point you to other sections as needed.

Remember, the index may be your best starting point, as every important word is included. Looking for a drug, but don't know its exact spelling? Start your search in the index. As long as you have the first few letters correct, you'll be able to spot the word there. All drugs are listed both by their generic (chemical) name, as well as all possible brand names. Every name for each disease can be found in the index, along with every word in the glossary and each medical abbreviation. It's all there for you!

If you're simply feeling overwhelmed, flip through the book for motivating words of encouragement. These are scattered throughout to remind you of the incredible potential you have for positive change in yourself and your clients. Be well informed as well as inspired with *The Essential Massage Companion*!

*Stress is neither good nor bad—
It's simply a part of life. Our
ability to handle stress molds and
shapes us and controls our
quality of life.
The good or bad lies in each of us.*

*You are a member of a noble
profession. By helping others
improve their ability to handle
life's stresses, you make
a positive change
that can last a lifetime.*

Chapter 1

Stress and the Healing Response

Stress

There are three kinds of stress: Physical, mental and chemical. These come in two different intensities: Macrotrauma and microtrauma. Macrotrauma is like a guillotine. It's subtle like a train wreck. It is the obvious injury, accident, or fall, a significant trauma that occurs in a single event.

Microtrauma is the subtle stresses we subject our body to over the course of a lifetime: The *"death by a thousand cuts."* Poor posture, airborne chemical toxins, and mental stress are all examples of microtrauma. They are often considered insignificant and forgotten in the big health picture. Microtrauma and macrotrauma must be combined for a complete stress evaluation.

Physical

Physical stress includes anything that acts upon our body, from lifting heavy objects to incorrect posture. It includes poor shoes, soft beds and bad work ergonomics, as well as accidents, sprains, strains and other injuries.

Mental

Numerous studies have linked stress with decreased immune response. For example, when laboratory animals are physically restrained, exposed to inescapable electric shocks, or subjected to overcrowding, loud noises, or maternal separation, they show decreased immune system activity. Researchers have reported similar findings for humans.

It is well documented that mental stress affects our physical body; indeed, it is the type of stress we think of when we are "under stress".

Chemical

GIGO is a computer acronym for Garbage In, Garbage Out. It applies equally to the human body. In the 2004 documentary *"Super Size Me,"* filmmaker Morgan Spurlock set out to eat only fast food for thirty days. He was given a clean bill of health by a team of physicians and monitored frequently throughout the month. Before the month was out his doctors called his condition "obscene" and "outrageous," comparing the liver damage that Spurlock had begun to suffer to that of an alcoholic. This occurred in less than thirty days!

A lack of nutrition is as chemically traumatic as toxic chemicals. One must consider both in evaluating chemical stress.

Davis' Law

Increased stress to the tissues of the body stimulates growth of that tissue. This is a fundamental law. We typically refer to Davis' law in its opposite: *"If you don't use it, you lose it!"* If you increase stress to any tissue, it will grow, and if you stop all stress to a tissue it atrophies and dies. This is our normal body maintenance in action, from calluses on our feet to skeletal muscle strength.

Wolff's Law

"Bone is rebuilt more if there are stresses on the bone, less if there are not." This affects the tissues providing structure for the body. Wolff's law explains the effects of stress on the bones, causing both osteoporosis in an inactive limb and bone spurring in a hyperactive or overstressed ligament.

*Work your magic
to help your client relieve stress,
and know that you play
a significant role
in improving
their quality of life!*

The Healing Response

Tissue inflammation and repair occurs in three phases: The inflammatory phase, the proliferation (repair) phase, and the maturation (remodeling) phase.

Phase One -- The Inflammatory Phase

Acute inflammation is a protective response. The moment a trauma occurs, the body responds with vasoconstriction to limit blood loss. This lasts from seconds to minutes depending upon the severity of the trauma.

In the next fifteen minutes, the body releases chemicals causing capillary vasodilation and cellular infiltration. The swollen cells provide a "cast" of the area and limit the spread of possible infection. White blood cells and clotting agents are deposited.

The body maintains this state for the first three days after the onset of trauma, unless the area is further exacerbated. If additional trauma or infection occurs, this "timer" is reset and acute inflammation increases as a response to the new level of injury.

There are four components of the inflammatory response:

> ➢ Redness
>
> ➢ Swelling
>
> ➢ Heat
>
> ➢ Pain

The result is a loss of function for the inflamed tissues. If you sprain your ankle, the swelling prevents you from using it. Likewise, nephritis inhibits the proper functioning of the inflamed kidney.

Inflammation is ever-present and a vital friend of all circulatory massage techniques. Even LIGHT techniques cause tissues to be torn on a microscopic level. The body reacts with inflammation to begin the healing process. When the inflammation is visible or can be felt by the therapist, all circulatory massage is contraindicated.

P.R.I.C.E.

There are five action steps involved in expediting the inflammatory phase of healing.

Protect
Protecting the area is crucial in order to move on with the healing process. This consists of bandaging open wounds to keep the area moist and free of infection, as well as preventing additional mechanical injury through outside forces.

Rest
Resting is different from protection. Even "normal" motion or activity may exacerbate the trauma and prevent the tissue from moving to the repair phase.

Ice
Ice therapy during acute inflammation can dramatically increase the speed of the healing process. It increases the movement of healing fluids, and encourages the removal of debris. Most importantly, though, is the significant neurological benefit ice has. (See the section on hydrotherapy for more information.)

Compression
The vasodilation is controlled by the pressure nerve endings in the tissues immediately surrounding the damaged area. Adding mild compressive force to the area (as in an elastic wrap) stimulates these nerve endings and limits the infiltration of fluid into the cells. This provides for a more flexible area and assists in the circulation. Care must be taken not to stop the flow of fluids in or out of the area with too much pressure.

Elevation
The injured area should be kept raised so that gravity assists the flow of fluids towards the heart.

Phase Two -- The Proliferation (Repair) Phase

In the second phase, cellular inflammation is reduced and circulation is largely restored in the tissue surrounding the injury. Any disruption of the skin has been patched. Tissue repair and regeneration depends on three factors:

> ➢ elimination of debris,

> ➢ regeneration of cells and blood vessels,

> ➢ and the production of *fibroblasts*, which compose connective tissue and form the basis of scar tissue.

Typically, in a traumatic event, injured blood vessels become deprived of oxygen and die. Before repair and regeneration can occur, debris must be removed. Stimulated by a lack of oxygen, capillary buds begin to form in the walls of the intact vessels. From these buds grow immature vessels that form connections with other vessels.

Primary Healing
With an injury that has even and close edges held together, minimal scar tissue is formed and the original tissues knit together.

Secondary Healing
Secondary healing happens when there are open wounds or tissue loss. The extra space is filled in with scar tissue.

LIGHT techniques during this phase are encouraged. The increased circulation speeds the formation of the capillary beds and aids in the elimination of debris. Care must be taken not to damage the fragile tissue. If a re-injury occurs at this stage, it stimulates additional scar tissue formation.

Phase Three -- The Maturation (Remodeling) Phase

This phase lasts for two to twelve months with the wound reaching maximal strength at one year. Portions of the protein fibers in the scar tissue orient themselves in the direction of increased stress. (It is unrealistic to expect a majority of the fibers to be in alignment with the original tissue, because the weaker scar tissue requires the three-dimensional webbing for strength.) The protein matrix matures and the numbers of cells decrease, causing the scar to contract. *Mature scar tissue* has a tensile strength that is only 30 percent of normal skin.

More pressure can be applied to the injured area during this phase. Care must be taken not to exacerbate the scar itself. The goal for creating maximum flexibility would be to ensure the removal of adhesions in the tissue surrounding the injury. These are unavoidable consequences of the reduced activity in the area during the last two phases of healing, and can make a dramatic difference years later in the mobility and function of the area.

Strains

A *strain* is an injury sustained by a muscle and/or tendon that has been exposed to excessive tensile stress. Muscle strains most commonly occur at the musculotendinous junction (where the muscle attaches to the tendon). An excessive stretch on a relaxed muscle can cause a strain, however, they occur most often from tensile force while the muscle is contracted. They are also referred to as *pulled* or *torn* muscles.

First Degree
A first-degree strain is a tearing of less than 25 percent of the tendon. This is characterized by mild pain and may not be felt until the day after the injury. Healing time may be as little as a week or two.

Second Degree
A second-degree strain is a tearing of 25 percent to 75 percent of the tendon. The pain is more severe and is felt immediately. Bruising may be visible. This will require weeks to months to heal and may require surgery.

Third Degree
A third-degree strain is a complete rupture of the muscle or tendon. This will require immediate medical attention and eventually surgery. It can take up to 12 months to fully heal.

Strain Precautions

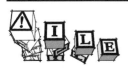 **Restrict massage to Incremental, Light and Energy techniques in the affected area(s). Your full technique range is encouraged for the rest of the body.**

 Pain that is moderate or severe in nature is a clear warning. Stop massage locally if this level of pain occurs, and have the client consult their physician.

 Avoid deep pressure massage and intense stretching, as there is an increased chance of bruising or tearing. Soft tissues are extra fragile with long-term oral steroid use or any time after an injection.

 Warning: Begin massage cautiously, and use your own sense of appropriate pressure. Avoid relying entirely upon the client's perception of appropriate intensity; both medications and their internal endorphins can mask the true intensity.

 Analgesic medications, muscle relaxants and anti-inflammatory medications are all used extensively. Ask before each visit what they are currently taking, and adjust your massage appropriately.

 Ice therapy is especially helpful throughout the healing process. Use ice massage only when the acute inflammation phase has passed.

Improving the body's ability to function will have a positive effect on the client's overall quality of life.

Sprains

A *sprain* is an injury to a ligament. Every joint has ligaments that hold the two bones together and prevent excess movement. They can also be called *joint capsules*.

There are two kinds of ligament fibers. *White ligaments* have a high collagen matrix for strength, whereas *yellow ligaments* have high elasticity. Examples of "white" ligaments with a high strength/low elasticity ratio are the ligaments preventing extension of the knee; hyperextending the knee even once tears the ligaments and forces a lengthy rehabilitation. An example of a high elasticity/low strength ratio "yellow" ligament is the pinkie finger; you can stretch that joint backwards far beyond its passive range of motion without any damage.

When ligaments are subjected to repetitive overloading stress or a traumatic injury, the ratio of yellow and white fibers is altered. The body creates a more flexible ligament with more yellow fibers compared to white fibers to withstand the stress. This is a normal adaptation response and although the ligament is less likely to tear with future trauma, the joint is weaker and more susceptible to dislocation and arthritic degeneration.

This adaptation is altered in the opposite fashion also. When less stress is placed upon the ligament over time, that ligament adapts by decreasing the yellow, flexible fibers and becoming more brittle. This can be seen when over-restrictive knee braces are habitually used, when rigid orthotics are worn in the shoe, or with a disease process called *adhesive capsulitis*.

Stretching a joint beyond its normal passive range of motion is rarely recommended. Stretching should be limited to the muscle and tendon; if the stretch is felt in the joint and not the muscle or tendon, it should be avoided.

The good news is that our body is constantly adapting to current stresses. If we prevent excessive stress on the weakened joint while maintaining *normal* stresses in the normal range of motion, our body will repair the correct white-to-yellow ligament ratio given enough time. This is the rehabilitation process and the time is determined by the severity of the sprain.

First Degree

A first-degree sprain is where ligaments are overstretched but not torn, and pain and swelling are minimal. The joint has normal function but the client is tentative and guarded. This will take weeks to months to heal.

Second Degree

A second-degree sprain is where the ligament is partially torn and pain and swelling are greater. Bruising may be visible. This will require months to heal and may require surgery.

Third Degree

The ligament is completely torn in third-degree sprains and frequently requires surgery. It requires a long period of rehabilitation to fully heal, often 12 to 18 months or more.

In an acute sprain with associated inflammation, do not massage directly on the joint. Encourage the client to P.R.I.C.E. the area using ice therapy at home. Massage on either side of the joint, massaging away from the area. The more severe the sprain, the farther away from it you begin work. Begin working directly upon the region only when the swelling and pain level has been reduced enough that you are certain the tissue can handle the technique. No stretching or mobility exercises until the client is well into the maturation phase of healing.

Ice massage during the maturation phase will speed the healing. Use active/passive stretching and exercise after the ligament damage is significantly healed. Keep in mind however, the time frame for healing different degrees of a sprain, and avoid rushing the healing process.

Sprain Precautions

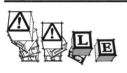 **Restrict massage to Light and Energy techniques in the affected area(s). Your full technique range is encouraged for the rest of the body.**

 Pain that is moderate or severe in nature is a clear warning. Stop massage locally if this level of pain occurs, and have the client consult their physician.

Sprain precautions, cont'd.

 Soft tissues are extra fragile with long-term oral steroid use or any time after an injection. Avoid deep pressure massage and intense stretching, as there is an increased chance of bruising or tearing.

 Warning: Remember that ligaments adapt due to stress. Avoid taking the joint past the appropriate range of motion and be on guard for their limits as the healing tissue will be more fragile.

 Warning: Begin massage cautiously, and use your own sense of appropriate pressure. Avoid relying entirely upon the client's perception of appropriate intensity; both medications and their internal endorphins can mask the true intensity.

 Analgesic medications, muscle relaxants and anti-inflammatory medications are all used extensively. Ask before each visit what they are currently taking, and adjust your massage appropriately.

 Ice therapy is especially helpful throughout the healing process. Use ice massage only when the acute inflammation phase has passed.

Communicating and
coordinating your care
with other healthcare providers
is seen as wisdom by the client,
rather than an
admission of weakness.

Hydrotherapy

Hydrotherapy is the use of hot and/or cold temperatures to maintain and restore health. It is a general term to describe a multitude of techniques to change the temperature of a portion of the body or the body as a whole. This book will use either Ice therapy or Heat therapy to differentiate the two main categories of hydrotherapy.

Ice Therapy

Physiological Effects

Ice therapy (also called *cryotherapy*) produces extended vasoconstriction and anesthesia. It often has the additional effect of reducing muscular contractions in skeletal muscle.

Have you ever felt an ice pack burn or tingle? This is an example of a physiological phenomenon called the *Hunting Effect*. When ice is first applied to the skin, the nerves sense the cold and react by constricting blood vessels and reducing blood supply to the area. This helps protect the body's core temperature. After a few minutes, however, the body senses that the local tissue temperature is lower than desired. It reverses the initial reaction by dilating the blood vessels in order to bring the tissue temperature back to normal. This will be held for a few minutes, and then the vasoconstriction will kick in again.

This has the beneficial effect of "squeezing the sponge," forcing blood from the area then bringing in fresh blood and nutrients, which accelerates the healing process. The body alternates vasoconstriction and vasodilation until the sensory nerves in the local area become numb and cease sending information. Sensory (*afferent*) nerves fatigue before motor (*efferent*) nerves, which is why you can have numb hands from throwing a snowball and still be able to move your fingers.

If the ice is applied continuously to the area until the sensory nerves fatigue, they will be less sensitive when they warm back to normal body temperature and for a short time thereafter. This calming effect is one of the most powerful, yet overlooked effects of ice therapy. A second ice treatment can begin as soon as the tissue has warmed to body temperature. If it is applied while the sensory nerves are still sedated, it will further reduce the hypersensitive "set point." This can be repeated until the sensory nerves have been calmed to near normal sensitivity.

The sedating Hunting Effect is negated if heat is applied. Heat will stimulate the nerves. Thus, the protocol of short-term ice therapy immediately followed by heat therapy is far less effective. The sensory nerves actually become more sensitized when alternating the two therapies. Ice then heat eliminates the long-term anesthetic effects of ice therapy alone. The Hunting Effect actively increases the ebb and flow of blood in the local area as well.

Precautions
How long should ice be applied? The old standard has been 20 minutes on, then off for anywhere from 20 minutes to an hour. This, however, would be insufficient for the anesthetic effect to take place for a larger body part such as the knee or spine. Likewise, 20 minutes may be too long for a small body part like a bruised finger.

It is very important to protect the most superficial layers of skin when applying ice. A common mistake with many ice packs is to apply them directly to the skin without a protective layer. The plastic can get colder than 32 degrees F, and when it contacts the skin, it can freeze cells in the first few layers. This may cause the plastic to "stick". There is damage to the skin cells, and if the ice pack is removed before the skin thaws, it could tear away those frozen layers.

Applying ice (i.e. frozen water) directly to the skin is considered safe, because the water melting from the ice provides the protective layer. This is the reason why your tongue never sticks to an icicle but can traumatically stick to a frozen metal object. A single layer of paper or fabric toweling provides the same protection. Multiple layers are not necessary and may make the treatment less effective by insulting the body.

Another important caution is to avoid leaving the ice on the skin after it has become numb. If the local area is cooled for too long a period, you risk *"supercooling"* the area. This happens when the motor nerves begin to lose function from the extreme temperature. They will increase vasodilation, flooding the area with blood until the body part is back to normal skin temperature. The body's intent is to avoid frostbite. The result, however, is that you now have more inflammation than when you began ice therapy.

Types
There are four main ways to apply ice:

1. a rubber, plastic or fabric bag with ice inside,

2. a plastic container with a non-water substance (like a gel),

3. a disposable, chemical "instant" ice pack,

4. and ice (frozen water) directly applied to the skin.

Using a bag or container to hold ice requires a thin absorbent layer to protect the skin. Care must be taken with this type of application because it can stay cold for longer than the body can handle, creating the supercooling effect as mentioned above. Add a moderate amount of salt to the ice (up to a quarter cup) along with just enough water to dissolve the salt. This will lower the freezing point of the water and keeps a consistent temperature until the ice is melted.

Gel packs are carefully designed to prevent the supercooling effect. They do not stay cold as long as ice alone, and they are more flexible and comfortable than ice and water. Be sure to use a protective layer unless one is specifically built into the pack.

Disposable ice packs are made up of an outer plastic bladder filled with one chemical, and an inner, fragile bladder filled with a different chemical. Breaking the inner bladder mixes the two chemicals and the reaction that occurs drops the temperature of the mixture dramatically. These are convenient for an unexpected need, but they rarely provide a cold temperature long enough for the body part to achieve numbness. These do not typically need a protective layer between the skin and the bag.

Ice massage can combine the effects of ice therapy and massage therapy for conditions that allow pressure massage. Water frozen in a styrofoam cup provides insulation for your fingers, allowing you to hold the ice cup and massage the area at the same time. Peel away the lip of the cup to reveal more ice as it melts, and continually move the ice over the area with light pressure until numbness has been achieved. Be cautious with firm pressure as the client will be unable to sense pressure and pain accurately.

Contraindications

Cold therapy should never be applied to already chilled skin. The supercooling effect occurs more rapidly and can damage tissue. Wait until the body has warmed enough so that the skin feels like it is back to normal temperature. Applying ice again at that time is safe and effective.

Another contraindication is when there is insufficient circulation to the local area even at normal temperatures. Diabetes is one example of a condition requiring caution before deciding to apply ice therapy. Another example is degenerative arthritis in the hands. Poor circulation and poor joint lubrication cause joint pain for these conditions, and they would not benefit from ice therapy.

Any condition or medication that creates a decreased sensory perception is of concern and may contraindicate ice therapy. It does not automatically prevent you from applying ice. The prudent protocol may be to actively monitor and remove the ice within 20 minutes.

Heat Therapy

Physiological Effects
Applying heat produces local, superficial vasodilation and has an analgesic effect. Heat also relaxes smooth and skeletal muscle tension and allows connective tissues to stretch more easily. The analgesia occurring from heat therapy is local and temporary, lasting only a few minutes after the heat source is removed.

There is a myth about *"deep heat."* The sensation of deep heat comes from the stimulation of heat sensing nerve endings at the surface of the skin. This relaxes smooth muscle tension in the blood vessels, which produces vasodilation. When additional blood is allowed to surface from the body's core, it has a temperature of 98.6° F (less than six degrees cooler than the hottest hot tub). It washes into the area and stimulates deeper heat-sensing nerve endings. This produces the sensation that the heat is going deep, when in fact it is drawing heat from the depths of your body.

Precautions
The integumentary system has a much larger capacity to withstand cold temperatures than hot. For example, the body handles temperatures over 60 degrees colder than the core temperature for long periods without skin damage. On the other hand, a thirty-second exposure to water heated to 130° F will result in third degree burns. Even water heated to 120° F will scald in less than 10 minutes. If you have ever experienced a *hot tub* you can recall how hot it felt; hot tubs are kept at or below 104° F to prevent scalding.

Our body can often acclimate to a temperature that will eventually burn if left on long enough. Consider how easy it is to become sunburned without sensing it. Medications both topical and oral can also reduce your perception of heat. Before applying any heat therapy, care must be taken to ensure that the temperature is appropriate, and that nothing has been taken or applied that will compromise the client's ability to determine their limits.

Types
There are many different ways to transfer heat to the body. A popular massage technique is called *hot stone therapy*, where stones are heated up to a maximum of 125° F and then placed on the client's skin at strategic points. Others are used as hand tools to assist in the massage. Other hot therapies and tools include *mineral baths, paraffin wax, hydrocollator pads, sitz*

baths, electric heating pads (such as the *Thermophore®*), *heating wraps, steam baths, saunas, hot water bottles* and *hot compr*esses.

There are also a number of ointments, creams, lotions, etc. on the market designed to chemically stimulate the heat-sensing nerve endings and produce vasodilation and an analgesic effect (see Topical Analgesics.)

Contraindications

Any acute inflammation contraindicates heat therapy. If an abundance of fluid is present in the area as a protective mechanism against further injury, applying heat will force additional fluid into cells causing them to rupture. The interstitial fluid pressure can also become great enough to collapse veins. This further compromises proper circulation and inhibits healing.

Any condition or medication that creates a decreased sensory perception is of concern and may contraindicate heat therapy. Other specific conditions are as follows: Do not apply heat to burned skin, regardless of the severity of the burn. Pregnant women should avoid general heat therapies like hot tubs, where the body temperature may be affected. Local application of heat is fine for a normal pregnancy with the exception of the abdomen. Care must be taken with multiple sclerosis not to overstimulate the client, which can result in painful and uncontrolled muscle spasms. Symptoms also may be exacerbated by heat. Always check with the treating physician when uncertain of any client's condition. (Specific precautions are listed with the individual condition.)

Teaching your clients tools for active healing gives them control. They in turn give you their respect and loyalty.

Analgesic and Anti-Inflammatory Medications

NSAIDS (Non-Steroidal Anti-Inflammatory Drugs)

Non-steroidal anti-inflammatory drugs are some of the most common medications used today. These drugs all have pain-relieving properties (analgesic).

Despite their constant presence in our daily lives, they do pose a risk. Both *The New England Nournal of Medicine* and the *Pain Journal* state that "On average, 1 in 1,200 patients taking NSAIDs for at least two months will die from gastroduodenal complications who would not have died had they not taken NSAIDs."

 If the client has recently developed any of the following, avoid massage and call the physician immediately: An unexplained skin rash, severe headache, increased difficulty breathing, ringing in the ears, recent muscle weakness, unusual bleeding or bruising or swelling of the lips, tongue, or face. (This is a massage-specific list; refer to the documentation that was included with the medication for a complete list of side effects.)

 Avoid all heat therapies or use with extreme caution (including hot stone massage, heat pads, etc), as the client's ability to sense heat is compromised.

 Warning: Begin massage cautiously, and use your own sense of appropriate pressure. Avoid relying upon the client to determine their limits. The client is likely to have a reduced perception of pressure and pain as a result of this medication.

 Side Effects: Headaches, stomach pain, constipation, nausea and vomiting can all be side effects of the medication. Adjust your massage therapy accordingly to take these into account. Recommend they seek medical advice if side effects persist or worsen.

 Postural hypotension can occur as a side effect of this class of medication. Help the client to change positions and be on guard for dizziness or blacking out.

NSAID Precautions, cont'd.

 NSAID medications include: <u>diclofenac</u> (APO-Diclo, Arthrotec, Cataflam, Voltaren, Voltarol), <u>diflunisal</u> (Dolobid), <u>etodolac</u> (Imbrilon), <u>etoricoxib</u> (Arcoxia), <u>fenoprofen</u> (Fenopron, Nalfon), <u>floctafenine</u> (Idarac), <u>flurbiprofen</u> (Froben, Vicoprofen), <u>ibuprofen</u> (Aches-N-Pain, Advil, Apsifen, Dimetapp, Dolgesic, Genpril, Haltran, Ibifon, Ibren, Ibumed, Ibuprin, Ibupro, Ibutex, Ifen, Medipren, Midol, Motrin, Novoprofen, Nuprin, Paxofen, Pedia, Ro-Profen, Rufen, Saleto, Sine-Aid, Trendar), <u>indomethacin</u> (Indameth, Indocid, Indocin, Novomethacin, Nu-Indo), <u>ketoprofen</u> (Alrheumat, Keto, Orudis, Oruvail, Rhodis), <u>ketorolac</u> (Toradol), <u>meclofenamate</u> (Meclofen, Meclomen), <u>mefenamic</u> <u>acid</u> (Ponstel), <u>meloxicam</u> (Mobic), <u>nabumetone</u>, <u>naproxen</u> (Aleve, Anaprox, Naprelan, Naprosyn, Naxen, Novonaprox, Synflex), <u>oxaprozin</u> (Daypro), <u>phenylbutazone</u> (Alka-Butazolidin, Alkabutazone, Brufen, Butacote, Butazone, Cotylbutazone, Novobutazone, Phenylone), <u>piroxicam</u> (Feldene, Novopirocam, Nu-Pirox), <u>sulindac</u> (Clinoril, Novo-Sundac), <u>tenoxicam</u> (Mobiflex), <u>tiaprofenic</u> <u>acid</u> (Tiafen, Surgam), <u>tolmetin</u> (Tolectin).

Acetaminophen

Acetaminophen is a specific medication used to treat mild to moderate pain and to reduce fever. It does not relieve joint swelling or tissue inflammation.

 If the client reports any of the following serious side effects, stop or avoid all massage and seek emergency medical attention: A severe headache, difficulty breathing, closing of the throat, swelling of the lips, tongue, or face, or hives. (This is a massage-specific list; refer to the documentation that was included with the medication for a complete list of side effects.)

 Avoid all heat therapies or use with extreme caution (including hot stone massage, heat pads, etc), as the client's ability to sense heat is compromised.

Acetaminophen Precautions, cont'd.

 Warning: Begin massage cautiously, and use your own sense of appropriate pressure. Avoid relying upon the client to determine their limits. The client is likely to have a reduced perception of pressure and pain as a result of this medication.

 Be alert for symptoms of anemia with long-term use of this medication, including low endurance, headaches, lightheadedness and fatigue. Stop circulatory massage if these become apparent and recommend they consult their physician at their earliest convenience.

 Acetaminophen is most commonly known as Tylenol. Acetaminophen has become too prolific to create a complete list of brand names. Please refer to the active ingredients of the medication in question.

Salicylates

Aspirin was first brought to market by the Bayer company in 1899. It has become the single most popular and available medication in the world. As little as 10 grams— about 30 regular-strength tablets— can be fatal in adults. In 1996, aspirin ranked eighth among all drugs as a cause of overdose and poisoning.

Aspirin is a specific **NSAID** used to treat mild to moderate pain, reduce inflammation and to reduce fever. Aspirin inhibits the elimination of uric acid, which may precipitate an attack of gout. It is commonly prescribed in daily doses between 81 and 325mg to treat heart conditions.

 If the client has recently developed any of the following, avoid massage and call the physician immediately: An unexplained skin rash, increased difficulty breathing, ringing in the ears, sudden severe headache, recent muscle weakness, severe abdominal cramping or pain, unusual bleeding or bruising or swelling of the lips, tongue, or face. (This is a massage-specific list; refer to the documentation that was included with the medication for a complete list of side effects.)

Salicylate Medication Precautions, cont'd.

 Avoid all heat therapies or use with extreme caution (including hot stone massage, heat pads, etc), as the client's ability to sense heat is compromised.

 Reduce your normal massage pressure as the client is more likely to bruise. Aspirin inhibits blood clotting. Even one baby aspirin can inhibit the platelet function for up to 10 days, and repeated doses become more dangerous as aspirin accumulates in the body.

 Warning: Begin massage cautiously, and use your own sense of appropriate pressure. Avoid relying upon the client to determine their limits. The client is likely to have a reduced perception of pressure and pain as a result of this medication.

 If the client is on another anticoagulant (see anticoagulants and/or thrombolytics) and has taken aspirin, be extremely cautious about any pressure massage. The combined effect of these medications creates potentially severe internal bleeding and bruising.

 Salicylate medications include: acetylsalicylic acid (Aspirin, Anacin, Bayer, Bufferin and others too numerous to list), choline magnesium salicylate (Tricosal, Trilisate), choline salicylate (Arthropan, Teejel), magnesium salicylate (Doan's, Mobidin, Momentum), salsalate (Argesic-SA, Artha-G, Disalcid, Monogesic, Salflex, Salgesic, Salsitab), and sodium thiosalicylate (Rexolate).

Steroids (Systemic)

(also called adrenocorticosteroids, corticosteroids)

This class of drugs mimics the hormone cortisol to produce anti-inflammatory and pain relieving effects. They also actively suppress the immune system. This is beneficial in treating autoimmune conditions, but will make the client more susceptible to infection. Steroids have a deteriorating effect on tissue strength and sensitivity, and the client will heal more slowly than expected.

Systemic means that the drug effects are distributed throughout the entire body. A systemic medication means that the medication has gone through some portion of the digestive tract, either by ingesting it or as a suppository. A *steroid injection* has a dramatic deteriorating effect on the joint or local tissue by disrupting granular and connective tissue formation necessary for proper tissue strength. Although the steroid is usually injected locally into the joint capsule, it also has a significant systemic effect.

Systemic Steroid Precautions

 If the client has recently developed any of the following, avoid massage and call the physician immediately: An unexplained skin rash, increased difficulty breathing, ringing in the ears, sudden severe headache, recent muscle weakness, unusual bleeding or bruising or swelling of the lips, tongue, or face. (This is a massage-specific list; refer to the documentation that was included with the medication for a complete list of side effects.)

 Avoid all heat therapies or use with extreme caution (including hot stone massage, heat pads, etc), as the client's ability to sense heat is compromised.

 Steroid injection: Avoid deep pressure or stretching techniques to the area for six weeks after being administered. Steroid injections remain in the tissues for an extended period of time.

 Long-term or ongoing steroid use: Avoid deep pressure massage and stretching techniques. There is an increased likelihood of trauma with long-term oral steroid use, as the soft tissues become increasingly fragile. Long-term use of steroids also predisposes the client to advanced osteoporosis. Consider limiting the session to LIGHT and ENERGY techniques if there is concern about bone stability.

 Warning: Postponing the session is recommended if the therapist is unwell. The client's immune system is compromised from this medication.

 Warning: Begin massage cautiously, and use your own sense of appropriate pressure. Avoid relying upon the client to determine their limits. The client is likely to have a reduced perception of pressure and pain as a result of this medication.

Systemic Steroid Precautions, cont'd.

 Side Effects: Peripheral edema, cold extremities and joint pain, back pain, nausea and/or vomiting all can occur with this class of medication all can occur with this class of medication. Take these into consideration as they may limit your ability to achieve your client's massage goals.

 Postural hypotension can occur as a side effect of this class of medication. Help the client to change positions and be on guard for dizziness or blacking out.

 Healing time will be extended while taking this medication because it is an immune suppressant; adjust your treatment schedules and goals to account for the slower than normal time frame.

 Systemic steroid medications include: <u>betamethasone</u> (Celestone), <u>budesonide</u> (Entocort), <u>cortisone</u> (Cortone), <u>dexamethasone</u> (Decadron, Dexameth, Dexone, Hexadrol), <u>hydrocortisone</u> (Anucort, Anumed, Anusol, Cortef, Dermol, Hemril, Hydrocortone, Proctocort), <u>methylprednisolone</u> (Medrol, Meprolone), <u>prednisolone</u> (Delta-Cortef, Orapred, Pediapred, Prelone), <u>prednisone</u> (Deltasone, Liquid Pred, Meticorten, Orasone, Panasol, Prednicen, Prednisone Intensol Concentrate, Sterapred), <u>triamcin-olone</u> (Aristocort, Atolone, Kenacort).

Steroids (Topical)

(also called corticosteroids, adrenocorticosteroids)

Topical steroid medications produce localized anti-inflammatory and pain relieving effects. Steroids have a deteriorating effect on tissue strength and sensitivity especially if used in high doses or for long periods of time. They also actively suppress the immune system. Topical steroids have a deteriorating effect on tissue strength and sensitivity, and the client will heal more slowly than expected.

Topical Steroid Precautions

 If the client has recently developed any of the following, avoid massage and call the physician immediately: An unexplained skin rash, increased difficulty breathing, ringing in the ears, sudden severe headache, recent muscle weakness, unusual bleeding or bruising or swelling of the lips, tongue, or face. (This is a massage-specific list; refer to the documentation that was included with the medication for a complete list of side effects.)

 Avoid all heat or cold therapies in the areas that topical pain medications have been applied within the last six hours (including hot stone massage, heat pads, etc).

 Long-term or ongoing steroid use: Avoid deep pressure massage and stretching techniques to the area where the client routinely applies the topical medication. Local soft tissues become fragile with long-term topical corticosteroid use.

 Warning: Begin massage cautiously, and use your own sense of appropriate pressure in the areas that topical pain medications have been applied. Avoid relying upon the client to determine their limits. The client is likely to have a reduced perception of pressure and pain as a result of this medication.

 Healing times will be extended because this medication is an immune suppressant; adjust your treatment schedules and goals to account for the slower than normal time frame.

 Topical steroid medications include: alclometasone (Aclovate), amcinonide (Cyclocort), beclomethasone (Beconase, Propaderm, Vancenase), betamethasone (Alphatrex, Betaderm, Betalene, Betamethacort, Betatrex, Celestoderm, Maxivate, Diprolene, Diprosone, Prevex, Teladar, Topisone, Topilenem, Valisone), clobetasol (Cormax, Dermovate, Embeline, Olux, Temovate), clobetasone (Eumovate), clocortolone (Cloderm), desonide (DesOwen, Tridesilon), desoximetasone (Topicort), dexamethasone (Aeroseb, Decaderm, Decadron), diflorasone (Florone, Maxiflor, Psorcon), diflucortolone (Nerisone), flumethasone (Locacorten), fluocinolone (Capex, Fluonid, Flurosyn, Synalar, Synemol), fluocinonide (Fluonex, Lidex, Lonide), (continued next page)

Topical Steroid Precautions. cont'd.

 flurandrenolide (Cordran), fluticasone (Cutivate), halcinonide (Halciderm, Halog), halobetasol (Utravate), hydrocortisone (Acticort, Allercort, Alphaderm, Anucort, Caldecort, Carmol, Cortaid, Cortdome, Cortenema, Cortifair, Cortiment, Cortisol, Cortoderm, Cortril, Dermacort, DermiCort, Dermolate, Dermtex, Emocort, Gynecort, Hycort, Hyderm, Hydrocream, Hytone, LactiCare, Lanacort, Lemoderm, Locoid, McCort, Nupercainal, Orabase, Pandel, Penecort, Penecort, Preparation-H, ProctoCream, Rederm, Rhulicort, Sential, Synacort, Unicort, Westcort), methylprednisolone (Medrol, Meprolone), mometasone (Elocon), pimecrolimus (Elidel), prednicarbate (Dermatop), triamcinolone (Aristocort, Delta-Tritex, Flutex, Kenalog, Kenonel, Triacet, Triderm).

Topical Analgesics and Anesthetics

Many creams, ointments, gels and lotions are on the market to produce a pain relieving effect. They stimulate the hot and cold nerve endings to produce vasoconstriction and vasodilation near the surface. An evaporating agent (such as alcohol) stimulates cold nerve endings and produces a localized superficial vasoconstriction. Other ingredients stimulate the heat sensing nerve endings and produce superficial vasoconstriction. The sensation of deep heat can be felt due to the additional core-temperature blood drawn to the area.

 If the client has recently developed any of the following, avoid massage and call the physician immediately: An unexplained skin rash, itching, or swelling, increased difficulty breathing, ringing in the ears, sudden severe headache, recent muscle weakness, unusual bleeding or bruising or swelling of the lips, tongue, or face. (This is a massage-specific list; refer to the documentation that was included with the medication for a complete list of side effects.)

 Avoid all heat therapies in the areas that topical pain medications have been applied within the last six hours (including hot stone massage, heat pads, etc).

Topical Analgesics and Anesthetic Precautions, cont'd.

 Warning: Begin massage cautiously, and use your own sense of appropriate pressure in the areas that topical pain medications have been applied. Avoid relying upon the client to determine their limits. The client is likely to have a reduced perception of pressure and pain as a result of this medication.

 Analgesic medications include: <u>bupivacaine</u> (Duocaine Marcaine, Sensorcaine), <u>chloroprocaine</u> (Nesacaine), <u>etidocaine</u> (Duranest), <u>lidocaine</u> (Anestacon, Dentipatch, EMLA, Lidoderm, Oraqix, Xylocaine), <u>mepivacaine</u> (Carbocaine, Polocaine), <u>prilocaine</u> (Citanest), <u>procaine</u> (Novocaine), <u>ropivacaine</u> (Naropin), and <u>tetracaine</u> (Pontocaine.)

 Partial list of analgesic ointments include: Absorbine, Alocane, Arnica, Aspercreme, Banalg, Ben Gay, Biofreeze, Blue-Stop, Blue-Emu, Bodyglide, Boiron, Boroleum, Capsaisin, DiabetAid, Flexall, Heet, Icy-Hot, Joint-Ritis, Mentholatum, Mineral-Ice, MyoRx, NatraBio, Phiten, Sloan's, Stopain, Thera-Gesic, Tiger-Balm, Ultra Blue, Unguentine, Watkins, Zostrix.

COX-2 Inhibitors

Two enzymes called cyclooxygenase are present in the body. COX-1 is virtually everywhere, and contributes to vital functions like protecting the stomach lining. COX-2 appears to be present mostly during times of inflammation. COX-2 inhibitors were designed to reduce arthritic pain without causing stomach ulcers. Recent studies however, have linked a higher incidence of heart attack and stroke with long-term use of COX-2 inhibitors.

 If the client has recently developed any of the following, avoid massage and call the physician immediately: Chest pain, unexplained arm or neck pain, cold sweats, shortness of breath, sudden severe headache, skin rash, increased difficulty breathing, ringing in the ears, recent muscle weakness, unusual bleeding or bruising or swelling of the lips, tongue, or face. (This is a massage-specific list; refer to the documentation that was included with the medication for a complete list of side effects.)

COX-2 Inhibitor precautions, cont'd.

 Avoid all heat therapies or use with extreme caution (including hot stone massage, heat pads, etc), as the client's ability to sense heat is compromised.

 Warning: Begin massage cautiously, and use your own sense of appropriate pressure. Avoid relying upon the client to determine their limits. The client is likely to have a reduced perception of pressure and pain as a result of this medication. In addition, all side effects are increased if they are taking other NSAIDS along with this medication.

 COX-2 Inhibitor medications include: <u>celecoxib</u> (Celebrex), etori-coxib (Arcoxia), <u>rofecoxib</u> (Vioxx) and <u>valdecoxib</u> (Bextra).

Barbiturates

Barbiturates reduce the likelihood of seizures in epilepsy. They are also prescribed for pain relief, in the treatment of anxiety, and as a temporary sleep aid.

 If the client has recently developed any of the following, avoid massage and call the physician immediately: An unexplained skin rash, increased difficulty breathing, ringing in the ears, sudden severe headache, recent muscle weakness, unusual bleeding or bruising or swelling of the lips, tongue, or face. (This is a massage-specific list; refer to the documentation that was included with the medication for a complete list of side effects.)

 Avoid all heat therapies or use with extreme caution (including hot stone massage, heat pads, etc), as the client's ability to sense heat is compromised.

 Avoid stretching techniques as the sensory feedback is depressed. Reduce and closely monitor pressure intensity and duration to avoid damaging tissue.

Barbiturate Precautions, cont'd.

 Warning: Begin massage cautiously, and use your own sense of appropriate pressure. Avoid relying upon the client to determine their limits. The client is likely to have a reduced perception of pressure and pain as a result of this medication. In addition, all side effects are increased if they are taking other NSAIDS along with this medication.

 Postural hypotension can occur as a side effect of this class of medication. Help the client to change positions and be on guard for dizziness or blacking out.

 Barbiturate medications include: amobarbital (Amytal), aprobarbital (Alurate), amobarbital with secobarbital (Tuinal), butabarbital (Buta-lan, Butisol, Sarisol), mephobarbital (Mebaral), pentobarbital (Nembutal), phenobarbital (Bellatal, Solfoton), and secobarbital (Seconal).

Narcotics

(also called opiates)

Narcotics raise the pain threshold and reduce the brain's perception of pain. They also cause drowsiness, depress the respiratory, vasomotor, and cough reflex centers.

 If the client has recently developed any of the following, avoid massage and call the physician immediately: An unexplained skin rash, increased difficulty breathing, ringing in the ears, sudden severe headache, recent muscle weakness, unusual bleeding or bruising or swelling of the lips, tongue, or face. (This is a massage-specific list; refer to the documentation that was included with the medication for a complete list of side effects.)

 Avoid all heat therapies (including hot stone massage, heat pads, etc). Normal heat dissipation is compromised with medications that suppress the CNS and burns may occur.

Narcotic Precautions, cont'd.

 Avoid stretching techniques as the sensory feedback is depressed. Reduce and closely monitor pressure intensity and duration to avoid damaging tissue.

 Warning: Begin massage cautiously, and use your own sense of appropriate pressure. Avoid relying upon the client to determine their limits. The client is likely to have a reduced perception of pressure and pain as a result of this medication. In addition, all side effects are increased if they are taking other NSAIDS along with this medication.

 Side Effect: Constipation is common but does not respond well to massage due to the suppressed smooth muscle in the intestines.

 Postural hypotension can occur as a side effect of this class of medication. Help the client to change positions and be on guard for dizziness or blacking out.

 Medications include: <u>anileridine</u> (Leritine), <u>buprenorphine</u> (Buprenex, Suboxone, Temgesic), <u>butalbital</u> (Alagesic, Amaphen, Americet, Anolor, Anoquan, Arcet, Axotal, B-A-C, Butace, Endolor, Esgic, Ezol, Fioricet, Fiorgen, Fiorinal, Fiortal, Fortabs, Isollyl, Lanorinal, Marnal, Medigesic, Pacaps, Repan, Tencet, Zebutal), <u>butorphanol</u> (Stadol), <u>codeine</u> (Paveral), <u>hydrocodone</u> (Alor, Anexsia, Azdone, Bancap, Ceta-Plus, Co-gesic, Damason, Dolacet, Duocet, Hy-Phen, Hydrocet, Hydrogesic, Lorcet, Lortab, Margesic, Maxidone, Norco, Panacet, Stagesic, T-Gesic, Vanacet, Vicodin, Zydone), <u>hydromorphone</u> (Dilaudid, Hydrostat), <u>levorphanol</u> (Levo-Dromoran), <u>meperidine</u> (Demerol), <u>methadone</u> (Dolophine, Methadose), <u>morphine</u> (Astramorph, Avinza, Duramorph, Epimorph, Kadian, MSIR, OMS Concentrate, Oramorph, Rescudose, Roxanol, RMS, Statex), <u>nalbuphine</u> (Nubain), <u>opium</u> (Pantopon), <u>oxycodone</u> (Endocet, Endodan, OxyFAST, OxyContin, Oxydose, Panasal, Percocet, Percodan, Percolone, Roxicet, Roxicodone, Roxiprin, Roxilox, Supeudol, Tylox), <u>oxymorphone</u> (Numorphan), <u>pentazocine</u> (Fortral, Talwin), and <u>propoxyphene</u> (Cotanal, Darvocet, Darvon, E-Lor, Genagesic, Propacet, Wygesic).

Aminosalicylates

Aminosalicylates have a local anti-inflammatory effect in the intestines. They are chemically similar to aspirin, but unlike aspirin, these medicines are effective if topically applied to the intestinal lining. As such they are typically administered as suppositories.

 If the client has recently developed any of the following, avoid massage and call the physician immediately: An unexplained skin rash, increased difficulty breathing, ringing in the ears, sudden severe headache, recent muscle weakness, unusual bleeding or bruising or swelling of the lips, tongue, or face. (This is a massage-specific list; refer to the documentation that was included with the medication for a complete list of side effects.)

 Side Effects: Headaches, abdominal pain, back pain and/or extremity pains and chronic diarrhea can occur with this class of medication.

 Aminosalicylate medications include: balsalazide (Colazal), mesalamine (5-ASA, Asacol, Canasa, Pentasa, Rowasa) and olsalazine (Dipentum).

Biologic Response Modifiers

Biologic response modifiers work by inhibiting a chemical that causes protective inflammatory reactions against bacteria. This chemical, called *tumor necrosis factor* (TNF), causes extensive tissue damage when overproduced. This appears in conditions like rheumatoid arthritis.

 If the client has recently developed any of the following, avoid massage and call the physician immediately: An unexplained skin rash, increased difficulty breathing, ringing in the ears, sudden severe headache, recent muscle weakness, unusual bleeding or bruising or swelling of the lips, tongue, or face. (This is a massage-specific list; refer to the documentation that was included with the medication for a complete list of side effects.)

 Side Effects: Nausea, constipation, diarrhea, and aching muscles can be side effects leaving the client weak and fatigued. Limit the duration and intensity of the session if reported and have the client contact the physician.

Biologic Response Modifier Precautions, cont'd.

 Biologic response modifier medications include: <u>etanercept</u> (Enbrel) and <u>infliximab</u> (Remicade).

Disease Modifying Antirheumatic Drugs (DMARDs)

This class of medication acts in various ways to prevent the immune reaction that causes conditions like rheumatoid arthritis, Crohn's disease and other inflammatory conditions.

 Serious side effects are common and include: Sudden back, muscle or joint pain, unexplained skin rash or hives, rapid heart rate, diarrhea, vomiting, excessive fatigue, mouth sores, blood in stool or urine and dizziness. Avoid massage and call the treating physician immediately if any of these are reported. (This is a massage-specific list; refer to the documentation that was included with the medication for a complete list of side effects.)

 Warning: Postponing the session is recommended if the therapist is unwell. The client's immune system is compromised from this medication.

 Healing time will be extended while taking this medication because it is an immune suppressant; adjust your treatment schedules and goals to account for the slower than normal time frame.

 Disease modifying antirheumatic drugs include: <u>auranofin</u> (Ridaura), <u>aurothioglucose</u> (Solganal), <u>azathioprine</u> (Azasan, Imuran), <u>gold sodium thiomalate</u> (Aurolate), <u>hydroxychloroquine</u> (Plaquenil), <u>leflunomide</u> (Arava), <u>sulfasalazine</u> (Azulfidine, Azulfidine EN-tabs, Sulfazine EC).

Central Nervous System Analgesics

These drugs work directly on the central nervous system to help control pain.

 Chest pain, rapid heart rate, vision changes, numbness, torso, back or leg cramps, difficulty urinating or uncoordinated movements are all signs of a medical emergency. Stop massage and call physician or emergency assistance. (This is a massage-specific list; refer to the documentation that was included with the medication for a complete list of side effects.)

 Avoid all heat therapies (including hot stone massage, heat pads, etc). Normal heat dissipation is compromised with medications that suppress the CNS and burns may occur.

 Warning: Begin massage cautiously, and use your own sense of appropriate pressure. Avoid relying upon the client to determine their limits. The client is likely to have a reduced perception of pressure and pain as a result of this medication.

 Side Effects: Nausea, constipation, and sleeplessness are common, leaving the client weak and fatigued. Limit the duration and intensity of the session.

 Central analgesics include <u>tramadol</u> (Ultracet, Ultram).

Ergot Derivatives

These drugs are administered for headaches that do not respond to milder analgesics. It acts as a vasoconstrictor for certain blood vessels in the brain.

 Chest pain, rapid heart rate, vision changes, muscle pain, numbness, torso, back or leg cramps, difficulty urinating or uncoordinated movements are all signs of a medical emergency. Stop massage and call physician or emergency assistance. (This is a massage-specific list; refer to the documentation that was included with the medication for a complete list of side effects.)

Ergot Derivative Precautions, cont'd.

 Avoid all heat therapies or use with extreme caution (including hot stone massage, heat pads, etc), as the client's ability to sense heat is compromised.

 Warning: Begin massage cautiously, and use your own sense of appropriate pressure. Avoid relying upon the client to determine their limits. The client is likely to have a reduced perception of pressure and pain as a result of this medication.

 Side Effects: Nausea, constipation, and sleeplessness are common, leaving the client weak and fatigued. Limit the duration and intensity of the session.

 Ergot derivative medications include: <u>dihydroergotamine</u> (DHE injection, Migranal), <u>ergotamine</u> (Ergomar), <u>ergotamine</u> <u>tartrate</u> <u>and</u> <u>caffeine</u> (Cafatine, Cafergot, Cafetrate, Ercaf, Ergo-Caff, Migergot, Wigraine).

Serotonin Receptor Agonists

(also called Triptans)

Triptans are the newest class of medications used to treat migraine and cluster headaches by constricting blood vessels and moderating central nervous system chemicals.

 Chest pain, rapid heart rate, vision changes, numbness, torso, back or leg cramps, difficulty urinating or uncoordinated movements are all serious side effects of this class of medication. Stop or avoid massage and call the client's physician or emergency assistance. (This is a massage-specific list; refer to the documentation that was included with the medication for a complete list of side effects.)

 If the client has recently developed any of the following, avoid massage and call the physician immediately: An unexplained skin rash, increased difficulty breathing, ringing in the ears, sudden severe headache, recent muscle weakness, unusual bleeding or bruising or swelling of the lips, tongue, or face.

Serotonin Receptor Agonist Precautions, cont'd.

 Avoid all heat and cold therapies as these medications cause peripheral vasoconstriction. Normal heat dissipation is compromised and burns may occur with heat therapy. The smooth muscle may spasm with cold therapy and produce a painful loss of blood to the area (called *ischemia*).

 Warning: Begin massage cautiously, and use your own sense of appropriate pressure. Avoid relying upon the client to determine their limits. The client is likely to have a reduced perception of pressure and pain as a result of this medication.

 Serotonin receptor agonist medications include: almotriptan (Axert), eletriptan (Relpax), frovatriptan (Frova), methysergide (Sansert), naratriptan (Amerge), rizatriptan (Maxalt), sumatriptan (Imitrex), and zolmitriptan (Zomig).

Muscle Relaxants

These medications act on the central nervous system to reduce skeletal muscle tension.

 If the client has recently developed any of the following, avoid massage and call the physician immediately: An unexplained skin rash, increased difficulty breathing, ringing in the ears, sudden severe headache, recent muscle weakness, unusual bleeding or bruising or swelling of the lips, tongue, or face. (This is a massage-specific list; refer to the documentation that was included with the medication for a complete list of side effects.)

 Avoid all heat therapies (including hot stone massage, heat pads, etc). Normal heat dissipation is compromised with medications that suppress the CNS and burns may occur.

 Avoid deep pressure massage, as muscle tone is abnormally flaccid. Reduce the duration of massage to each area to prevent bruising.

 Avoid stretching techniques as the sensory feedback is depressed. Reduce and closely monitor pressure intensity and duration to avoid damaging tissue.

Muscle Relaxant Precautions, cont'd.

 Postural hypotension can occur as a side effect of this class of medication. Help the client to change positions and be on guard for dizziness or blacking out.

 Muscle relaxant medications include: baclofen (Lioresal), carisoprodol (Rela, Soma, Vanadom), chlorphenesin (Maolate), chlorzoxazone (Paraflex, Parafon Forte, Relaxazone, Remular), cyclobenzaprine (Cycloflex, Flexeril), metaxalone (Skelaxin), dantrolene (Dantrium), methocarbamol (Carbacot, Robaxin, Skelex), orphenadrine (Antiflex, Banflex, Disipal, Flexoject, Mio-Rel, Myolin, Myotrol, Norflex, Orfro, Orphenate), and tizanidine (Zanaflex).

Benzodiazepines

The benzodiazepines are central nervous system depressants used in a variety of conditions to control muscle spasms, panic, anxiety, insomnia, seizures, and vomiting.

 If the client has recently developed any of the following, avoid massage and call the physician immediately: An unexplained skin rash, increased difficulty breathing, ringing in the ears, sudden severe headache, recent muscle weakness, unusual bleeding or bruising or swelling of the lips, tongue, or face. (This is a massage-specific list; refer to the documentation that was included with the medication for a complete list of side effects.)

 Avoid deep pressure massage, as muscle tone is abnormally flaccid. Reduce the duration of massage to each area to prevent bruising.

 Avoid stretching techniques as the sensory feedback is depressed. Reduce and closely monitor pressure intensity and duration to avoid damaging tissue.

 Side Effect: Constipation is common but does not respond well to massage due to the suppressed smooth muscle in the intestines.

 Postural hypotension can occur as a side effect of this class of medication. Help the client to change positions and be on guard for dizziness or blacking out.

Benzodiazepine Precautions, cont'd.

 Benzodiazepine medications include: <u>alprazolam</u> (Xanax), <u>brom-azepam</u> (Lectopam), <u>chlordiazepoxide</u> (Librium, Mitran, Reposans, Sereen), <u>clobazam</u> (Frisium, Mystan), <u>clonazepam</u> (Ceberclon, Clon-apam, Klonopin, Rivotril), <u>clorazepate</u> (ClorazeCaps, ClorazeTabs, GenENE, Tranxene), <u>diazepam</u> (Diastat, Diazemuls, Dizac, Valium, Valrelease, Vivol), <u>estazolam</u> (ProSom), <u>flurazepam</u> (Dalmane, Somnol), <u>halazepam</u> (Paxipam), <u>ketazolam</u>, <u>lorazepam</u> (Ativan), <u>midazolam</u>(Versed), <u>nitrazepam</u> (Berk, Mogadon, Nitrados, Rem-nos, Roche, Unisomnia, Unigreg), <u>oxazepam</u> (Novoxapam, Serax), <u>prazepam</u> (Centrax), <u>quazepam</u> (Doral), <u>temazepam</u> (Restoril), and <u>triazolam</u> (Halcion, Triolam).

Treat your client, not the medication. Massage has a lot to offer in their quest for an enhanced quality of life.

Chapter 2

Cancer

What is Cancer?

Cancer is an abnormal and excessive growth of new cells. These cell types are not normally found in humans and have no function to support the body. These new types of cells are called *neoplasms.* They grow outside the nervous system control, and they will continue to grow until the host is consumed. Neoplastic cells need a small fraction of the *growth factor* that a normal cell requires before it replicates, which allows them to multiply far faster.

Precancerous tissue is called *dysplastic,* because it is also outside the nervous system control. The cellular makeup has become disorganized due to mutation, and the cells no longer provide a useful function for the body. Dysplastic cells are also persistent and will not die off unless the body takes action and eliminates them.

Over one million people get cancer each year. Approximately one out of every two American men and one out of every three American women will have some type of cancer at some point during their lifetime.

There are two kinds of neoplasms, which are differentiated by their cellular characteristics. *Benign neoplasms* (tumors) typically are well differentiated, which means they look similar to the tissue from which they originated. *Malignant neoplasms* (tumors) are totally undifferentiated and do not follow a well-defined progression of maturation. They look foreign when compared to any normal cell type.

Normal cells will stop growing when they contact an adjacent cell. They only grow when they have an anchor point, and when they are separated from that anchor they stop replicating and self-destruct. Malignant neoplastic tissue can exist and replicate while suspended in fluid and does not need an anchor point for survival. This is what makes it possible for live malignant cells to infiltrate distant tissue sites by being transported via blood and lymph pathways.

Benign neoplasms will continually pressure the surrounding tissues as they grow and expand. This pressure causes trauma that results in normal tissue malfunction and death. Malignant neoplasms, on the other hand, secrete enzymes, called *collagenases*, which destroy the matrix holding healthy cells together. This creates gaps through which malignant cells invade surrounding tissue. This is one avenue by which malignancies reach lymph and blood vessels and spread. This is called *metastasis*. Benign neoplasms do not metastasize.

Benign neoplasms have a pattern of slow growth, which allows the body time to wall off (*encapsulate*) the neoplastic cells from the surrounding healthy tissue. The encapsulation does not slow the growth process. The body will also attempt to encapsulate malignant neoplasms, but they replicate too quickly. Malignant cells can continue to multiply while suspended in a liquid medium and do not require an anchor point to thrive.

Angiogenesis is the process of creating new blood vessels. After puberty is complete, the body does not create new blood vessels; it only repairs those created during maturity. Malignant neoplasms have the ability to induce new capillary growth. Within months of angiogenesis the malignant neoplasm can expand to over a billion cells.

Causes of Cancer

Besides heredity and aging, scientific studies point to the existence of three main categories of factors that contribute to the development of cancer: chemicals (e.g., from smoking or diet), radiation, and viruses or bacteria.

Cancer is not considered an inherited illness because most cases of cancer, perhaps 80 to 90 percent, occur in people with no family history of the disease. However, a person's chances of developing cancer can be influenced by inheriting alterations in the DNA.

There is a pre-programmed lifespan for each cell. When the cell has reached a certain state of age or malfunction it self-destructs without stimulating the inflammatory response. This is called *apoptosis*. Genes in some malignancies inhibit apoptosis, forcing the "normal cells" to live beyond their normal lifespan. This is considered to be a factor in increased cellular mutation as a person ages. Because cancer usually requires a number of mutations, the chances of developing cancer increase as a person gets older because more time has been available for mutations to accumulate.

A specific listing of the foods and chemicals that cause cancer would be both exhausting and controversial. Currently there are numerous studies being conducted regarding foods as well as toxins occurring in our daily lives. Virtually every substance one can think of will have proponents claiming that it causes cancer and studies reporting that it does not (and vice versa). Of all the toxins we encounter, tobacco smoking is most agreed upon as the greatest risk of developing cancer. Cigarette smoke contains more than two dozen different chemicals capable of causing cancer. Suffice it to say that as a general rule, the amount of chemical toxin your body ingests, coupled with your ability to eliminate those toxins will determine your risk of developing cancer.

Prolonged or repeated exposure to certain types of radiation causes cancer. The ability of ultraviolet radiation from the sun to cause cancer is most common in people who spend long hours in strong sunlight. As the radiation intensity increases it takes less time to mutate cells with radiation. Electromagnetic radiation from power lines, cell phones, and microwave ovens is also suspect.

Infectious agents are becoming more suspect as causes of cancer, although little concrete scientific data is yet available. The bacterium *H. pylori*, which can cause stomach ulcers, has been associated with the development of stomach cancer. In the case of viruses, some have been implicated in cervical cancer, liver cancer, lymphomas, leukemias, and sarcomas. These include the human papillomavirus (HPV) and the hepatitis B virus.

How Tumors Are Named

Benign Tumors
The prefix for a benign tumor contains the tissue type in which it originated. Benign tumors tend to have the suffix -oma, so that a benign muscle tumor is called a *myoma*, one formed primarily of bone cells is an *osteoma* and one consisting primarily of glandular tissue is an *adenoma*.

Malignant Tumors

Malignant tumors are also named based on the type of cell from which they originate: *Adenocarcinomas* originate in glandular tissue; *blastomas* originate in embryonic tissue of organs; *carcinomas* originate in epithelial tissue; *leukemias* originate in tissues that form blood cells; *lymphomas* originate in lymphatic tissue; *myelomas* originate in bone marrow; and *sarcomas* originate in connective or supportive tissue (e.g., bone, cartilage, or muscle).

Common Cancers by Area of Origin

Adrenal Cancer

Adrenal cancer is a rare disease that originates in the adrenal glands.

Bladder Cancer

Bladder cancer accounts for approximately 90 percent of cancers of the urinary tract (kidney, ureter, bladder, and urethra). Bladder cancer is the fourth most common type of cancer in men in the United States, and the eighth most common type in women.

Brain Cancer

Brain cancer is the leading cause of cancer-related death in patients younger than 35 years of age in the United States. Secondary brain cancer (where the cancer originated elsewhere and spread to the brain) occurs in 20–30 percent of patients with metastatic disease.

Breast Cancer

Breast cancer is the second most common type of cancer in women and the second leading cause of cancer-related death in women in the United States.

Cervical Cancer

Cervical cancer develops in the tissues lining the cervix. Cancer of the cervix is the second most common cancer in women worldwide.

Colorectal Cancer

Colon carcinomas may occur any where in the large intestine, from the ileo-cecal valve to the rectum, but the majority of colon cancers occur in the ascending colon. Colorectal cancer currently occurs in one out of every 20 individuals at some point in their lifetimes in the United States.

Endometrial Cancer

Endometrial cancer originates in the endometrial lining of the uterus. It is the fourth most common cancer in women in the United States.

Kaposi's Sarcoma

Once a rare disease, currently the vast majority of cases of this cancer have developed in association with infection by the human immunodeficiency virus (HIV). Skin lesions appear as raised blotches or nodules that may be purple, brown, or red.

Kidney Cancer

Several types of cancer can develop in the kidneys. In the United States, kidney cancer accounts for approximately 3 percent of all adult cancers.

Leukemia

Leukemia is a form of cancer that begins in the blood-forming cells of the bone marrow. It causes more deaths than any other cancer among children under age 20 in the United States.

Liver Cancer

Approximately 1 million new cases of liver cancer are diagnosed around the globe every year. They are relatively rare in the United States as primary cancers.

Lung Cancer

Sometimes called *bronchogenic cancer*, lung cancer in the United States is the leading cause death by cancer in men.

Lymphoma

Lymphomas are cancers in which the malignant tumor originates in the lymph system. 90 percent of lymphomas are a collective grouping of similar cancers known as *Non-Hodgkin's lymphomas* (NHLs). Non-Hodgkin lymphoma is the sixth most common cancer in the United States. *Hodgkin's lymphoma* will represent about 12 percent of all lymphomas diagnosed in 2004. The lymphatic tissue in Hodgkin's disease contains specific cells called *Reed-Sternberg cells* that distinguish this disease from other lymphomas.

Ovarian Cancer

Ovarian cancer is a disease produced neoplastic growth of the ovaries. In the United States ovarian cancer is the leading cause of gynecologic cancer deaths.

Pancreatic Cancer

Cancer of the pancreas is the fifth leading cause of cancer deaths following breast cancer, lung cancer, colon cancer, and prostate cancer.

Prostate Cancer

Prostate cancer is the most common type of cancer in men in the United States, according to the American Cancer Society.

Testicular Cancer

Testicular cancer is treated successfully in more than 95 percent of cases. The disease is most prevalent in men between the ages of 18 and 32.

Cancer Staging and Grading

There is no universal standard for describing the severity of every kind of cancer. This book focuses on the four most common methods of classifying cancer: *grading*, *numerical staging*, *summary staging*, and *TNM staging*.

For an accurate description of a specific type of cancer and it's grading or staging, a reliable source is the National Cancer Institute's website, www.Cancer.gov. There you will find extensive information tailored to the specific condition.

Grading

Grading involves examining tumor cells that have been obtained through biopsy under a microscope. The abnormality of the cells determines the grade of the cancer.

Grade 1

The cells listed as grade one are slightly abnormal and well differentiated. Differentiated tumor cells resemble normal cells and tend to grow and spread at a slower, normal rate.

Grade 2

These cells appear more abnormal and are moderately differentiated. These cells tend to grow more rapidly than Grade 1 cells.

Grade 3

Grade three cells are very abnormal when compared to the naturally occurring cells around them, and they appear poorly differentiated.

Grade 4

These cells are fully undifferentiated and abnormal. These cells grow most aggressively.

Numerical Staging

A numerical system is also used to classify the extent of cancers.

Stage 0   Cancer in situ, i.e. pre-invasive tumor limited to surface cells.

Stage I   Cancer limited to the tissue of origin, with evidence of tumor growth.

Stage II   Limited tumor growth with local invasion of cancerous cells.

Stage III Extensive tumor growth with local and regional invasiveness; no metastasis.

Stage IV   Extensive tumor growth with local and regional invasiveness and metastasis (spread to non-adjacent tissues).

Summary Staging

This system can also be used for all types of cancer. It groups cancer cases into five main categories:

In situ

This category classifies early cancer that is present only in the layer of cells in which it began.

Localized

Localized cancer is cancer that is limited to the organ in which it began, without evidence of spread.

Regional

This category classifies cancer that has spread beyond the original (primary) site to nearby lymph nodes, organs or tissues.

Distant

The distant classification is cancer that has spread from the primary site to distant organs or distant lymph nodes.

Unknown

Unknown is used to describe cases for which there is not enough information to indicate a stage.

TNM Staging

The tumor, node, metastasis (TNM) system is the most complex and specific method of classifying solid cancers. They separate the classifications into three categories: Tumor size (T), degree of regional spread or node involvement (N), and distant metastasis (M).

Tumor (T)

Tx   Primary tumor cannot be assessed.

T0   No evidence of tumor.

Ti.s. Cancer in situ, i.e. pre-invasive tumor limited to surface cells.

T1   A tumor that is 2 cm or less with no invasion into surrounding tissue.

T2   A tumor between 2 cm and 5 cm with no invasion into surrounding tissue.

T3   A tumor larger than 5 cm with no invasion into surrounding tissue.

T4   Tumor of any size with invasion into surrounding tissue.

Node (N)

Nx   Lymph nodes cannot be assessed.

N0   No lymph node involvement.

N1   Lymph node involvement on the ipsilateral side (same side as primary tumor).

N2   Lymph node involvement on the ipsilateral side and fixed to other structures.

N3   Lymph node involvement on both the ipsilateral and contralateral side (opposite side as primary tumor).

Metastasis (M)

M0   No evidence of metastasis (spread to non-adjacent tissues).

M1   Evidence of metastasis.

How the Body Fights Cancer

The human immune system contains several cell types capable of fighting cancer cells. These include some types of *killer T cells, macrophages* and natural killer cells. Some of the *immunoglobulins* (*antibodies*) may also participate in these immune activities against cancer cells.

Malignancies, however, can escape the surveillance of the immune system. This may happen because a person has a genetic predisposition toward developing a certain type of cancer, because the immune system has been suppressed (through the use of some types of drug) or because the surface antigens of cancer cells have been modified to appear similar to normal tissue. This is an increasingly important area of research.

The most important factor in the body's ability to fight any disease, including cancer and AIDS, is the extent to which the immune system is compromised. The nervous system (which is the master system, controlling all other systems) MUST be able to communicate with every part of the body through the spinal cord and nerves. The brain "manages" the immune system, controlling the extent to which it fights disease in the body. Therefore, the first step in boosting the immune system is to remove all nervous blockages and pressures allowing the brain to efficiently utilize its resources. Massage therapists have much to offer the client battling cancer. The next section specifically discusses the benefits and concerns.

Cancer Treatments
and Their Effects

Surgery

Before surgery, ENERGY techniques can boost your client's strength and have a calming effect on their anxiety. They may be approved soon after surgery also. Be clear in your communication to the physician that you are avoiding traditional massage (i.e. pressure) techniques. This will ensure the greatest chance of approval. Avoid touch near any wound, suture, or medical device attached to the skin. Review and adhere to the Standard/Universal precautions (detailed in the integumentary system chapter).

LIGHT techniques may be acceptable as soon as the client is released from the hospital. Obtain prior approval from the physician for any technique other than ENERGY techniques, however, as the specific condition being treated, the surgery, the anesthesia and other medications all cause chaos and instability in the client's ability to regulate blood clotting.

Avoid all pressure techniques near surgical sites for 6 weeks after being released from the hospital. Remember that your techniques will have an effect on deep body parts, and avoid placing those hidden tissues under stress as well. This may include client positioning as well as your techniques. ENERGY techniques are encouraged, as long as there is absolutely no possibility of infecting the client (i.e. no touch to the client's skin around the sutures). Those who have had one marrow or stem cell transplant procedures require extra time before introducing pressure massage. Use ENERGY techniques exclusively for the first four months and obtain approval from their physician before introducing pressure techniques.

To minimize blood clots the client is usually on one or more anticoagulant medications. Even gentle pressure can result in bruising. The risk of blood clots is increased with any trauma to sensitive blood vessels, which is another reason for limiting the session to gentle therapies. Medications will reduce or eliminate the client's ability to give you reliable feedback on pressure, stretching and appropriate duration.

Wait at least two months after the oncologist has stated that the client is in complete remission before introducing INCREMENTAL massage techniques designed for treatment or therapeutic effect. Remember that the maturation phase of healing is not complete for up to twelve months after surgery.

Radiation Therapy

During the radiation treatment regime use ENERGY techniques only. The medication, treatment and side effects make even LIGHT techniques too traumatizing for the client. As an example, the lightest touch sends nerve signals to improve circulation to the area touched as well as any reflexive areas. This forces additional blood through the capillary beds and increases the toxin load being eliminated. The immune-challenged cancer patient should not be subjected to this increased stress.

The skin around the radiation entry site (called the *entry portal*) as well as the exit site (the *exit portal*) will be fragile and may be highly sensitive. One or both may be marked by tattoos for identification during the treatments, as well as a reminder for future therapies. Avoid techniques that stretch or pressure the skin to these areas and always avoid applying any cream, lotion, gel, etc., unless specifically directed by the physician.

Skin exposed to radiation therapy may continue to form scar tissue even years or decades after the treatment has concluded. There will be some permanent lymph system scarring, depending upon the intensity of the radiation treatments. This reduced function may or may not be visually apparent. Note in the client's file that lighter pressure and intensity is necessary for these areas as a permanent precaution.

Chemotherapy

LIGHT and ENERGY techniques may be acceptable during, as well as after the chemotherapy treatment, to provide relief from the side effects of the medication. A pilot study has found that massage administered before and after chemotherapy reduced nausea, vomiting, and diarrhea in test patients. Honor the client's wishes as always, as they may be too overwhelmed to handle even ENERGY techniques.

Before each session, obtain a complete list of the client's current medications. This is especially important for the specific chemotherapy drug names. Read the precautions for each before proceeding, as they may have unique, time-sensitive concerns.

A comprehensive listing of the current medications and specific precautions follows, but here is a general list of common symptoms resulting from chemotherapy: Hair loss (*alopecia*); skin dryness, fragility, cracking, discoloration and sensitivity to touch; anemia associated with loss of platelets, easy bruising, nosebleeds and fatigue; nerve symptoms in hands and feet (peripheral neuropathy), including burning, tingling, pins and needles, electric shock sensations, and a general loss of touch, pressure and pain senses; edema; diarrhea, nausea, vomiting, loss of appetite and weight loss; depression, confusion, and emotional fragility with frequent mood swings.

Remember:
Your healing energy is unlimited
because it flows
through you,
not simply from you.

Concerns Regarding Massage and Cancer

Accepting a client who is battling cancer is no insignificant decision. Massage therapists must consider a number of factors when deciding what therapies and techniques are best for the client with cancer:

 Recent treatments that may contraindicate massage,

 The client's reduced ability to perceive pressure, pain and temperature changes,

 The tissue fragility in the local area surrounding the tumor(s),

 The client's tissue general strength and resiliency,

 Generalized weakness and lack of endurance,

 The threat of infection from the therapist,

 All secondary conditions and their precautions,

 The emotional state of the client.

Recent Treatments

Be sure to take into consideration all treatments in the last six months and the precautions for each procedure. Document each procedure in a chronological fashion to better estimate the timetable for your sessions. Chemotherapy techniques differ, as do radiation therapy and surgery. Investigate each medication to discover what challenges they bring to massage.

Reduced Perception

Pain medications as well as chemotherapy and radiation all reduce the client's perception of heat, cold, pressure and pain. There can be a generalized loss of sensation, complicated on certain days by the medications the client has ingested in the last 24 hours. Be sure to ask before each session and have reference material handy to check side effects.

Local Tissue Fragility

Local pressure on a malignant neoplasm can induce large numbers of cells to "shed" and be driven into circulation. Once in circulation the cells may lodge in the lymph nodes, lying dormant or creating an inflammatory reaction.

Gayle MacDonald, in her book *Medicine Hands: Massage Therapy for People with Cancer*, states, *"Gentle massage does not increase lymphatic circulation any more than the activities of daily life such as exercising, shopping, and caring for children."* The general consensus is that light, comfort-oriented massage has a minimal effect in the spread of dislodged neoplastic cells to distant parts of the body through the lymph or circulatory systems.

Moderate to intense pressure can rupture tissue surrounding the tumor. This provides openings for increased tumor growth. Pressure massage stimulates vasodilation to the capillary beds in and around the tumor. Increased pressure from circulation combined with external massage pressure stimulates the inflammatory response, which increases growth capillary production. Again, circulatory massage in the local area where a tumor is suspected should be light and comforting in nature.

General Tissue Strength

Consider past treatments as well. For example, long-term corticosteroid use (both systemic and steroid injection) weakens tissue strength and leaves the body permanently more brittle. Healing time will be significantly longer.

All treatments for cancer can permanently damage the lymph system. Chemotherapy and radiation both cause scarring of the lymph system, and these tissues become highly sensitive to trauma. Surgical removal of lymph nodes and lymph drainage systems also devastates lymph circulation. A cancer survivor can be untouched by lymphedema and have no apparent swelling despite having a compromised lymph system, only to have it flare from something as common as moderate touch massage. Other factors such as physical trauma and infection can trigger lymphedema also. Permanent restrictions are in place with gentle massage techniques only in treated areas (as well as the lymph system supporting that tissue) to prevent the possibility of lymphedema.

Generalized Weakness

The therapist is charged first and foremost with the health of the client. Always focus your goals towards compassionate relaxation with cancer survivors. Factors including diet, mental stress and lifestyle situations must all be considered when estimating the amount and type of massage a client can endure and benefit from. Guard your client's general energy level and never allow your touch to deplete them. They must have energy to continue healing once your massage session is concluded.

Infection Susceptibility

The therapist should take a critical look at their own immunity, and cancel for that day if they have the slightest infection. Remember that symptoms of an infection are a clue that your immune system is struggling to stay ahead. Spreading even a mild infection from you to the client may be life threatening for them.

Secondary Conditions

Those battling cancer likely have additional diseases or conditions that massage therapists must be aware of. Research every condition the client is suffering from. Make a list in the client's file of the permanent precautions first, then list the precautions that are temporary or are linked to certain medication usage. As you proceed with subsequent sessions, update this list as needed to avoid having to look up each condition and drug on every visit.

Emotional Climate

Keep in mind that the most appropriate, compassionate action in some cases may be avoiding massage entirely. Even ENERGY techniques can be emotionally overwhelming to the client.

Imagine this perspective: You are massaging the client's psyche as a whole, and their body in thoughtful, measured portions. It is not necessary to massage the whole body, and to even attempt such can be extremely damaging in certain cases. Consider the bruised psyche of a client overworked by an eager therapist. Recognize that your exuberance for all that massage can bring is fed by your inner health, and they haven't the nourishing wellspring you enjoy.

Medications for Cancer Treatment

Alkylating Medications

This class of chemotherapy drug is commonly used in chemotherapy. It works by preventing the DNA from unzipping and replicating by locking the two strands together.

 If the client has recently developed any of the following, avoid massage and call the physician immediately: An unexplained skin rash, increased difficulty breathing, ringing in the ears, sudden severe headache, recent muscle weakness, unusual bleeding or bruising or swelling of the lips, tongue, or face. (This is a massage-specific list; refer to the documentation that was included with the medication for a complete list of side effects.)

 Postponing the session is recommended if the therapist is unwell. The client's immune system is compromised from this medication.

 Warning: These medications have been proven to exit the body through the sweat. The chemical may accumulate on the therapist's hands and can burn their skin. Therapists should be gloved and avoid skin touch when administering massage within 24 hours of treatment.

 Warning: Begin massage cautiously, and use your own sense of appropriate pressure due to the peripheral neuropathy associated with this class of medication. Avoid relying upon the client to determine their limits. The client is likely to have a reduced perception of pressure and pain as a result of this medication.

 Warning: Alkylating medications tax the respiratory system. A reduction in the normal oxygen intake and carbon dioxide elimination makes body tissues more fragile. Reduce the duration to each area, and limit your session in general.

 Side Effects: Headaches, dizziness, and diarrhea can occur with this class of medication. Adjust your massage therapy accordingly to take these into account.

 Postural hypotension can occur as a side effect of this class of medication. Help the client to change positions and be on guard for dizziness or blacking out.

Alkylating Medication Precautions, cont'd.

 Alkylating medications include: <u>busulfan</u> (Myleran), <u>carboplatin</u> (CBDCA, Paraplatin), <u>carmustine</u> (BCNU, BiCNU), <u>chlorambucil</u> (Leukeran), <u>cyclophosphamide</u> (Cytoxan, Endoxana, Neosar, Procytox), <u>dacarbazine</u> (DTIC), <u>ifosfamide</u> (Ifex, Isophosphamide, Mitoxana), <u>lomustine</u> (CCNU, CeeNu), <u>mechlorethamine</u> (Mustargen, Nitrogen Mustard), <u>melphalan</u> (Alkeran, L-PAM), <u>streptozocin</u> (Zanosar) and <u>thiotepa</u> (Thioplex).

Chemotherapy Medications

This is a loose grouping of medications all utilized in chemotherapy. Individual medications may be specific to certain kinds of cancers, while others have a more widespread usage.

 If the client has recently developed any of the following, avoid massage and call the physician immediately: An unexplained skin rash, increased difficulty breathing, ringing in the ears, sudden severe headache, recent muscle weakness, unusual bleeding or bruising or swelling of the lips, tongue, or face. (This is a massage-specific list; refer to the documentation that was included with the medication for a complete list of side effects.)

 Postponing the session is recommended if the therapist is unwell. The client's immune system is compromised from this medication.

 Avoid deep pressure massage, and reduce the duration of massage to each area to prevent bruising, as soft tissues are extra fragile.

 Side Effects: Headaches, muscle pain, back, torso or abdominal pain, peripheral neuropathy, nausea, vomiting, diarrhea, weakness and fatigue are all common side effects. Take these into consideration as they may limit your ability to achieve your client's massage goals.

 Postural hypotension can occur as a side effect of this class of medication. Help the client to change positions and be on guard for dizziness or blacking out.

Chemotherapy Medication Precautions, cont'd.

 Chemotherapy medications include: <u>alemtuzumab</u> (Campath), <u>arsenic trioxide</u> (Trisenox), <u>bevacizumab</u> (Avastin), <u>bortezomib</u> (Velcade), <u>busulphan</u> (Myleran), <u>capecitabine</u> (Xeloda), <u>cetuximab</u> (Erbitux), <u>cisplatin</u> (Platinol), <u>clodronate</u> (Bonefos), <u>crisantaspase</u>, <u>epirubicin</u> (Ellence, Pharmorubicin), <u>gefitinib</u> (Iressa), <u>gemtuzumab ozogamicin</u> (Mylotarg), <u>goserelin</u> (Zoladex), <u>hexamethylmelamine</u> (Altretamine, Hexalen), <u>IFL</u> (Irinotecan, Fluorouracil, and Leucovorin), <u>imatinib</u> (Gleevec, Glivec), <u>irinotecan</u> (Campto, Camptosar), <u>oxaliplatin</u> (Eloxatin), <u>pamidronate</u> (Aredia), <u>pemetrexed</u> (Alimta), <u>porfimer sodium</u> (Photofrin), <u>procarbazine</u> (Matulane), <u>raltitrexed</u> (Tomudex), <u>tegafur</u> with <u>uracil</u> (Uftoral), <u>temozolomide</u> (Temodar), <u>topotecan</u> (Hycamtin), <u>trastuzumab</u> (Herceptin), <u>triptorelin pamoate</u> (Trelstar), <u>vindesine</u> (Eldisine), <u>vinorelbine</u> (Navelbine), and <u>zoledronic acid</u> (Zometa).

Interferon Medications

The mechanism by which interferon works is still unknown, but it appears that it activates immune system cells like macrophages and killer T cells.

 If the client has recently developed any of the following, avoid massage and call the physician immediately: Numbness in their extremities, unexplained skin rash, increased difficulty breathing, ringing in the ears, sudden severe headache, recent muscle weakness, unusual bleeding or bruising or swelling of the lips, tongue, or face. (This is a massage-specific list; refer to the documentation that was included with the medication for a complete list of side effects.)

 Avoid deep pressure massage, and reduce the duration of massage to each area to prevent bruising, as soft tissues are extra fragile.

 Side Effects: Severe mood swings, rash, skin itching, stomach pain, dizziness and diarrhea all can occur with this class of medication. Adjust your massage therapy accordingly to take these into account.

Interferon Medication Precautions, cont'd.

 Postural hypotension can occur as a side effect of this class of medication. Help the client to change positions and be on guard for dizziness or blacking out.

 Interferon medications include: <u>interferon</u> (Actimmune, Alferon N, Avonex, Betaseron, Infergen, Intron A, Rebif, Roferon-A, Veldona), <u>interferon beta-1a</u> (Avonex), <u>high-dose/frequency</u> <u>interferon beta-1a</u> (Rebif), <u>interferon beta-1b</u> (Betaseron), <u>glatiramer</u> (Copaxone), and <u>mitoxantrone</u> (Novantrone).

Antiemetic Medications

Nausea and vomiting are common symptoms in clients being treated for cancer. Antiemetic medication reduces nausea and helps prevent vomiting. Some of these medications may also be prescribed for motion sickness.

 If the client has developed an unexplained skin rash, ringing in the ears, sudden severe headache, tremors, insomnia, excitement, or significant restlessness, avoid massage and have them call their doctor immediately. These drug side effects are considered very serious and require medical attention. (This is a massage-specific list; refer to the documentation that was included with the medication for a complete list of side effects.)

 Postponing the session is recommended if the therapist is unwell. The client's immune system is compromised from this medication.

 Avoid all heat therapies (including hot stone massage, heat pads, saunas, steam rooms, etc.) as the client's ability to control their body temperature is compromised.

 Avoid local massage to prevent an increase in circulation and absorption if the medication is administered through the skin. Transdermal skin patches and ointments carefully administer medicine for an extended time.

Antiemetic Medication Precautions, cont'd.

 Side Effects: Drowsiness and fatigue, dizziness, urine retention, constipation, upset stomach, nervousness or a fast pulse all can occur with this class of medication.

 Postural hypotension can occur as a side effect of this class of medication. Help the client to change positions and be on guard for dizziness or blacking out.

 Antiemetic medications include: <u>aprepitant</u> (Emend), <u>chlorpromazine</u> (Thorazine), <u>dexamethasone</u> (Decadron, Dexameth, Dexone, Hexadrol), <u>diphenhydramine</u> (Altryl, Banophen, Beldin, Belix, Benadryl, Benylin, Diphedryl, Diphenhist, Genahist), <u>dimenhydrinate</u> (Calm-X, Dimetabs, Dinate, Dramamine, Dramanate, Dymenate, Hydrate, Triptone), <u>dolasetron mesylate</u> (Anzemet), <u>dronabinol</u> (Marinol), <u>granisetron</u> (Kytril), <u>droperidol</u> (Inapsine), <u>haloperidol</u> (Haldol), <u>hydroxyzine</u> (Atarax, Vistaril), <u>meclizine</u> (Antivert, Antrizine, Bonine, Dizmiss, Meni-D, Ru-Vert-M, Vergon), <u>metoclopramide</u> (Apo-Metoclop, Clopra, Maxeran, Maxolon, Octamide, Reclomide, Reglan), <u>ondansetron</u> (Zofran), <u>palonosetron</u> (Aloxi), <u>phenothiazines</u> (Promethazine, Trimeprazine), <u>perphenazine</u> (Trilafon), <u>prochlorperazine</u> (Compazine). <u>scopolamine</u> (Barbidonna, Buscopan, Kinesed, Transderm-Scop), <u>thiethylperazine</u> (Torecan), and <u>trimethobenzamide</u> (Benzacot, Tigan, Trimazide).

Be steadfast in your confidence in the power that emanates from simple human touch.

Antimetabolite Medications

These drugs work by disrupting the RNA and DNA synthesis reducing cell replication. This alters the body's inflammatory process. They are most effective against the cells that proliferate rapidly, such as cancer or blood cells, and they are effective with autoimmune conditions like irritable bowel disease.

 If the client has developed an unexplained skin rash, ringing in the ears, sudden severe headache, tremors, insomnia, excitement, or significant restlessness, avoid massage and have them call their doctor immediately. These drug side effects are considered very serious and require medical attention. (This is a massage-specific list; refer to the documentation that was included with the medication for a complete list of side effects.)

 Postponing the session is recommended if the therapist is unwell. The client's immune system is compromised from this medication.

 Avoid deep pressure massage, and reduce the duration of massage to each area to prevent bruising, as soft tissues are extra fragile.

 Warning: Begin massage cautiously, and use your own sense of appropriate pressure due to the peripheral neuropathy associated with this class of medication. Avoid relying upon the client to determine their limits. The client is likely to have a reduced perception of pressure and pain as a result of this medication.

 Side Effects: Headaches, weakness and body aches are common side effects of antimetabolites. Take these into consideration as they may limit your ability to achieve your client's massage goals.

 Antimetabolite medications include: <u>cytarabine</u> (Cytosar), <u>floxuridine</u> (FUDR, Fluorodeoxyuridine), <u>fludarabine</u> (Fludara), <u>fluorouracil</u> (Adrucil, Carac, Efudex, Fluoroplex), <u>gemcitabine</u> (Gemzar), <u>hydroxyurea</u> (Droxia, Hydrea), <u>mercaptopurine</u> (6-MP, Purinethol), <u>methotrexate</u> (Folex, Matrex, Mexate, Rheumatrex, Trexall) and <u>thioguanine</u> (6-TG, Lanvis, TG, Tabloid).

Antitumor Antibiotic Medications

These antibiotics also have been found to disrupt or bind to the DNA, much like the alkylating and antimetabolite medications.

 If the client has recently developed any of the following, avoid massage and call the physician immediately: Red urine or sweat, unexplained skin rash, increased difficulty breathing, ringing in the ears, sudden severe headache, recent muscle weakness, unusual bleeding or bruising or swelling of the lips, tongue, or face. (This is a massage-specific list; refer to the documentation that was included with the medication for a complete list of side effects.)

 Postponing the session is recommended if the therapist is unwell. The client's immune system is compromised from this medication.

 Avoid deep pressure massage, and reduce the duration of massage to each area to prevent bruising, as soft tissues are extra fragile.

 Warning: Begin massage cautiously, and use your own sense of appropriate pressure due to the peripheral neuropathy associated with this class of medication. Avoid relying upon the client to determine their limits. The client is likely to have a reduced perception of pressure and pain as a result of this medication.

 Side Effects: This class of medication taxes the respiratory system. A reduction in the normal oxygen intake and carbon dioxide elimination makes body tissues more fragile.

 Antitumor antibiotic medications include: bleomycin (Blenoxane), dactinomycin (Actinomycin), daunorubicin (Cerubidine, Dauno-mycin, DaunoXome, Rubidomycin), doxorubicin (Adriamycin, Caelyx, Doxil, Hydroxydaunomycin, Hydroxydoxorubicin, Lipo-somal Doxorubicin, Rubex), idarubicin (Idamycin, Zavedos), mito-mycin (Mitomycin-C, Mutamycin), mitoxantrone (Novantrone, Onkotrone), pentostatin (Deoxycoformycin, Nipent), and plicamycin (Mithracin, Mithramycin).

Cancer ✤ **79**

Hormonal Inhibitory Medications

Some tumors depend on hormones produced by the body to proliferate (like testosterone and estrogen). These drugs may reduce the production of the hormone or limit the hormone's ability to bind with the tumor.

 If the client has recently developed any of the following, avoid massage and call the physician immediately: Lower leg pain, edema, swelling or cramping, unexplained skin rash, increased difficulty breathing, ringing in the ears, sudden severe headache, recent muscle weakness, unusual bleeding or bruising or swelling of the lips, tongue, or face. (This is a massage-specific list; refer to the documentation that was included with the medication for a complete list of side effects.)

 Postponing the session is recommended if the therapist is unwell. The client's immune system is compromised from this medication.

 Side Effects: Headaches, nausea, vomiting, or breast tenderness all can occur with this class of medication. Adjust your massage therapy accordingly to take these into account.

 Postural hypotension can occur as a side effect of this class of medication. Help the client to change positions and be on guard for dizziness or blacking out.

 Hormonal inhibitory medications include: aminoglutethimide (Cytadren), anastrozole (Arimidex), bicalutamide (Casodex), exemestane (Aromasin), flutamide (Euflex, Eulexin), fulvestrant (Faslodex), goserelin (Zoladex), letrozole (Femara), megestrol (Megace), mitotane (Lysodren), nilutamide (Nilandron), tamoxifen (Nolvadex), and toremifene (Fareston).

Interleukin Medications

Interleukin works by stimulating certain immune system cells. These cells recognize the tumor cells as "foreign" and destroy them.

 If the client has recently developed any of the following, avoid massage and call the physician immediately: Yellowing of the skin, unexplained skin rash, increased difficulty breathing, ringing in the ears, sudden severe headache, recent muscle weakness, unusual bleeding or bruising or swelling of the lips, tongue, or face. (This is a massage-specific list; refer to the documentation that was included with the medication for a complete list of side effects.)

 Postponing the session is recommended if the therapist is unwell. The client's immune system is compromised from this medication.

 Avoid deep pressure massage, and reduce the duration of massage to each area to prevent bruising, as soft tissues are extra fragile.

 Side Effects: Headaches, back, torso or abdominal pain, muscle pain, increased sweating, nausea, vomiting, diarrhea, weakness, anxiety, and fatigue are all common side effects. Take these into consideration as they may limit your ability to achieve your client's massage goals.

 Interleukin medications include aldesleukin (IL-2, Interleukin-2, Proleukin).

Tubulin Inhibitor Medications

These drugs act specifically to inhibit cell division by rendering the mitotic spindle ineffective in separating the DNA strands.

 If the client has recently developed any of the following, avoid massage and call the physician immediately: A change in bowel habits for the last two days, unexplained skin rash, increased difficulty breathing, ringing in the ears, sudden severe headache, recent muscle weakness, unusual bleeding or bruising or swelling of the lips, tongue, or face. (This is a massage-specific list; refer to the documentation that was included with the medication for a complete list of side effects.)

Tubulin Inhibitor Medication Precautions, cont'd.

 Postponing the session is recommended if the therapist is unwell. The client's immune system is compromised from this medication.

 Warning: Begin massage cautiously, and use your own sense of appropriate pressure due to the peripheral neuropathy associated with this class of medication. Avoid relying upon the client to determine their limits. The client is likely to have a reduced perception of pressure and pain as a result of this medication.

 Side Effects: Headaches, muscle aches, and diarrhea all can occur with this class of medication. Adjust your massage therapy accordingly to take these into account.

 Tubulin inhibitor medications include: <u>docetaxel</u> (Taxotere), <u>etoposide</u> (Etopophos, Toposar, VP-16, VePesid), <u>paclitaxel</u> (Taxol), <u>teniposide</u> (Vumon), <u>vinblastine</u> (Velban, Velsar), <u>vincristine</u> (Oncovin, Vincasar).

Chemoprotectants

These medications protect against the harmful effects of the cancer-fighting drugs.

 If the client has recently developed any of the following, avoid massage and call the physician immediately: A change in bowel habits for the last two days, fever or chills, severe nausea or vomiting, unexplained skin rash, increased difficulty breathing, ringing in the ears, sudden severe headache, recent muscle weakness, unusual bleeding or bruising or swelling of the lips, tongue, or face. (This is a massage-specific list; refer to the documentation that was included with the medication for a complete list of side effects.)

 Postponing the session is recommended if the therapist is unwell. The client's immune system is compromised from this medication.

 Side Effects: Diarrhea, nausea, vomiting, and hiccups all can occur with this class of medication. Adjust your massage therapy accordingly to take these into account.

Chemoprotectant Medication Precautions, cont'd.

 Chemoprotectant medications include: <u>allopurinol</u> (Alloprim, Zyloprim), <u>amifostine</u> (Ethiofos, Ethyol), <u>dexrazoxane</u> (Zinecard), leucovorin (Wellcovorin), and <u>mesna</u> (Mesnex).

*People surviving cancer
don't always look to you for
answers or solutions. Often they
just want a safe place to express
their fears and anxieties and to
be themselves. They don't
necessarily want to be alone.
They want someone to listen,
to care without trying to
fix them, or make light
of their concerns.
Control your urge to make a
comment, add to a story or offer
advice. Don't analyze, compare,
criticize, or cheer them up.
Simply listen.*

Chapter 3

Musculoskeletal System

Osteopenia and Osteoporosis

Osteopenia results when the formation of bone is not enough to offset normal bone loss. The World Health Organization (WHO) defines osteopenia as a *bone density* between one standard deviation (SD) and 2.5 SD below the bone density of a normal young adult on a bone density test. Osteoporosis is defined as 2.5 SD or more below that reference point.

Osteoporosis is a widespread disease that results from a loss of calcium in the bones, creating fragile, brittle bones. Many think it is due to an insufficient intake of calcium. It is far more commonly due to one or more of the following: An unbalanced diet high in protein, smoking, habitual alcohol consumption, overuse of acid blocking or reducing medication, and the hormonal imbalances brought on as a result of chronic stress.

Osteopenia and Osteoporosis Precautions

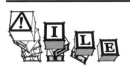 **Restrict massage to Incremental, Light and Energy techniques. Limit massage to light pressure over the torso and pelvis.**

 If there has been a recent history of falling (in the last few weeks), avoid massage until the client has consulted a physician. Do not trust that all fractures are accompanied by pain, as there may be medications or other conditions (such as peripheral neuropathy) that mask the discomfort.

 Avoid deep tissue massage techniques for those with a history of osteoporosis, and be especially careful with pressure on the torso. There are no visible signs to determine if a client has bone loss. Because it is so hidden and so common, extra care should be taken with men and women over 50 years of age.

Osteopenia/Osteoporosis precautions, cont'd.

 Medications to improve bone density are prescribed for this condition. Check all medications for additional precautions.

 Help your client understand the need to remain active to maintain the bone strength. Encourage them to take quality dietary calcium supplements.

Osteogenesis Imperfecta (OI)

(also called brittle bone disease)

OI is caused by a genetic defect that affects the body's production of collagen. The result is fewer or weakened collagen fibers. The client with OI may have only a few fractures, or may have hundreds. Fractures can begin in the birthing process and occur throughout their lifetime. Those with a mild to moderate form of OI may have a relatively normal activity level and a normal lifespan.

Osteogenesis Imperfecta Precautions

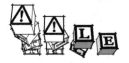 **Restrict massage to Light and Energy techniques.**

 If there has been a recent history of falling (in the last few weeks), avoid massage until the client has consulted a physician. Do not trust that all fractures are accompanied by pain, as there may be medications or other conditions (such as peripheral neuropathy) that mask the discomfort.

 Only LIGHT and ENERGY techniques should be performed because of the extremely unstable condition of the bones and connective tissues.

 Be sure to ask about current medications and check their precautions.

Osteogenesis Imperfecta precautions, cont'd.

 Your compassionate touch may be the best gift you give the client with this condition. Be an emotionally strong reservoir and watch your client thrive!

Osteomalacia and Rickets

Osteomalacia involves a softening of the bones due to deficiency of vitamin D in the bones. The childhood form of this is called rickets. This can be due to inadequate absorption or metabolism of vitamin D, inadequate sunlight, phosphates in the diet (e.g. from carbonated beverages) blocking vitamin D from binding in the bones, and side effects from seizure medication. Stress on softened bones can result in greenstick fractures. (see fractures). Unless complicated by medication this condition is usually resolved within a 12 month period.

Osteomalacia and Rickets Precautions

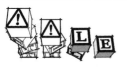 **Restrict massage to Light and Energy techniques.**

 If there has been a recent history of falling (in the last few weeks), avoid massage until the client has consulted a physician. Do not trust that all fractures are accompanied by pain, as there may be medications or other conditions (such as peripheral neuropathy) that mask the discomfort.

 Only LIGHT and ENERGY techniques should be performed during the acute stage of this disease due to the unstable condition of the bones.

 Be sure to ask about current medications and check their precautions, including those for seizures.

Osteomalacia and Rickets Precautions, cont'd.

 Guiding your client with nutritional support in addition to your massage skills can hasten their recovery.

Paget's Disease

(also called Osteitis Deformans)

This is a common disease of the skeletal system where areas of bone are replaced by a soft fibrous material. Over time, the body compensates by creating excess periosteum over the affected bones, creating a deformed bony appearance upon x-ray. This can sometimes be seen or palpated by the therapist. Paget's disease is the second-most common bone disorder (following osteoporosis) in people age 50 and older.

Paget's Disease Precautions

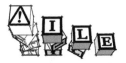 **Restrict massage to Incremental, Light and Energy techniques. Limit massage to light pressure over the torso and pelvis.**

 If any of the following symptoms occur, avoid massage and call the physician immediately: An unexplained skin rash, increased difficulty breathing, swollen face or lower extremity, recent muscle weakness, unusual bleeding or bruising.

 Avoid the inflamed joints during the acute stages. Limit the duration to short massages in the affected areas to avoid an exacerbation.

 Warning: Begin massage cautiously, and use your own sense of appropriate pressure. Avoid relying upon the client to determine their limits. The client is likely to have a reduced perception of pressure and pain as a result of this medication. Colchicine is a specific anti-inflammatory medication used for gout and Paget's disease. It often causes numbness or tingling in the hands and feet.

Paget's Disease Precautions, cont'd.

 Be sure to ask about current medications and check their precautions, especially those taken in the last 24 hours.

 Your compassionate touch may be the best gift you give the client with this condition. Be an emotionally strong reservoir and watch your client thrive!

Fractures

A fracture is defined as any interruption of outer layer of the bone (called the periosteum). Fractures take up to 12 months to heal and possibly much longer if infection has set in (see Osteomyelitis). It is a common misconception that when the cast is removed, the fracture is healed. This is far from the truth! To limit the joint stiffness and deterioration due to immobility the physician removes the cast when the *callous* has finished forming. The callous is the body's internal cast, stabilizing the fragments until they can heal. The callous is strongest along the long axis of the bone, yet weakest perpendicular to the bone. It can be cracked with sufficient direct pressure. The callous will be fully absorbed once the fracture is completely healed.

Precautions for fractures during the casting period:

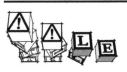 **Restrict massage to Light and Energy techniques above and below the cast. Your full technique range is encouraged for the rest of the body.**

 Insensitive, inflamed, or discolored tissues below (distal) to the cast are signs of trouble. Avoid massage and have client contact their physician immediately.

Precautions for fractures during the casting period, cont'd.

 Circulatory massage above and below the cast (working in the direction of flow towards the heart) is very helpful to limit edema and to stimulate the nervous system pathways. The body will be compensating for the injured body part, so your full range of techniques to the rest of the body will also be beneficial.

 Be sure to ask about current medications on each visit and check their precautions.

 Teach your client techniques they can use daily to maintain their circulation and control the inflammation.

Precautions for fractures after the cast has been removed:

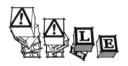 **Restrict massage to Light and Energy techniques in the affected limb. Your full technique range is encouraged for the rest of the body.**

 Deep pressure should be avoided until a physician can determine by x-ray examination that there is complete union. As the healing progresses, do passive and active exercise with the client (including resistive exercise) to restore the muscle strength and flexibility.

 Continue to work above and below the site. You may be able to perform LIGHT techniques over the fracture, but remember that the callous is weakest perpendicular to the bone. Always monitor the client's tolerance, and be aware of the potential for going beyond their healing capacity.

 Be sure to ask about current medications (especially non-prescription pain medicines) and check their precautions.

 Your skills in this area have the ability to dramatically improve their healing and limit atrophy.

Types of Fractures

Closed/Simple F.   Any type of fracture that does not break the skin. This can include one or more descriptive fracture types listed below.

Open/Compound F.   This type of fracture has penetrated the skin. The word compound refers to the added complexity caused by a risk of infection on the skin being drawn into the wound.

Avulsion F.   This type of fracture is where a small part of the bone has been pulled or torn away, leaving an island of bone. A common example of an avulsion would be a *Clay Shoveler's Fracture*, where the combined muscles of the neck and upper shoulder pull the spinous process of C-7 away from the body. Avulsions are not castable, and usually are not surgically removed unless they pose an ongoing instability or a risk of further trauma.

Comminuted F.   This is where the bone is splintered or crushed.

Complete F.   A fracture is said to be complete when the bone is separated into at least two pieces.

Compression F.   A compression fracture occurs when a short bone is pushed inward on itself. The most common site for a compression fracture is in the body of the thoracic vertebra. Osteoporosis affects the body more than the posterior aspect of the vertebra, and when the stress becomes too great for the remaining bone it collapses inward. *Breaking your back* is a common phrase associated with compression fractures. They pose no threat to the spinal cord or peripheral nervous system.

Depressed F.	This type of fracture happens in the bones of the cranium when they are pushed inward towards the brain.
Greenstick F.	When the bones are soft they do not fracture completely. Rather, the bone resembles a green stick when you try to break it; the inside of the curve bends and the outside is shredded. This type of fracture is considered incomplete, because the bone is still in one piece. This type of fracture is associated with rickets and osteomalacia.
Impacted F.	This traumatic fracture is where one broken end is wedged into the other broken end. This is typically used to describe long bones.
Incomplete F.	An incomplete fracture is a partial fracture in which the bone is still intact at some point. Greenstick fractures are incomplete, and others like stress or spiral fractures may be considered incomplete also.
Pathological F.	This is a broad category describing fractures that were caused by an underlying disease. A compression fracture can be considered pathological if caused by advanced osteoporosis, and Paget's disease can result in a pathological complete fracture.
Spiral F.	A fracture, sometimes called a torsion fracture, in which a bone has been twisted apart.
Stress F.	This is a fracture characterized by multiple traumas over time rather than one traumatic event. For example, stress or *"fatigue"* fractures can be diagnosed in the bones of the foot due to excess in training for a sporting event like long-distance running.

Scheuermann's Disease

(also known as juvenile kyphosis or vertebral epiphysitis.)

This disease is a common disorder of adolescents ages 13 to 17, more commonly found in males than females. It is a disorder of unknown etiology, once thought to be due to ischemic necrosis of the vertebral body growth plate. This has since been disproved and is now speculated to be somehow due to trauma, resulting in a stoppage of growth and advanced localized osteoporosis.

The areas most likely affected by Scheuermann's disease are the middle to lower thoracic vertebral bodies. Vertebral wedging due to compression fractures are common as well as a stooped posture. Torso range of motion will be reduced.

Scheuermann's Disease Precautions

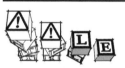 **Restrict massage to Light and Energy techniques in the affected area(s). Your full technique range is encouraged for the rest of the body.**

 If there has been a recent history of falling (in the last few weeks) with pain in the spinal area, avoid massage until the client has consulted a physician.

 Warning: The client may be unable to comfortably lie prone. Consider seated or side-lying massage as alternatives. Use only LIGHT and ENERGY techniques for the affected area of the spine.

 Be sure to ask about current medications and check their precautions, including non-prescription pain medicines.

 Guidance in improving your client's postural habits can lead to longer lasting results from your therapy as well as a grateful and loyal client.

Osteomyelitis

Any time a broken bone has been exposed to air it can become infected. This is called osteomyelitis. It can occur in compound fractures, gunshot wounds, and especially open heart surgery (where they cut through the sternum to gain access to the heart). For example, before planned heart surgery the patient is placed on high doses of systemic antibiotics to limit the possibility of infection once the surgery commences. Captured and treated early, osteomyelitis responds well and can be resolved within 12 to 18 months. Chronic osteomyelitis is much more challenging, with acute recurrences over years.

Osteomyelitis Precautions

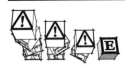 **Energy techniques only. Avoid all pressure and circulatory massage techniques on the affected limb. Osteomyelitis of the torso prohibits massage to the entire body.**

 If lymph nodes become swollen, tender, and hard, or if you see red streaks from the infected area to the armpit or groin, with throbbing pain and a fever, avoid massage and seek immediate medical attention.

 Osteomyelitis is an internal infection. It can be spread inside the client's body with improper massage, but it cannot be transported from one client to the next through massage (i.e. it's not contagious). If there has been a recent history of falling or increased pain in the area, avoid massage until the client has consulted a physician.

 Avoid all pressure techniques in the infected limb and any areas that would flow blood or lymph through the joint. Osteomyelitis of the torso prohibits massage to the entire body. ENERGY techniques are encouraged.

 Long-term antibiotic use along with medications to control pain are common. Be sure to ask about current medications and check their precautions.

 Massage within the above guidelines will stimulate their emotional strength as well as the healing response.

Osteoarthritis

(also called spondylosis, degenerative joint disease, DJD)

Among the over 100 different types of arthritic conditions, osteoarthritis is the most common, affecting over 20 million people in the United States. *Primary osteoarthritis* has no distinct cause, but is considered to be a function of aging. Water loss in the joint capsule allows more friction and decay in the cartilage.

When there is a distinct cause for the arthritic condition it is called *secondary osteoarthritis*. This group may include obesity, trauma, surgery or hormonal disorders.

Osteoarthritis Precautions

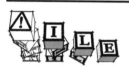 **Restrict massage to Incremental, Light and Energy techniques in the affected joint(s). Your full technique range is encouraged for the rest of the body.**

 If there is severe or extreme pain with a recent history of trauma, or if there is significant loss of function, avoid all pressure techniques to the area until the client has consulted a physician. ENERGY techniques are encouraged.

 Avoid any acutely inflamed joint. Concentrate on the muscles supporting that joint for maximum relief.

 Be sure to ask about current medications and check their precautions, especially those taken in the last 24 hours.

 Osteoarthritis is often diagnosed with finality, as if there were no hope for improvement. Although the condition is non-reversible, you have the power to improve circulation, stimulate healing, and bring relief and hope.

Infective Arthritis

(also called septic arthritis)

This is an acute bacterial infection of one or more joints, most commonly caused by *Staphylococcus Aureus* or *Neisseria Gonorrhea*. The client usually also has a high fever.

Infective Arthritis Precautions

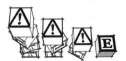 **Energy techniques only. Avoid all pressure and circulatory massage techniques.**

 Discuss your client's condition and current status with their physician before agreeing to perform massage.

 Avoid pressure techniques for the entire body until the infection is gone. ENERGY techniques are encouraged.

 Warning: After the infection has cleared, reduce your overall massage time to guard against overwhelming the client. Begin with LIGHT and ENERGY techniques and increase your intensity and duration in subsequent sessions.

 The client will likely be on intensive antibiotics and anti-inflammatory medications such as NSAIDS, COX-2 inhibitors or corticosteroids. Be sure to get a complete list and check for additional precautions.

 Your healing energy goes beyond your techniques; accept the limitations imposed by this temporary condition and know that your presence alone is beneficial.

Lyme Disease

This disease only became apparent in 1975, when a group of children who lived near each other in Lyme, Connecticut were all diagnosed with juvenile rheumatoid arthritis. Upon further testing, the bacterial spirochete *Borrelia Burgdorferi* was discovered which eventually lead to the naming of the new disease. It causes extreme inflammation and possible degeneration of one, two or three joints, most commonly the knees or shoulders. It often produces a characteristic *"bull's eye" rash* at the site of the tick bite. Some clients respond well to antibiotics, while others have chronic symptoms lasting years.

Lyme Disease Precautions

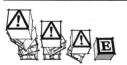 **Energy techniques only. Avoid all pressure and circulatory massage techniques.**

 Anyone suspected of Lyme disease should be treated without delay. Avoid massage and have the client seek immediate medical attention. Complications to the heart, joints and nervous system can occur if left untreated. Young children with fever and severe headache should see a doctor immediately, because these may be their only symptoms.

 Avoid pressure techniques in the limbs affected by this condition. It can be spread inside the client's body with improper massage, but it cannot be transported from one client to the next through massage (i.e. it's not contagious).

 Long-term antibiotic use is standard. NSAIDS, COX-2 inhibitors, muscle relaxants and corticosteroids are all possible medications used to manage this condition. Keep an updated list of the client's medications and their precautions to massage.

 Lyme disease is emotionally as well as physically taxing. Consistent, compassionate massage within the above guidelines will stimulate the client's emotional strength and healing response.

Rheumatoid Arthritis (RA)

(also called rheumatoid disease, juvenile rheumatoid arthritis (JRA), Still's disease.)

RA is an autoimmune disorder that attacks the synovial membranes of joints and other organs of the body. Clients with RA have antibodies in their blood that target their own body tissues. This is a chronic degenerative condition in which there are acute exacerbations followed by (possibly lengthy) periods of normalcy.

Rheumatoid Arthritis Precautions

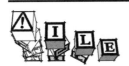 **Restrict massage to Incremental, Light and Energy techniques in the affected area(s). Your full technique range is encouraged for the rest of the body.**

 Have the client consult their physician if there has been a dramatic change in symptoms or if the client has a persistent fever and severe fatigue.

 Avoid pressure massage on acutely inflamed joints or lesions.

 NSAIDS are common, often replaced during exacerbations with corticosteroids or COX-2 inhibitors. Other medications can include antimetabolites. See these sections for precautions. Be sure to ask about current medications and check their precautions.

 Rheumatoid arthritis is an emotionally as well as physically challenging condition. Even though it is progressively degenerative, you have the power to improve circulation, stimulate healing, and bring significant relief.

Psoriatic Arthritis

(also called psoriasis)

Psoriasis is an *autoimmune* condition. Autoimmune conditions are illnesses that occur when the body's tissues are attacked by its own immune system. There is a genetic predisposition for this disease but the cause is unknown. It produces red, irritating skin patches with loose, whitish scales. In about 15 percent of the cases it damages the joints much like rheumatoid arthritis, producing progressive, chronic degeneration.

Psoriatic Arthritis Precautions

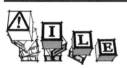 **Restrict massage to Incremental, Light and Energy techniques in the affected area(s). Your full technique range is encouraged for the rest of the body.**

 Have the client consult their physician if there has been a dramatic change in symptoms or if the client has a persistent fever and severe fatigue.

 Avoid pressure massage on acutely inflamed joints or lesions.

 Warning: Any pressure massage on skin lesions stimulates the body's growth and cleaning response, and will likely aggravate the condition. If you and the client both agree that massage is warranted, preapprove any lubricant with the client and test for irritation on a small area of skin. Using linen as an alternate to lubricants may be preferred.

 Medications vary frequently with clients as they build resistance. Immunosuppressants, anti-inflammatory and pain medications are common and ever changing. Ask before each visit what topical and oral medications are currently being used.

 Keep foremost in your mind the mental benefits of touch when helping clients with this condition.

Gouty Arthritis

(also called gout)

Gout is an inflammatory arthritis caused by too much *uric acid* in the body. Uric acid is a by-product of protein metabolism. When the kidneys become unable to eliminate all the uric acid, a condition known as *hyperuricemia* results. Acute joint inflammation is precipitated by deposits of uric acid crystals in the joint fluid (*synovial fluid*) and joint lining (*synovial lining*). Intense joint inflammation occurs as white blood cells engulf the uric acid crystals and release lysosomal enzymes.

It is believed that gout primarily affects the foot and lower extremity joints because the lower body temperature encourages the crystals to form. Crystals can also form in the kidneys, causing kidney stones.

Gouty Arthritis Precautions

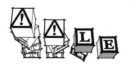 **Restrict massage to Light and Energy techniques in the affected area(s). Your full technique range is encouraged for the rest of the body.**

 If any of the following symptoms occur, avoid massage and call the physician immediately: An unexplained skin rash, increased difficulty breathing, swollen face or lower extremity, recent muscle weakness, unusual bleeding or bruising.

 Avoid the inflamed joints during the acute stages. When the inflammation has subsided, light techniques may be helpful in increasing the circulation to the area. Limit the duration to short massages in the affected areas to avoid an exacerbation.

 Warning: Begin massage cautiously, and use your own sense of appropriate pressure. Avoid relying upon the client to determine their limits. The client is likely to have a reduced perception of pressure and pain as a result of this medication. Colchicine is a specific anti-inflammatory medication used for gout and Paget's disease. It often causes numbness or tingling in the hands and feet.

Gouty Arthritis Precautions, cont'd.

 Be sure to ask about current medications and check their precautions, especially those taken in the last 24 hours.

 Aspirin inhibits the elimination of uric acid, which may precipitate an attack of gout. If they are taking aspirin, have them consult with their physician to be sure it is appropriate.

 Encourage your client to drink plenty of water daily, and to eliminate alcohol and caffeine. Educate them about limiting their consumption of foods high in *purines*, including meats, mushrooms, lentils, asparagus and spinach.

Systemic Lupus Erythematosus

(also called lupus, SLE)

Lupus is an autoimmune disease that attacks the tissues of the body, most commonly the musculoskeletal system. Other systems potentially affected are the urinary system (glomerulonephritis) and the cardiovascular system (atherosclerosis, thrombophlebitis) among others. Symptoms commonly include fatigue, muscle aches, arthritis, facial rash (*butterfly rash*), and poor circulation to the fingers and toes with cold exposure (see Raynaud's Syndrome). The condition is debilitating but rarely fatal; the 10-year survival rate for lupus clients exceeds 85 percent.

Systemic Lupus Erythematosus Precautions

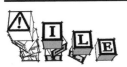 **Restrict massage to Incremental, Light and Energy techniques.**

 Avoid all pressure massage during any stage of glomerulonephritis. ENERGY techniques that do not stimulate the circulatory system are encouraged. Only consider light pressure massage when the client's physician has given approval.

Systemic Lupus Erythematosus Precautions, cont'd.

 Avoid using ice or cold therapies as this may aggravate the circulatory challenges of this condition.

 Warning: Begin massage cautiously, and use your own sense of appropriate pressure. Avoid relying upon the client to determine their limits. The client is likely to have a reduced perception of pressure and pain from the circulatory complications.

 Reduce your overall massage time to guard against overwhelming the client.

 Be sure to ask about current medications and check their precautions.

 Your ability to improve circulation can be a welcome relief for clients with this condition. Keep focused on what you can do to best support the client.

Myasthenia Gravis (MG)

Myasthenia gravis is a chronic autoimmune disease caused by a defect in the transmission of nerve impulses to muscles. It is not directly inherited nor is it contagious.

Symptoms include muscle weakness that increases during periods of activity and improves after periods of rest. Muscles that control eye and eyelid movements, facial expression, chewing, talking, and swallowing are often involved. The muscles that control breathing and neck and limb movements may also be affected. Flare-ups are a result of emotional stress, an infection, fever, becoming overheated, or an adverse reaction to medication.

Although there is no known cure, those afflicted with MG can live nearly normal lives with current medical treatment. One treatment is called plasmapheresis. In autoimmune conditions, the body's immune system mistakenly turns against itself, attacking its own tissues, in part by producing substances known as *autoantibodies. Plasmapheresis* is a process in which autoantibody-filled plasma is filtered from the blood. It unfortunately filters out supportive antibodies also, which leaves the client extremely vulnerable to other diseases and infections.

In rare cases a *myasthenic crisis* can occur. This is when the muscles that control breathing weaken to the point that ventilation is inadequate, creating a medical emergency and requiring a respirator for assisted ventilation.

Myasthenia Gravis Precautions

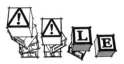 **Restrict massage to Light and Energy techniques.**

 Talk with the physician and rehabilitation team before attempting any therapy other than ENERGY techniques.

 Postponing the session is recommended if the therapist is unwell. The client's immune system is compromised, especially if they are on medication and/or plasmapheresis.

 Avoid all heat therapies (including hot stone massage, heat pads, etc), as this condition may worsen if the client becomes overheated.

 Avoid overstimulating the client. Limit your massage to LIGHT and ENERGY techniques, and limit the duration of massage.

 Medications frequently include antimyasthenics and immuno-suppressants and are utilized on and off throughout the course of this disease. Be sure to ask about current medications and check their precautions.

 Your work in reducing their stress can be a deciding factor in the quality of your client's lifestyle.

Healing energy is best
when presented with a smile.

Ankylosing Spondylitis

(also known as ankylopoietica, Bechterew's disease, Marie-Strumpell disease, rheumatoid spondylitis)

This is a systemic disorder that causes inflammation of the spine and the large joints in the extremities. Seen as early as 16 years of age, the disease progressively fuses the affected joints. Men are five times more likely than women to be affected. Pain is nocturnal and recurrent, and clients often assume a bent over posture. Complications may include irritable bowel disease and heart disease.

Ankylosing Spondylitis Precautions

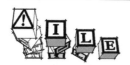 **Restrict massage to Incremental, Light and Energy techniques.**

 If there has been a recent history of falling (in the last few weeks), avoid massage until the client has consulted a physician. Do not assume that all fractures require significant stress. Fractures may not be painful, as there may be medications or other conditions (such as peripheral neuropathy) that mask the discomfort.

 Avoid acutely inflamed joints. Range of motion is severely limited in the spine and may also affect other joints. Massage and range of motion techniques are encouraged. They should be done lightly, cautiously, and should be limited to pain relief and relaxation.

 Gentle abdominal massage can be very helpful, however, the client will have low endurance and a reduced tolerance for pressure. Be brief and light in your technique to prevent an inflammatory reaction.

 NSAIDS, muscle relaxants, corticosteroids and other pain medications may be used for joint pain, possibly on a long-term basis. Be sure to ask about current medications and check their precautions.

 Heat therapies are especially beneficial for ankylosing spondylitis, as long as no other drug or condition prohibits its use.

Subluxation

(also called vertebral subluxation complex)

In a nutshell, a subluxation is a loss of normal joint mobility coupled with a nervous system deficit. It takes less than the weight of a dime (or 10 mm Hg) to reduce the nerve flow by more than 50 percent. This causes significant disruption in both sensory and motor nerve function. It not only can cause pain, but also frequently disrupts the muscular balance and proper organ function as well. The medical community occasionally uses the word subluxation to refer to an incomplete dislocation, rather than a functional condition.

Chiropractic physicians remove the adhesions that form between the spinal joints when the joint is immobilized due to inflammation. Massage is incredibly helpful in restoring the proper muscle function and mobility impeded by this condition.

Subluxation Precautions

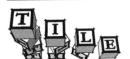 **Tolerance, Incremental, Light and Energy techniques are all encouraged.**

 Low back pain or pain in the lower ribs coupled with fever and/or painful urination can be due to a kidney infection. Avoid massage and call the physician immediately.

 Ask the client if there has been any loss of sensation or function in either the upper or the lower limbs that has not been discussed with their physician. If so, avoid pressure massage to the affected areas and have the client consult their physician without delay.

 Warning: Be cautious of range of motion techniques in the part of the spine affected by the subluxation, as it may increase the pressure against the nerve. If pain increases, discontinue motion.

 Warning: Be extra cautious with deep pressure, as the client may not be able to accurately determine their limits. When the nerve supply is compromised, the pain threshold can be reached without warning.

Subluxation Precautions, cont'd.

 Clients may self-medicate; ask before each visit what medications they have taken in the last 24 hours and check the precautions for each.

 Teamwork between a massage therapist and a chiropractic physician will have a synergistic effect on the healing capacity of the client.

 General massage therapy is recommended for clients being treated for a subluxation. In cases of medical use of the term subluxation, consider the loss of function of the affected joint and alter your approach accordingly.

 Ice therapy is especially helpful throughout the healing process. Use ice massage only when the acute inflammation and bruising has passed.

Low Back Pain

Massage is effective in reducing or eliminating many of the causes of low back (lumbar spine) pain. All forms of massage are highly recommended, assuming the cause of the pain is not a condition mentioned elsewhere in this guide. (See the following sections for specific information: Subluxation, disc herniation, sacroiliac pain.)

Low Back Pain Precautions

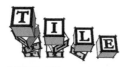 **Tolerance, Incremental, Light and Energy techniques are all encouraged.**

 Low back pain or pain in the lower ribs coupled with fever and/or painful urination can be due to a kidney infection. Avoid massage and call the physician immediately.

Low Back Pain Precautions, cont'd.

 Ask the client if there has been any loss of sensation or function in the lower limbs that has not been discussed with their physician. If so, avoid pressure massage to the low back and affected areas, and have the client consult their physician without delay.

 Warning: Be cautious of torso and leg range of motion techniques both supine and prone, and stop if the client experiences any increase in pain. (e.g., A common orthopedic test to diagnose low back pain has the same motion as a supine hamstring stretch.)

 Avoid pressure on the vertebra immediately above and below as well as directly on any painful spinal segment, as it is likely to increase pressure on the nerve root.

 Clients may self-medicate; ask before each visit what medications they have taken in the last 24 hours and check the precautions for each.

 Ice therapy is especially helpful during all stages of back pain, both passive and ice massage. Encourage the client to wear supportive shoes to minimize the stress on the leg and back muscles.

Sciatica

The roots of the sciatic nerve come from the fourth and fifth lumbar nerves, and the first through the third sacral nerves. They unite to form a trunk that is almost an inch in diameter and supplies sensory and muscular function to most of the leg. It can be found just lateral to the ischial tuberosity (the "sitting bone").

Sciatic pain (called *sciatica*) occurs when persistent pressure is applied to any portion of the nerve. Nerve entrapment from a subluxation or disc herniation is by far the most common cause, followed occasionally by a *piriformis syndrome*, where a tight, spastic piriformis muscle can strangle the largest nerve in the body.

Chiropractic treatments focus on the proper functioning of the spine and the elimination of the nerve pressure. Medical treatments focus on alleviating the pain and inflammation through oral medication and possibly corticosteroid injections. Surgery is an option if there is unrelenting disc pressure (see disc conditions, this chapter). Massage can benefit the client, regardless of their choice of treatment for sciatica.

Sciatica Precautions

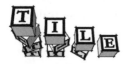 **Tolerance, Incremental, Light and Energy techniques are all encouraged.**

 Ask the client if there has been any loss of sensation or function in the lower limbs that has not been discussed with their physician. If so, avoid pressure massage to the low back and affected areas, and have the client consult their physician without delay.

 Warning: Be careful with deep pressure lateral to the ischial tuberosity, as direct pressure on the nerve trunk can cause a painful inflammatory response.

 Warning: Stretching the hamstring muscle with a trapped nerve root may also cause a painful inflammatory reaction; stop the stretch if it increases the client's symptoms.

 Be sure to ask if their condition has ever been treated by injection, and refer to the section on steroids if necessary. Ask about all current medications and check their precautions also.

 Your techniques are just "what the doctor ordered" if in fact a piriformis syndrome exists, and even if the entrapment is higher, releasing muscle tension in the posterior gluteal region is sure to bring welcome relief.

Look deep within your client
to find the real person
behind their mask of pain.

Spondylolysis and Spondylolisthesis

Spondylolysis (spon-di-lo-LI-sis) is a break in the bridge between the joints in the spine (the *pars interarticularis*). This usually results in a spondylolisthesis (spon-di-lo-lis-THEE-sis), a forward slipping of the vertebral body. 95 percent of the time this occurs at one of the last two lumbar vertebrae. The most common cause is due to stress fracture from repetitive trauma. *Baby walkers*, *bouncers*, early walking devices and certain sports like *diving* and *gymnastics* are linked to an increased prevalence of spondylolisthesis.

As the vertebral body is anteriorly displaced, it pulls on the individual lumbar nerve roots and the spinal cord itself. The spinal cord after L-1 separates into individual strands for the remaining lumbar and sacral nerve roots called the *cauda equina*(translated: *horses tail*), and pressure from this condition is called a *cauda equina syndrome*. Symptoms can include back and leg pain, weakness and loss of sensation in a random pattern.

Spondylolysis and Spondylolisthesis Precautions

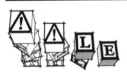 **Restrict massage to Light and Energy techniques over the affected spinal area. Your full technique range is encouraged for the rest of the body.**

 Ask the client if there has been any loss of sensation or function in the lower limbs that has not been discussed with their physician. If so, avoid pressure massage to the low back and affected areas, and have the client consult their physician without delay.

 Avoid all but light pressure on the spinal segments immediately above and below as well as directly on the affected segment, as this increases the possibility of forward slippage.

 Avoid low back stretching or assisted stretching techniques; be sensitive to increased symptoms with hamstring stretches as this may stress the joint also.

 Clients may self-medicate; ask before each visit what prescription and non-prescription medications they have taken in the last 24 hours.

Spondylolysis and Spondylolisthesis Precautions, cont'd.

 Ice therapy is especially helpful as an ongoing tool to control pain. Encourage the client to wear supportive shoes to minimize the extra stress on the leg and back.

 Strongly encourage the client to learn proper seated posture, utilizing supportive pillows to relieve the muscle stress. Poor posture will create more frequent and severe flare-ups.

Disc Herniation

(also called an intervertebral disc syndrome, slipped disc, bulging disc, disc protrusion, disc prolapse)

The *nucleus pulposus* is a jellylike material surrounded by a thick ligamentous material called the *annulus fibrosus*. Combined, these form an intervertebral disc, the shock absorber between your spinal bones. The disc is welded to the vertebral body above and below. Like a jelly doughnut, when pressure is applied to one edge, the jelly will be pushed to the open side. This pressure can come from a hidden subluxation (see subluxation) where the pressure builds for an extended period of time, or it can occur due to some significant traumatic event. If the nucleus remains pressed to one side of the disc it cannot function properly to absorb shock, and any additional pressure pushes the disc into the spinal nerve, or rarely, the spinal cord itself.

If the nucleus is still contained by the surrounding annulus it is considered herniated. A *hernia* (simplified) is any body part in an opening where it isn't meant to be. In this case, the disc is herniated into the *intervertebral foramen* (the opening between two spinal segments) that allows the nerve root to exit the spinal canal. Chiropractic and massage work well together to assist the client in healing disc herniations.

Disc Herniation Precautions

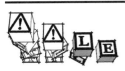 **Restrict massage to Light and Energy techniques over the affected spinal area. Your full technique range is encouraged for the rest of the body.**

 Low back pain or pain in the lower ribs coupled with fever and/or painful urination can be due to a kidney infection. Avoid massage and call the physician immediately.

 If the client has undergone recent surgery, consult with the treating physician before any circulatory massage. Ask about appropriate positions and precautions to massage.

 Ask the client if there has been any loss of sensation or function in either the upper or the lower limbs that has not been discussed with their physician. If so, avoid pressure massage to the affected areas and have the client consult their physician without delay.

 Avoid pressure on the vertebra immediately above and below as well as directly on the affected segment, as this increases the possibility of disc pressure on the nerve root.

 Avoid low back or neck stretching or assisted stretching techniques as this may stress the disc. For low back conditions, be sensitive when performing hamstring stretches and stop if symptoms increase.

 Warning: Be extra cautious with deep pressure, as the client may not be able to accurately determine their limits. When the nerve supply is compromised, the pain threshold can be reached without warning.

 Prescriptions for pain, inflammation and spasms are many and varied. Clients may also self-medicate; ask before each visit what medications they have taken in the last 24 hours and check the precautions for each.

 Teamwork between a massage therapist and a chiropractic physician will have a synergistic effect on the healing capacity of the client.

 Ice therapy is especially helpful as an ongoing tool to control pain. Encourage the client to wear supportive shoes to minimize the extra stress on the spine.

Sacroiliac Pain

(also called sacroiliitis)

Sacroiliac joint motion plays an important role in the normal gait cycle. Sacroiliac subluxation, gracilis or sartorius muscle imbalances and/or chronic ankle overpronation during the gait cycle are just a few of the possible causes of malfunction at this joint. It produces a sharp, frequently severe pain whenever the client attempts to move the pelvis. The pain is typically local and does not radiate to other areas.

Sacroiliac Pain Precautions

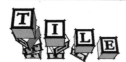 **Tolerance, Incremental, Light and Energy techniques are all encouraged.**

 Ask the client if there has been any loss of sensation or function in the lower limbs that has not been discussed with their physician. If so, avoid pressure massage to the low back and affected areas, and have the client consult their physician without delay.

 Warning: Be sensitive when performing hamstring stretches and stop if symptoms increase.

 Clients may self-medicate; ask before each visit what medications they have taken in the last 24 hours and check the precautions for each.

 Encourage the client to use ice aggressively to limit the joint inflammation. Ice therapy is particularly effective with sacroiliac conditions.

*Hope combined with action is
one of your most powerful gifts.*

Scoliosis

(also called idiopathic scoliosis)

Scoliosis is a side-to-side curvature of the spine beginning during puberty. It has no symptoms in the vast majority of cases until it has progressed to a severe stage. This makes it very difficult for the parent to discover that their child has scoliosis and understand their child's need for early treatment. There are a number of causes of scoliosis. Idiopathic scoliosis is the most common, accounting for 80 percent of all cases. In females, the sacral base grows unevenly, skewing the lumbar vertebrae and forcing the body to compensate by curving back towards center. The other possibility is an untreated subluxation in any area creating an uneven base for the spine above it. Other diseases such as neurofibromatosis and muscular dystrophy also cause scoliosis.

Sometimes a restrictive brace (called a *Milwaukee brace*) is used during puberty. The client must stay in the brace for 23 hours a day, removing it only to wash. This may seem drastic, but it may be the only non-surgical option left if conservative treatment was sought too late or was ineffective in stopping the progression.

The last resort is a major surgery to fuse spinal segments using a combination of bone grafts and steel *Harrington rods* screwed into the spine. Failing to stop the progression of the curvature places extreme pressure on the heart, lungs and other organs and causes early organ failure and death.

Scoliosis Precautions

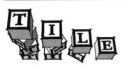 **Tolerance, Incremental, Light and Energy techniques are all encouraged.**

 If the client has undergone recent surgery, consult with the treating physician before any circulatory massage. Ask about appropriate positions and precautions to massage.

 If the client is wearing a brace, contact the physician for permission to remove it during massage. Enquire about additional precautions.

Scoliosis Precautions, cont'd.

 Many clients with this condition will have strict limitations on what stretches they may perform. Assisting them with these specific stretches can be helpful to your client.

 A variety of medications may be utilized in severe cases; ask about medications if they complain of symptoms. or are being treated by a medical physician.

 Scoliosis causes chronic, recurring muscle spasms. Having a compassionate therapist to rely on can be emotionally as well as physically comforting to the client with scoliosis. Be sure to encourage the use of ice for pain control.

Neck Pain

Massage is effective in reducing or eliminating many of the causes of neck (cervical spine) pain. All forms of massage are highly recommended, assuming the cause of the pain is not a condition mentioned elsewhere in this guide.

Neck Pain Precautions

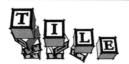 **Tolerance, Incremental, Light and Energy techniques are all encouraged.**

 Neck pain accompanied by fever, confusion, light sensitivity, severe headache and/or nausea or vomiting can be acute encephalitis or meningitis. Avoid massage and call the physician immediately.

 Ask the client if there has been any loss of sensation or function in the neck or upper limbs that has not been discussed with their physician. If so, avoid pressure massage to the affected areas and have the client consult their physician without delay.

Neck Pain Precautions, cont'd.

 Avoid pressure on the vertebra immediately above and below as well as directly on any painful spinal segment, as it is likely to increase pressure on the nerve root.

 Avoid neck stretching techniques if the client shows a decreased, painful neck range of motion.

 NSAIDS, muscle relaxants, corticosteroids and other pain medications may be used for joint pain, possibly on a long-term basis. Clients may self-medicate; ask before each visit what medications they have taken in the last 24 hours and check the precautions for each.

 Ice therapy is especially helpful as an ongoing tool to control pain.

Whiplash

(also called acceleration deceleration injury, cervical acceleration-deceleration, CAD)

In a whiplash accident, *hyperflexion* and/or *hyperextension* causes strain on the neck muscles and frequently sprains the cervical ligaments. The muscles remain tight in a reaction called *splinting* in order to provide protection and limit motion. The splinting causes fatigue and a buildup of lactic acid and can become too painful to even balance the head on the shoulders. A cervical collar is used in these situations. A properly fitted foam *cervical collar* will push down against the collarbone and trapezius muscles, and up against the mandible and mastoid, to minimize movement and support the head. When the brain senses the additional support the splinted muscles relax.

Whiplash Precautions

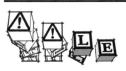 **Restrict massage to Light and Energy techniques in the neck and upper shoulders. Your full technique range is encouraged for the rest of the body.**

Whiplash Precautions, cont'd.

 Ask the client if there has been any loss of sensation or function in the neck or upper limbs that has not been discussed with their physician. If so, avoid pressure massage to the affected areas and have the client consult their physician without delay.

 Avoid all pressure massage in the acute stage. Reflexive work and ENERGY techniques are recommended. Be sure the client has healed sufficiently to handle the effects of the massage. LIGHT techniques can begin as soon as massage is tolerated and the client is past the acute stage.

 Avoid neck stretching techniques until the client has nearly normal, painless range of motion. Whiplash injuries potentially sprain cervical ligaments in addition to neck muscle strain. Refer to the precautions with sprains and strains.

 Prescriptions for pain, inflammation and spasms are many and varied. Clients may also self-medicate; ask before each visit what medications they have taken in the last 24 hours and check the precautions for each.

 Ice therapy is especially helpful as an ongoing therapy to control pain.

Whiplash injuries frequently include a significant emotional component. Be sensitive and understanding if the client releases that energy during your session.

Torticollis

(also called spasmodic torticollis, (ST), wry neck)

In Latin, tortus means "twisted," and "collum" means neck. This accurately describes the group of conditions called torticollis. There is an unyielding spasticity of the sternocleidomastoid (SCM) muscle on one side. It can range from having slept wrong and waking with a stiff neck or birth trauma to a (rare) congenitally absent sternocleidomastoid muscle on one side.

If the condition lasts for more than a day or two, the most common cause is compression of a nerve going to the SCM (from the cervical plexus, which originates from the first through the fourth cervical nerves). This causes a message to be sent to the neck muscle, telling it to contract.

Massage is an important solution if the nerve has proper function. This condition responds well in all cases (other than congenital abnormality) if chiropractic manipulative treatment for the traumatized nerve comes soon after the initial injury. Medical treatment to paralyze the nerve includes *Botox* injections (Botulinum Toxin Type A) or *selective peripheral denervation* (surgically cutting the nerve to the muscle).

Torticollis Precautions

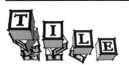 **Tolerance, Incremental, Light and Energy techniques are all encouraged.**

 Ask the client if there has been any loss of sensation or function in the neck or upper limbs that has not been discussed with their physician. If so, avoid pressure massage to the affected areas and have the client consult their physician without delay.

 Avoid neck stretching techniques and deep pressure if botox injections are administered or if the client is on medications such as muscle relaxants, as the stretch reflex has been eliminated and the muscle is prone to overstretching.

 Warning: Be extra cautious with deep pressure, as the client may not be able to accurately determine their limits. When the nerve supply is compromised, the pain threshold can be reached without warning.

Torticollis Precautions, cont'd.

 NSAIDS, muscle relaxants, corticosteroids and other pain medications may be used for joint pain, possibly on a long-term basis. Clients may self-medicate; ask before each visit what medications they have taken in the last 24 hours and check the precautions for each.

 Massage can be extremely helpful in providing relief and restoring normal function and can hasten recovery with torticollis. Ice therapy is especially helpful as an ongoing tool to control pain.

Thoracic Outlet Syndrome (TOS)

Have you ever fallen asleep with your arm over your head, and wake to find tingling or numbness in your arm or hand? You've experienced a temporary form of thoracic outlet syndrome. TOS is a group of disorders with a common theme: Each in their own way put pressure on the brachial nerve plexus or subclavian artery complex beneath the collarbone, resulting in varied shoulder and arm symptoms. In his book, *Thoracic Outlet Syndrome: A Common Sequela Of Neck Injuries*, Dr. Richard Sanders states that 95 percent of the time TOS occurs due to pressure on the nerves, and direct arterial pressure only occurs 5 percent of the time. Pressure can come from a jammed collarbone or rib, spastic scalene or pectoralis minor muscles, or inflammation due to injury or overuse.

Symptoms vary widely and can include any combination of the following: Numbness and tingling in the arm, hand or fingers; pain in the neck, shoulder, and arm; headaches; weakness of the arm, wrist and hand; and coldness and pale coloration of the hand. These often worsen at night or with activity, especially when raising the arm over shoulder height.

Conservative therapies (massage therapy, chiropractic, acupuncture, gentle strengthening exercises, stretching, and range of motion maneuvers) are considered effective in 89 to 90 percent of TOS cases. Surgery is rarely necessary and brings the risk of further nerve damage and scar formation.

Thoracic Outlet Syndrome Precautions

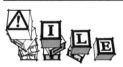 **Restrict massage to Incremental, Light and Energy techniques in the neck, shoulder and affected limb. Your full technique range is encouraged for the rest of the body.**

 Ask the client if there has been any loss of sensation or function in the neck or upper limbs that has not been discussed with their physician. If so, avoid pressure massage to the affected areas and have the client consult their physician without delay.

 Avoid aggressive stretching. Gentle movements and exercises are recommended. Keep the arm below the shoulder as much as possible.

 Clients may be taking pain or anti inflammatory medications for TOS. Check all medications for additional precautions.

 Various massage techniques including Alexander's technique and the Feldenkrais method have been successful in the improvement of TOS, and your client will surely benefit from your approach as well.

Carpal Tunnel Syndrome (CTS)

Carpal tunnel syndrome stems from pressure or irritation of the median nerve in the wrist. Symptoms include frequent burning, tingling, or itching numbness in the palm of the hand and the fingers, especially the thumb and the index and middle fingers. Decreased grip strength may make it difficult to form a fist or grasp objects.

The most common cause of CTS is repetitive stress to the wrist. When the wrist is subjected to awkward motion or position (e.g. angling the wrists while typing on a keyboard, or bending the wrists backward pushing off from an armchair), irritation and inflammation can build around the nerve. The eight *carpal bones* create a bridge, with the flexor ligament (the *flexor retinaculum*) forming the "tunnel" underneath. Often, a misalignment of the *lunate bone* collapses the bridge and prevents the pressure from releasing.

Steroid injections for the inflammation and surgically cutting the ligament are the medical treatments of choice if splinting the wrist proves ineffective. Conservative approaches including chiropractic and acupuncture to realign the carpals have achieved widespread success. Regardless of the treatment approach, success hinges upon the elimination of the repetitive trauma.

Since some fibers of the *median nerve* originate from the 6th and 7th cervical nerves, it's possible for the symptoms of carpal tunnel syndrome to be confused with nerve symptoms originating in the neck. When there is compression of the median nerve at the wrist as well as compression of the 6th and/or 7th cervical nerve as it exits the spine (see subluxation), the overlapping symptoms are called a *double crush syndrome*, and require attention to both the wrist and the neck. The nerve pressure in the neck can also arise from TOS (see thoracic outlet syndrome).

Carpal Tunnel Syndrome Precautions

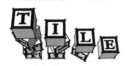 **Tolerance, Incremental, Light and Energy techniques are all encouraged.**

 If surgery or injections have been performed on the wrist in the last six weeks, avoid the wrist and hand until you have consulted with the physician and discussed specific precautions.

 Ask the client if there has been any loss of sensation or function in the neck or upper limbs that has not been discussed with their physician. If so, avoid pressure massage to the affected areas and have the client consult their physician without delay.

 Avoid range of motion exercises and stretching of the wrist to prevent irritation of the inflamed tissue. Wrist and hand massage is recommended unless there is sensory loss or irritation with pressure.

 Ask if they have a history of ever receiving a corticosteroid injection, and check current medications for additional precautions.

 Taking the time to discuss with the client possible wrist stresses in their daily activities can reveal vital solutions to a challenging condition.

TMJ Syndrome

(also called temporomandibular disorder, TMD)

The temporomandibular joint can be considered the most complex joint system in the entire body. Both the left and the right side of the jaw have to work as a team. Improperly fitting teeth, habitual grinding or clenching, muscle imbalances and joint inflammation among others can cause malfunction. Common symptoms include unusual jaw motion or sounds, a reduced opening of the mouth, muscle spasms, headaches, and pain on one or both sides of the jaw, which may radiate to the neck or head.

TMJ Syndrome Precautions

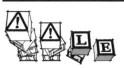 **Restrict massage to Light and Energy techniques for the face and entire jaw area on both sides. Your full technique range is encouraged for the rest of the body.**

 If your therapy goals include improving TMJ function, be sure the client is also actively being treated by a dentist for alterations to their bite.

 Warning: Rigorous or deep massage should only be attempted with proper training. External muscles such as the masseter, temporalis, and buccinator are easy to reach, but the internal muscles (lateral and medial pterygoids) can be overlooked, creating an imbalance and further exacerbating the condition.

 Warning: Caution should be exercised with regard to the nerves located in the region. Both the *trigeminal* and *facial nerves* (cranial nerves V and VII) exit near the TMJ, and undue pressure could instigate conditions such as Bell's palsy and trigeminal neuralgia (see the Nervous System).

 Be sure to ask about current medications and check their precautions. Clients may also self-medicate; ask before each visit what medications they have taken in the last 24 hours and check the precautions for each.

 Ice therapy is especially helpful as an ongoing tool to control pain. Cool water may be substituted if ice is too intense.

Dislocation

A dislocation is a complete separation of two joint surfaces. The *glenohumeral joint* of the shoulder is the most often dislocated joint in the body. It has one of the greatest ranges of motion, and that in part makes it more vulnerable. By contrast, the ball and socket *hip joint* is the least likely to dislocate, because it not only has a secure socket (the *acetabulum*), but it also has the *round ligament* (also called the *ligamentum capitis femoris*) attaching the femur head to the acetabulum.

A dislocation is both a sprain to the joint capsule and associated ligaments, and a strain to the tendons and muscles around the joint. The severity of the injury varies with the flexibility of the joint as well as the trauma. Refer to the sections on strains and sprains for more information.

There will be a lasting and possibly permanent apprehension on the client's part towards certain joint positions and motions. Indeed, the orthopedic test for an unstable glenohumeral joint is called *The Apprehension Test*. Placing the arm and hand in the " raised hand" position (palm facing forward) is a reasonable approximation of this test. It externally rotates the humerus, which places the supportive rotator cuff at a significant disadvantage. Discussing your session in advance will go a long way towards reassuring the client.

Dislocation Precautions

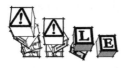 **Restrict massage to Incremental, Light and Energy techniques. Your full technique range is encouraged for the rest of the body.**

 Get approval from the treating physician before beginning stretching and mobility exercises after an acute dislocation.

 Avoid pressure directly on the joint in an acute dislocation. (Follow the precautions in the section on sprains.)

 Begin working directly upon the region only when the swelling and pain level has been reduced enough that you are certain the tissue can handle the technique. Ice massage at this stage can speed the healing.

Dislocation Precautions, cont'd.

 Use active/passive stretching and exercise after the ligament damage is significantly healed. Keep in mind however, the time frame for healing different degrees of a sprain, and avoid rushing the healing process.

 NSAIDS, muscle relaxants, corticosteroids and other pain medications may be used for joint pain, possibly on a long-term basis. Be sure to ask about current medications and check their precautions, especially those taken in the last 24 hours.

 Your skills and awareness of the body are invaluable in helping your client reach their full potential.

Shoulder Separation

A separation occurs most commonly in the *acromioclavicular joint,* which is the joint attaching the outer edge of the *collarbone* to the *scapula.* It can also refer to the *sternoclavicular joint* (the joint connecting the collarbone to the sternum). In both cases, it is a third degree sprain requiring months to years to heal. Since the healing process requires a lengthy time with the shoulder immobilized, a loss of shoulder mobility is common with adhesions forming in the shoulder girdle and space between the torso and the scapula.

Shoulder Separation Precautions

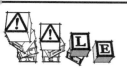 **Restrict massage to Light and Energy techniques for the affected shoulder. Your full technique range is encouraged for the rest of the body.**

 Get approval from the treating physician before beginning stretching and mobility exercises.

 Avoid all but light pressure directly on the joint in an acute shoulder separation. (Follow the precautions in the section on sprains.)

Shoulder Separation Precautions, cont'd.

 Begin working directly upon the region only when the swelling and pain level has been reduced enough that you are certain the tissue can handle the technique.

 Use active/passive stretching and exercise after the ligament damage is significantly healed. Keep in mind however, the time frame for healing different degrees of a sprain, and avoid rushing the healing process.

 NSAIDS, muscle relaxants, corticosteroids and other pain medications may be used for joint pain, possibly on a long-term basis. Be sure to ask about current medications and check their precautions, especially those taken in the last 24 hours.

 Use active/passive stretching and exercise after the ligament damage is significantly healed. Keep in mind however, the time frame for healing different degrees of a sprain, and avoid rushing the healing process.

Carefully consider how much support your client can benefit from, and how much may be overwhelming. Even Energy techniques can be physically and emotionally taxing.

Adhesive Capsulitis

(also called frozen shoulder)

When a shoulder remains injured longer than a few weeks, adhesions form in the joint capsule and in surrounding tissues. Ligaments gradually lose their yellow (flexible) fibers and become shortened and more brittle. The longer this continues the more severe the condition becomes, until the shoulder becomes entirely *frozen* or unable to move.

Rehabilitation for adhesive capsulitis is tedious, with progress measured in months and inches. Physical therapy is common, with home instructions for gentle, specific stretches.

Adhesive Capsulitis Precautions

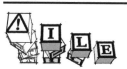 **Restrict massage to Incremental, Light and Energy techniques for the affected shoulder. Your full technique range is encouraged for the rest of the body.**

 Ask the client if there has been any loss of sensation or function in the neck or upper limbs that has not been discussed with their physician. If so, avoid pressure massage to the affected areas and have the client consult their physician without delay.

 Avoid acutely inflamed joints. The client's range of motion can be severely limited. Skin, fascia and muscle tissues will be weak and fragile from disuse atrophy and possibly from a history of corticosteroid use.

 Warning: Be very cautious with any stretching or range of motion techniques to the affected joint.

 Be sure to ask about current medications and check their precautions.

 Use heat therapy during sessions, and ice therapy for healing and pain control. Keep in mind the time frame for healing different degrees of a sprain, and avoid rush.ng the healing process.

Bursitis

Found in most large joints, a bursa is a fluid-filled sac that separates moving body tissues. The thin layer of fluid in a bursa creates a virtually friction-free surface for a tendon or ligament to glide over another body part. When traumatized, a bursa swells and places extra stress on those tendons and ligaments. It can be a long-term, chronic condition because of the frequent use of the joint unless aggressive ice therapy or other anti-inflammatory action is taken.

Bursitis Precautions

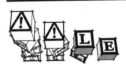 **Restrict massage to Light and Energy techniques directly on the bursa. Your full technique range is encouraged for the rest of the body.**

 Bursitis is a straightforward condition with no dangerous complications.

 Avoid all but light pressure directly on the bursa.

 Warning: Be very cautious about any stretching or range of motion techniques to the affected joint.

 NSAIDS, corticosteroids and other pain medications may be used for bursitis, possibly on a long-term basis. Be sure to ask about current medications and check their precautions.

 Encourage persistence with ice therapy, as it is especially helpful to turn the tide in the client's favor.

Dupuytren's Contracture

Dupuytren's contracture is a painless thickening of the fascia on the palms of the hands. This causes adhesions to the finger flexor tendons. More commonly affecting the last two digits, the fingers are unable to completely extend. The cause is unknown, but it is suggested that it is more common with repetitive trauma.

Dupuytren's Contracture Precautions

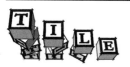 **Tolerance, Incremental, Light and Energy techniques are all encouraged.**

 Massage is only restricted if there is acute inflammation. If there has been recent trauma, refer to the sections covering sprains and strains for precautions pertaining to the specific stage of healing that fits your client's condition.

 If surgery or injections have been performed in the last six weeks, avoid the wrist and hand until you have consulted with the physician and discussed specific precautions.

 Massage and stretching techniques are beneficial in stabilizing this condition and helping the client gain flexibility.

 Ask if they have a history of ever receiving a corticosteroid injection, and check current medications for additional precautions.

 Teaching the client massage and stretching for the hands may prevent the progression of this condition and gives the client power to control stiffening between massage sessions.

Tendinitis and Tenosynovitis

(also called tenovaginitis, stenosing tenosynovitis, DeQuervain's stenosing tenosynovitis)

Certain tendons (most commonly in the wrist and hand) have a synovial sheath enveloping them, reducing friction on the surrounding tissues much like a bursa. When this tendon and sheath becomes inflamed it reduces the ability of the tendon to glide within the sheath. Long-term repetitive trauma can cause adhesions to form between the two tissues. In severe cases the synovial sheath may be surgically split.

DeQuervain's stenosing tenosynovitis occurs in the synovial sheaths of the abductor pollicis longus and the extensor pollicis brevis tendons of the thumb. The condition can be discovered by first making a fist with the thumb inside, and then stretching the thumb tendons away from the extended elbow (i.e. medial flexion).

Tendinitis and Tenosynovitis Precautions

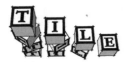 **Tolerance, Incremental, Light and Energy techniques are all encouraged.**

 Massage is only restricted if there is acute inflammation. Refer to the sections covering sprains and strains for precautions pertaining to the specific stage of healing that fits your client's condition.

 Warning: Be cautious if the client has had prior surgery, as the scar tissue will be more fragile than original tissue.

 Your full range of techniques are encouraged to help this condition. Cross fiber deep massage techniques are beneficial to eliminate the adhesions associated with this condition. Ice therapy will also be required to limit the inflammation response to the treatment.

 Be sure to ask about current and past medications. Corticosteroid injections may be administered in severe cases. Check precautions for past injections or long-term medication use.

Tendinitis and Tenosynovitis Precautions, cont'd.

 Massage therapists and bodyworkers who repeatedly utilize the thumb for heavy pressure techniques are especially at risk for DeQuervain's stenosing tenosynovitis. It is highly recommended that you routinely limit your thumb usage to light, sensitive work and use a handheld instrument or other body part to administer deep therapies.

Medial Tibial Stress Syndrome (MTSS)

(also called shin splints)

Overuse of the *tibialis anterior* and/or *peroneus* muscles can result in a rapid buildup of lactic acid. When the energy demand is greater than the available oxygen from the blood supply, the muscle switches from *aerobic energy* (which burns oxygen and fat) to *anaerobic energy* (which needs no oxygen, but burns muscle protein and produces lactic acid). Lactic acid chemically prevents a muscle contraction, so as it builds in the muscle it decreases the muscle function and causes increased pain upon contraction.

Shin splints hurt in the front of the lower leg and can be intensely painful during activity. A short rest from the activity will allow some of the lactic acid to be washed away by the blood supply, and the muscle will partially recover. If the shin pain persists for more than a short period of time, especially without action, it may indicate a more serious injury. Rarely, shin pain may be caused by periosteal or fascial tears, in which case it will be painful at rest and for an extended period of time.

The process of walking is called the *gait cycle*. The *stance phase* accounts for 60 percent of the gait cycle, beginning with the *loading response* (or *heel strike*), followed by the *midstance, terminal stance*, and *preswing* (or *toe off*). The *swing phase* accounts for 40 percent of the gait cycle. It begins with the *initial swing*, followed by the *midswing* and *terminal swing*. With a normal gait cycle, when one foot is in the loading response, the other foot is in preswing.

When the weight is on the heel during the loading response, the foot is in *supination*, a foot position in which the big toe is higher than the smallest toe. *Pronation* is the foot position that places the smallest toe higher than the big toe.

The most common cause of shin splints is from overpronation. This occurs when weak or absent shoe support causes the foot to pronate prematurely. One way to visualize overpronation is to view the ankle from the back while the client stands balanced. If the inside ankle bone (*medial malleolus*) appears larger than the outside ankle bone (*lateral malleolus*), the ankle has overstretched ligaments and is overpronated.

Medial Tibial Stress Syndrome Precautions

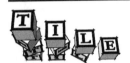 **Tolerance, Incremental, Light and Energy techniques are all encouraged.**

 Massage is only restricted if there is acute inflammation. Refer to the sections covering sprains and strains for precautions pertaining to the specific stage of healing that fits your client's condition.

 Warning: Be cautious if the client has had prior surgery, as the scar tissue will be more fragile than original tissue.

 Your full range of techniques are encouraged to help this condition.

 Massage is very effective in eliminating the lactic acid buildup as well as improving circulation to the area. This helps prevent shin splints from recurring. Ice massage is especially helpful for this condition. Refer to the section on ice therapy for specifics.

 Clients may self-medicate; ask before each visit what prescription and non-prescription medications they have taken in the last 24 hours.

 Take a look at the shoes they wear when they experience the pain. Encourage the client to wear supportive shoes, especially during healing and with activity.

Compartment Syndromes

(also called anterior compartment syndrome, anterior tibialis syndrome, growing pains)

Certain areas of the body have muscles encased in a tight, restrictive fascial compartment. Pain is produced when the muscle and fluids exceed the space causing pain. The most common compartment is the anterior compartment of the lower leg, which includes the anterior tibialis muscle. If it occurs in adolescents during the night (*nocturnal* pain), it is known as *growing pains*.

Compartment syndrome can also occur in an adult. This is a life-threatening reaction to blunt trauma to the area, causing massive inflammation and loss of circulation. *Necrosis* (tissue death) can occur in less than six hours due to the extreme pressure. A procedure called a *fasciotomy* is performed. A surgeon cuts through the fascia to release the pressure and buildup of excess fluids. Extreme pain out of proportion to the injury is a clear warning of traumatic compartment syndrome.

Compartment Syndrome Precautions

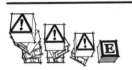 **Energy techniques only. Avoid all pressure and circulatory massage techniques to the limb. Your full technique range is encouraged for the rest of the body.**

 Extreme soft tissue pain out of proportion to the trauma should be considered a medical emergency. Avoid massage and have client seek medical attention immediately.

 Leg pain in children can sometimes be a sign of a serious condition, such as juvenile rheumatoid arthritis or Lyme disease. Contact a physician if any of the following symptoms accompany the pain: Fever, swelling of joints or muscles, exceptional fatigue, loss of appetite and weight loss and/or limping.

 Avoid all heat therapies (including hot stone massage, heat pads, etc), as an increase in fluid to the area would be counterproductive.

Compartment Syndrome Precautions, cont'd.

 Avoid pressure techniques locally as the compartment cannot handle an increase in pressure or fluids.

 NSAIDS may be administered for pain; Be sure to ask about current medications and check their precautions.

 A good source of calcium can be a lifesaver for children with growing pains. Have the client chew a calcium supplement immediately upon waking with pain. A daily supplementation program can minimize or eliminate the symptoms, with extra calcium taken during high activity days.

 Ice therapy is helpful whenever needed for pain control. If the client is an adolescent, adult supervision is recommended.

Osteochondritis Dissecans (OD)

(also called joint mice)

This condition is caused by a lack of blood supply producing inflammation and subsequent tissue death of an area of bone and cartilage. The affected piece of bone may break off and float around the joint. This can be referred to as *joint mice*. This can occur in children throughout puberty especially when active in sports. It also can occur in adults.

Osteochondritis Dissecans Precautions

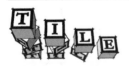 **Tolerance, Incremental, Light and Energy techniques are all encouraged.**

 Massage is only restricted if there is acute inflammation. If there has been recent trauma, refer to the sections covering sprains and strains for precautions pertaining to the specific stage of healing that fits your client's condition.

Osteochondritis Dissecans Precautions, cont'd.

 Warning: Range of motion in the affected joint may push the bone chip into the joint surface. Ask the client's permission and advice before proceeding, as they likely know the motions they consider safe.

 Clients may self-medicate; ask before each visit what prescription and non-prescription medications they have taken in the last 24 hours.

 Muscle spasms are common with this condition, and massage is very helpful within the client's limits.

Legg-Calve-Perthes Disease (LCP)

(also called Legg, Legg-Perthes, Perthes disease, coxa plana, juvenile osteochondrosis, and avascular necrosis of the femoral head.)

Legg-Calve-Perthes disease is caused by a loss of blood supply to the femur head leading to tissue death (*ischemic necrosis*). The cause of the permanent and crippling blood supply loss is unclear. Boys ages 4 to 10 are five times more likely to contract this than girls of the same age. 10 to 15 percent of the time it is bilateral, and can be of familial origin.

Destruction of the femur head usually progresses to the point where it requires hip replacement surgery. Materials used in joint replacement have progressed in the last decade, but frequently, repairs or replacements have to be made periodically. Consistent massage can help minimize the loss of mobility from the repeated scarring and limit muscle and tissue atrophy.

Legg-Calve-Perthes Disease Precautions

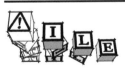 **Restrict massage to Incremental, Light and Energy techniques to the affected joints. Your full technique range is encouraged for the rest of the body.**

Legg-Calve-Perthes Disease Precautions, cont'd.

 If the client has undergone recent surgery, consult with the treating physician before any circulatory massage. Ask about appropriate positions and precautions to massage.

 If there has been a recent accident or injury, avoid all circulatory and mobility techniques to the limb until the client has had approval from their physician.

 Avoid stretching, range of motion exercises, and local deep pressure into the joint as they can exacerbate the condition.

 Warning: Be cautious if the client has had prior surgery, as the scar tissue will be more fragile than original tissue.

 Warning: The client may be unable to comfortably lie prone even with support. Consider seated or side-lying positions as alternatives.

 NSAIDS, muscle relaxants, corticosteroids and other pain medications may be used for joint pain, possibly on a long-term basis. Be sure to ask about current medications and check their precautions.

 Your ability to improve circulation can be a welcome relief for clients with this condition. Keep focused on what you can do to best support the client.

 Ice therapy is especially helpful as an ongoing tool to control pain.

You are unique and special.
Keep focused on what you do
best to support your client.

Osgood-Schlatter's Disease

(also called osteochondrosis)

Two authors, Robert Bayley Osgood and Carl Schlatter, working independently, were the first to describe the condition in 1903. This condition is caused by either repetitive flexion-extension trauma, or a singular significant traumatic event involving the muscular extension of the knee. The most common result is a partial tearing of the tibial patellar ligament as it attaches to the cartilage growth plate of the tibia. A total rupture is rare but possible. In this severe instance the quadriceps muscle and knee lose all function, and surgery is required to reattach the ligament.

Symptoms include pain at the tibial tuberosity that increases with activity and can be severe at times. The pain rarely travels (radiates) to the knee or into the leg. Muscle cramping is common in the affected leg as well as the other leg in a compensation reaction. Osgood-Schlatter's occurs most commonly in boys 10-15 years of age and is healed in all cases by the time puberty is complete.

Osgood-Schlatter's Disease Precautions

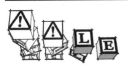 **Restrict massage to Light and Energy techniques to the local area(s). Your full technique range is encouraged for the rest of the body.**

 If there has been a recent accident or injury, avoid all circulatory and mobility techniques to the limb until the client has had approval from their physician.

 Avoid TOLERANCE and INCREMENTAL techniques to the tibial tuberosity and tibial patellar ligament. Avoid pressure or lateral movement of the patella.

 Common medications can include NSAIDS as needed for pain and inflammation. Watch for a reduced ability to gauge pain and pressure tolerance.

 Encourage the client to use ice therapy on an ongoing basis to speed the healing and control pain and inflammation. Massage with ice is not recommended.

Chondromalacia Patellae

(also called patellofemoral pain syndrome, PFS)

This is a common disease characterized by a softening and degeneration of the cartilage under the knee. Pain occurs when exerting force to straighten the knee when the knee is moderately to fully flexed, as in walking up steps. It also can occur with repetitive weight-bearing exercises like jogging. It is primarily due to an asymmetrical tension on the patella, causing erratic and abnormal tracking across the condyles.

This is the most common reason for *scoping the knee*, a slang term referring to *arthroscopic surgery*. The procedure scrapes the softened, uneven cartilage from the underside of the kneecap, providing almost instant relief. Long-term prognosis is poor, however, unless lifestyle changes are made to fix the instability causing the degeneration. Cartilage has no blood supply and will not regenerate. Thinning of the cartilage due to surgery will hasten the degeneration.

Chondromalacia Patellae Precautions

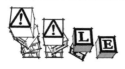 **Restrict massage to Light and Energy techniques to the affected knee. Your full technique range is encouraged for the rest of the body.**

 If there has been a recent accident or injury, avoid all circulatory and mobility techniques to the limb until the client has had approval from their physician.

 Avoid TOLERANCE and INCREMENTAL techniques to the tibial tuberosity and tibial patellar ligament. Avoid pressure on or lateral movement of the patella.

 NSAIDS, muscle relaxants, corticosteroids and other pain medications may be used for joint pain, possibly on a long-term basis. Be sure to ask about current medications and check their precautions.

Chondromalacia Patellae Precautions, cont'd.

 Watch the client walk and stand from behind. If you notice ankle pronation (with the medial ankle more prominent than the lateral), encourage the client to replace their shoes with those including firm counters and rigid shanks. Contrary to fashion, athletic shoes should be limited to athletics, and supportive shoes will help alleviate and eventually correct the condition with your therapy.

 Encourage the client to use ice therapy on an ongoing basis to speed the healing and control pain and inflammation. Massage with ice is not recommended.

Synovitis

Synovitis is the inflammation of a *synovial* (joint lining) membrane, usually painful with motion, and characterized by swelling, due to *effusion* (fluid collection) in the joint capsule. It isn't a disease per se, but rather a symptom of trauma, or an underlying condition such as osteoarthritis. See the section on sprains for more information.

Synovitis Precautions

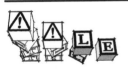 **Restrict massage to Light and Energy techniques to the affected knee. Your full technique range is encouraged for the rest of the body.**

 If there has been a recent accident or injury, avoid all circulatory and mobility techniques to the limb until the client has had approval from their physician. The rest of the body can benefit from all massage techniques.

 Avoid stretching, range of motion exercises, and local deep pressure into the joint as they can all exacerbate this condition.

Synovitis Precautions, cont'd.

 Clients may self-medicate; ask before each visit what prescription and non-prescription medications they have taken in the last 24 hours.

 Ice therapy is especially helpful as an aggressive tool for the client to control pain and stimulate healing. Focus your therapy on improving the circulation through the affected joint.

Baker's Cyst

(also called a popliteal cyst)

Baker's cyst is a pronounced swelling on the back of the knee, caused by the abnormal collection of fluid inside the popliteal bursa. A cyst doesn't actually grow on the back of the knee. Any fluid filled sac can be called a cyst. The symptoms are mild unless the cyst bursts or extends down into the calf muscles. Common causes of Baker's cyst include arthritis, infection, injury or repetitive trauma to the knee.

The inflammation may resolve with time. If not, cortisone injections, draining the bursa or even surgical removal are likely. Massage is very effective in reducing the inflammation associated with this condition.

Baker's Cyst Precautions

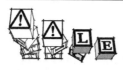 **Restrict massage to Light and Energy techniques to the affected knee. Your full technique range is encouraged for the rest of the body.**

 If there has been a recent accident or injury, avoid all circulatory and mobility techniques to the limb until the client has had approval from their physician. The rest of the body can benefit from all massage techniques.

 Avoid stretching, range of motion exercises, and local deep pressure into the joint as they can all exacerbate this condition.

Baker's Cyst Precautions, cont'd.

 Clients may self-medicate; ask before each visit what prescription and non-prescription medications they have taken in the last 24 hours.

 Ice therapy is especially helpful as an aggressive tool for the client to control pain and stimulate healing. Focus your therapy on improving the circulation through the affected joint.

Knee Trauma

The meniscus is a cartilage pad separating the femur from the tibia. Trauma can cause a portion of the meniscus to tear or break free. The meniscus is not accessible to the finger unless a torn portion protrudes. Clicking, locking, and often severe pain occurs when the torn piece is caught between the two bones, and the joint can be pain free at other times.

The *anterior cruciate ligament* (ACL) and the *medial collateral ligament* (MCL) are the most often ligaments injured, but the *posterior cruciate ligament* (PCL) or *lateral collateral ligament* (LCL) can also be injured. There may not be any pain with a grade one sprain after the initial injury. There may be a popping noise, and the leg can feel weak or buckle when standing or walking. With a tear or rupture, however, there is significant pain and loss of function.

Treatment initially includes **PRICE** therapy. If that fails to achieve satisfactory results alone, a steroid injection may be administered unless the instability is too severe. Arthroscopic surgery may be necessary based on the degree of knee instability. This type of surgery is desirable as it leaves minimal scar tissue while being effective in repairing the knee. A knee brace is usually recommended to limit specific range of motion during activity to avoid excess stress on the healing tissue. A certain level of activity is encouraged to stimulate growth and tissue repair. See the section on sprains for more information.

Knee Trauma Precautions

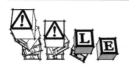 **Restrict massage to Light and Energy techniques.**

 If there has been a recent accident or injury, avoid all circulatory and mobility techniques to the limb until the client has had approval from their physician. The rest of the body can benefit from all massage techniques.

 Warning: Be cautious if the client has had prior surgery, as the scar tissue will be more fragile than original tissue.

 Assisting the client in range-of-motion exercises after knee repair has been shown to be more effective in promoting healing than simply keeping the joint immobile. Remember to work within the client's physical and emotional comfort level.

 Clients may self-medicate; ask before each visit what prescription and non-prescription medications they have taken in the last 24 hours.

 Massage and assisted mobility can give the client the relief and encouragement they often need to follow through with the rehabilitation of their knee.

Watch the client walk and stand from behind. If you notice excess pronation (with the medial ankle more prominent than the lateral), encourage the client to replace their shoes with those having firm counters and rigid shanks. Supportive shoes can make you a hero in their eyes!

Plantar Fasciitis and Calcaneal Periostitis

(also called a heel spur, stoned heel)

When too much stress is placed upon the tendon or fascia attached to the heel the tissue becomes inflamed. Pain on the heel or bottom of the foot can be severe with activity. The client may feel the most pain in the first 10 to 20 steps in the morning, as the inflammation is forced out of the tissues. Subsequently the client will alter their normal walking gait and other pains may develop. *Plantar fasciitis* is the pain, inflammation and hypersensitivity that comes from excessive physical stress to the bottom of the foot (see the section on stress for more information).

If the cause of the stress is not eliminated this can produce an unstable attachment at the heel. The body reacts by depositing calcium into the tendon to strengthen it, thereby producing a heel spur (*calcaneal periostitis*). The pain does not come directly from the spur. You would have to fracture the spur to cause the significant pain associated with this condition. Rather, the pain is caused by the overstressed tissues themselves.

Wearing non-supportive shoes is a common example of chronic trauma leading to plantar fasciitis and eventually heel spurs. Initial trauma from beginning an activity like running, followed by relatively normal activity without properly allowing the tissues to heal is another example.

Plantar Fasciitis and Calcaneal Periostitis Precautions

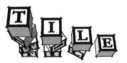 **Tolerance, Incremental, Light and Energy techniques are all encouraged.**

 If there has been a recent accident or injury that has caused acute inflammation, avoid all circulatory and mobility techniques to the foot until the client has had approval from their physician. The rest of the body can benefit from all massage techniques.

 Avoid stretching the plantar fascia and local deep pressure into the heel as they can both exacerbate these conditions.

Plantar Fasciitis and Calcaneal Periostitis Precautions, cont'd.

 Warning: Be cautious if the client has had prior surgery, as the scar tissue will be more fragile than original tissue.

 Be sure to ask about current medications and check their precautions. The client may have a history of cortisone (steroid) injections or oral medication. Check the precautions carefully before proceeding.

 Encourage the client to use ice therapy on an ongoing basis to speed the healing and control pain and inflammation. Massage with ice is not recommended.

*Empower the client by teaching
them massage techniques
they can use between sessions,
and encourage persistence
with ice therapy. Your guidance
can make all the difference!*

Muscular Dystrophy (MD)

(also called Duchenne muscular dystrophy, myotonic muscular dystrophy)

Muscular dystrophy is a group of nine genetic diseases involving progressive weakness and degeneration of the muscles that control movement. *Myotonic MD* is the most common form among adults, and *Duchenne MD* the most common form among children (affecting only boys). Muscular cramping and flexion contractures are the norm with all forms of MD leading to scoliosis and postural distortion.

The outlook for people with MD varies, depending on the type and severity of the disease. In mild cases, while incurable, the disease may progress slowly and the person may have a normal lifespan, while in more severe cases, there is a more swift degeneration of muscle weakness leading to fatality.

Muscular Dystrophy Precautions

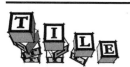 **Tolerance, Incremental, Light and Energy techniques are all encouraged within the client's limits.**

 Massage is not contraindicated, however, it may be best to consult with the physician for specific precautions as the severity and progression of MD varies widely.

 Warning: The client may have difficulty communicating their goals and limitations. Discuss verbal and nonverbal signals as well as physical goals and limitations with the client and/or guardian before your first session.

 Reduce your overall massage time to guard against overwhelming the client until you are certain about their limitations.

 Be sure to ask about current medications and check their precautions. Corticosteroids are commonly administered. Pay special attention to the precautions listed in those sections.

 Your ability to improve circulation and reduce spasms can be a welcome relief for clients with this condition. Your compassionate touch may be the best gift you give the client with this condition.

Polymyositis and Dermatomyositis

Polymyositis is an inflammatory muscle disease that causes progressive muscle atrophy. *Dermatomyositis* includes inflammation of the skin. These two related forms of myositis generally begin in the second decade of life and result from a disturbance in the body's immune system. These related conditions are not infectious and cannot be spread by contact.

Symptoms include muscle weakness and pain, usually affecting trunk muscles first and occasionally expands to include the extremities as the condition progresses.

Polymyositis and Dermatomyositis Precautions

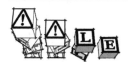 **Restrict massage to Light and Energy techniques.**

 Before any session including pressure techniques, consult with the physician to discuss the proper precautions for this client.

 Reduce your overall massage time to guard against overwhelming the client. Only LIGHT and ENERGY techniques should be performed because of the increasingly fragile tissue and compromised immune system.

 Be sure to ask about current medications and check their precautions. Corticosteroids are commonly administered on a long-term basis, as well as immunosuppressants and pain medications. Pay special attention to the precautions listed in those sections.

 Your compassionate touch may be the best gift you give the client with this condition. Be emotionally strong and supportive and recognize the healing benefits you provide are far more than simply physical.

Myositis Ossificans

(Also called fibrodysplasia ossificans progressiva, myositis ossificans circumscripta, myositis ossificans progressiva, soft tissue ossification)

There are two types of myositis ossificans, the hereditary form (*myositis ossificans progressiva*), and the inflammatory form (*myositis ossificans circumscripta*). The hereditary form is more severe, producing widespread calcium deposits beginning in the trunk and progressing to the extremities. It causes torticollis, scoliosis and kyphotic spinal curvatures. Chronic muscle spasms are common.

The non-hereditary form is a result of trauma. It can be a single traumatic event or repetitive mechanical injuries over time. Enough instability accumulates that the body enacts Wolff's Law, where increased stress produces calcium deposits to form. These are painless and may go unnoticed if the injury was not remarkable to the client.

Myositis Ossificans Precautions

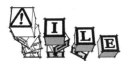 **Restrict massage to Incremental, Light and Energy techniques directly on the affected muscle. Your full technique range is encouraged for the rest of the body.**

 If there has been a recent accident or injury, avoid all pressure and mobility techniques to the limb until the client has had approval from their physician.

 Avoid deep local pressure permanently. Increased trauma to the area can result in increased calcium deposits. Massage in the surrounding areas is recommended however.

 Be sure to ask about current medications and check their precautions. The client may have a history of corticosteroid treatment and/or pain medication. Check the precautions carefully before proceeding.

 Spontaneous resorption of the calcium is rare but possible in a healthy individual. Proper, consistent massage can help create that environment.

Musculoskeletal Medications

NOTE: Most medications prescribed for musculoskeletal conditions are to reduce the symptoms and are found elsewhere in this guide. Please use the index to search for specific information about those medications.

Medications to Improve Bone Density

(also called bisphosphonates)

Bisphosphonates form a portion of bone that becomes resistant to the bone-consuming activity of *osteoclasts*. This results in increased bone mineral density.

 If the client has developed muscle weakness, persistent nausea, vomiting, constipation, or low energy, avoid massage and have them call their doctor immediately. These may be signs of too much calcium in the blood. These drug side effects are considered very serious and require medical attention. (This is a massage-specific list; refer to the documentation that was included with the medication for a complete list of side effects.)

 Side Effects: Increased blood pressure, muscle or bone pain, pain in extremities, mild leg cramps, swelling or edema, flushing, tenderness and/or tingling of the face, ears, hands, or feet can all occur with this class of medication. Take these into consideration as they may limit your ability to achieve your client's massage goals.

 Bisphosphonate medications include: <u>alendronate</u> (Fosamax), <u>ibandronate</u> (Boniva) and <u>risedronate</u> (Actonel).

Antimyasthenics

Antimyasthenics are given by mouth or by injection to treat myasthenia gravis by improving muscle strength. Sometimes neostigmine is given by injection to prevent or treat certain urinary tract or intestinal disorders.

 If the client has developed any of the following, stop or avoid all massage and have them call their doctor immediately: skin rash or hives, blurred vision, clumsiness or unsteadiness, confusion, convulsions (seizures), severe diarrhea, nausea or vomiting, increasing muscle weakness, severe muscle twitching or cramping, shortness of breath, or unusual tiredness. These drug side effects are considered very serious and require medical attention. (This is a massage-specific list; refer to the documentation that was included with the medication for a complete list of side effects.)

 Side Effects: Headaches, muscle aches, cramps or spasms, upset stomach, vomiting, diarrhea, dizziness, loss of balance and fatigue all can occur with this class of medication. Take these into consideration as they may limit your ability to achieve your client's massage goals.

 Postural hypotension can occur as a side effect of this class of medication. Help the client to change positions and be on guard for dizziness or blacking out.

 Medications include: ambenonium (Mytelase), edrophonium (Enlon, Reversol, Tensilon), neostigmine (Prostigmin), and pyridostigmine (Mestinon, Regonol, Timespans).

*Your compassionate touch
may be the best gift
you give your client.
Be emotionally strong and
supportive, and recognize
that the healing benefits you
provide are far more
than simply physical.*

Chapter 4

Cardiovascular System

Anemia

Anemia is a loss of oxygen-carrying capacity. This can be due to insufficient red blood cells (RBCs) and/or hemoglobin. *Hemoglobin* carries oxygen and can be found only in the red blood cells. In all cases, the symptoms produced are a result of the brain and body struggling with less oxygen than it needs for normal function.

Symptoms for all anemias are similar and include fatigue, tingling and numbness of hands and feet, shortness of breath, pallor (loss of normal skin coloring, tachycardia (rapid heart rate) and diarrhea.

The most common types of anemia are described below:

Aplastic Anemia
Aplastic anemia is a blood disorder caused by the destruction of the bone marrow due to chemicals (like arsenic or chemotherapy), radiation therapy or bone marrow diseases.

Sickle Cell Anemia
Sickle cell anemia is a hereditary, chronic condition caused by the presence of an abnormal type of hemoglobin occurring in people whose ancestors come from Africa, Central and South America and Mediterranean countries. Sickle cell anemia is characterized by the red blood cells taking a crescent or sickle shape. *Hemolytic anemias* like sickle cell have red blood cells that die prematurely. While the average lifespan of an RBC is 120 days, these cells die after only 10 to 20 days.

Iron Deficiency Anemia
Iron deficiency anemia results when the body has a greater demand for iron than what is utilized from the diet. Iron is required to produce hemoglobin. It is the most common type of anemia and affects approximately 18 million people in the US.

B12 and Folic Acid Anemias

Vitamin B12 (cobalamin) and folic acid (folate) are two B vitamins required for the rapid synthesis of DNA during cell division. This is especially important in tissues where cells like RBCs are dividing rapidly. While some fruits and vegetables contain folic acid, according to the Vegetarian Society there is no significant vegetarian source of vitamin B12. It can only be absorbed from an animal source. Chronic B12 anemia can be called *pernicious anemia* when it's due to a loss of *intrinsic factor*, a substance required for the absorption of vitamin B12.

Blood Loss Anemia

Trauma-related or blood loss anemia is due to red blood cells lost through injury.

Anemia Precautions (refer to description of specific type)

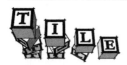 **Tolerance, Incremental, Light and Energy techniques are all encouraged within the client's limits.**

 Avoid all massage and have client contact their physician immediately if symptoms become severe or alarming. Symptoms include fatigue, tingling and numbness of hands and feet, shortness of breath, or increased heart rate.

 Warning: Take time before each session to ask about their fatigue and stress levels over the last few days. If these are elevated, a reduction in massage duration and intensity are recommended. Fatigue and endurance are factors in anemia, so limit the your massage to avoid overwhelming the client.

 Warning: Pressure techniques increase the flow of RBCs through the capillary beds. Be cautious with aggressive massage techniques.

 Antibiotics and immunosuppressants can be administered for some anemias. Avoid local injection and IV sites. Be sure to ask about current medications and check their precautions.

 Appropriate massage has the ability to improve RBC production, assuming the nutritional needs are also met.

Hemophilia

Hemophilia is due to low levels or the complete absence of a blood protein essential for clotting (called *clotting factors*). Hemophilia affects more than 20,000 people in the United States.

Clients with hemophilia experience excessive bruising and bleeding from seemingly minor trauma. There can be severe joint pain from bleeding in the joint cavities. Exercise extreme caution when working with clients afflicted with this condition.

Hemophilia Precautions

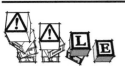 **Restrict massage to Light and Energy techniques.**

 Contact the client's physician before your first session to determine if any pressure techniques are acceptable as well as the suggested frequency of massage. Be sure to discuss precautions due to specific antihemophilia medications in your consultation.

 Avoid all massage and have the client contact their physician immediately if you determine there has been recent dramatic bruising, sudden loss of energy, or visible pallor.

 Avoid pressure massage other than LIGHT and ENERGY techniques, as there is an increased likelihood of excessive bruising and bleeding. Mobility and stretching techniques should be done with caution to avoid stress on the joints.

 Warning: Take time before each session to ask about their fatigue and stress levels over the last few days. If these are elevated, pressure techniques should be postponed and ENERGY techniques utilized as an alternative.

 Antihemophilia medications can be utilized. Refer to specific precautions listed by the physician or product labeling. Be sure to ask the client about all other medications and check their precautions also.

 Clients treasure the compassion in your attitude as much as they benefit from your techniques.

Thrombocytopenia

Thrombocytopenia refers to any disorder in which there are not enough platelets. This may be due to hereditary insufficiency, bone marrow dysfunction leading to reduced platelet production, or certain drugs causing the formation of antibodies against platelets.

The immune system is hampered by the reduced ability to form blood clots. Internal repairs take longer, and clients with thrombocytopenia experience excessive bruising and bleeding from seemingly minor trauma. There can be severe joint pain from bleeding in the joint cavities. Exercise extreme caution when working with clients afflicted with this condition.

Thrombocytopenia Precautions

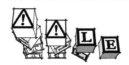 **Restrict massage to Light and Energy techniques.**

 Contact the client's physician before your first session to determine if any pressure techniques are acceptable as well as the suggested frequency of massage. Be sure to discuss precautions due to specific antihemophilia medications in your consultation.

 Avoid all massage and have the client contact their physician immediately if you determine there has been recent dramatic bruising, sudden loss of energy, or visible pallor.

 Avoid pressure massage other than LIGHT and ENERGY techniques, as there is an increased likelihood of excessive bruising and bleeding. Mobility and stretching techniques should be done with caution to avoid stress on the joints.

 Warning: Take time before each session to ask about their fatigue and stress levels over the last few days. If these are elevated, pressure techniques should be postponed; use only ENERGY techniques.

 Medications including steroids can be prescribed for long-term treatment of this condition. Be sure to ask about current medications and check their precautions.

 Your lightest techniques may be your best tools for health improvement in clients with this condition.

Peripheral Artery Disease (PAD)

(also called arteriosclerosis, atherosclerosis, hardening of the arteries, peripheral vascular disease, PVD)

Peripheral artery disease refers to narrowing of blood vessels outside the heart and brain. Fatty substances, cholesterol, cellular waste products, calcium and other substances build up in the inner linings of the artery walls and cause blockages. This buildup is called *plaque*. Plaque weakens the layers of the artery and encourages clotting (thrombus).

Coronary artery disease (CAD) is a specific type of PAD in which plaque builds in the arteries that supply blood to the heart muscle.

Often there are no symptoms to detect the buildup of plaque in the arteries. As the condition becomes more severe it may be detected by an optometrist when viewing your *retina* (back of the eye). *Intermittent claudication* is cramping or fatigue in the legs and buttocks during activity, caused by peripheral artery disease. If an *embolism* (floating blood clot) becomes lodged in a narrowed artery, an *infarction* results (tissue death from blood loss). If this occurs in the heart it is a *myocardial infarction* (MI) or *heart attack*. In the brain it is known as a *cerebrovascular accident* (CVA) or *stroke*.

Peripheral Artery Disease Precautions

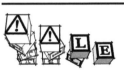 **Restrict massage to Incremental, Light and Energy techniques. Exercise caution when massaging near superficial arteries.**

 Any of the following symptoms are possible indications of a stroke. Sudden, severe headache with no known cause; Sudden numbness or weakness of the face, arm or leg, especially on one side of the body; Sudden confusion, trouble speaking or understanding; Sudden trouble seeing in one or both eyes; Sudden trouble walking, dizziness, loss of balance or coordination. Stop or avoid massage and call emergency services immediately.

Peripheral Artery Disease Precautions, cont'd.

 Techniques that aggressively increase circulation should be avoided with advanced PAD until you discuss with the physician the client's specific limits. LIGHT and ENERGY techniques are recommended and encouraged.

 Avoid vigorous or deep pressure in areas where an artery could become trapped against a bone. Of special concern are the following areas: The medial ankle, posterior knee, upper anterior thigh, abdomen, axillary region, anterior elbow, anterior wrist, anterior neck and the temporal area.

 Warning: Hypertension and other cardiovascular conditions often accompany this condition. Ask for and check all conditions for a complete understanding of massage precautions.

 Cardiovascular medications are common. Be sure to ask about current medications and check their precautions.

 Your client will benefit greatly from appropriate improvement in their circulation and energy. Be vigilant, however; with no symptoms to remind you, it is easy to forget the client's hidden limitations.

Raynaud's Syndrome

(also called Raynaud's Phenomenon, Raynaud's Disease)

Raynaud's is named after the French doctor Maurice Raynaud, who first described the condition in the mid-1800s. It is a condition in which the smallest arteries that bring blood to the fingers or toes constrict (go into spasm) when exposed to cold, emotional upset, or other triggers such as vibrations. Smoking also can cause these episodes. The result is that the fingers and/or toes lose their blood supply and become cold, numb and painful.

Certain medications and conditions (including lupus and diabetes) may increase the likelihood of contracting Raynaud's, but most often the cause is unknown. There is no cure, and treatment is usually limited to medication and protecting against the triggers that cause exacerbation.

Raynaud's Syndrome Precautions

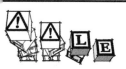

> **Restrict massage to Light and Energy techniques in the hands and feet. Your full technique range is encouraged for the rest of the body.**

 Ask your client what triggers their condition, and alter your sessions appropriately.

 Avoid all ice or cold therapies as they may trigger an attack.

 Warning: There may be tissue atrophy depending upon the severity and frequency of attacks. Be cautious in your application of pressure techniques to avoid tissue damage.

 Warning: Check all other conditions the client reports to gain a complete understanding of the precautions to take for this client.

 Calcium channel blockers are commonly prescribed and have significant side effects. Be sure to ask about current medications and check their precautions.

 Teach your client massage techniques they can use to increase circulation to their hands and they'll be grateful for life!

Aneurysm

An aneurysm is the abnormal bulging of an artery caused by weakness in the blood vessel wall. Aneurysms can form anywhere, but the most common location is in the *aorta*. They can also be found in the arteries of the brain (called *berry aneurysms*). Aneurysms often go undetected because they rarely produce symptoms. In certain cases the aneurysm may press on an adjacent body part and cause a malfunction.

Since the artery wall is subjected to constant blood pressure, aneurysms do not heal without surgery. Occasionally the physician may choose to avoid surgery because the client's other conditions make it too risky. Circulatory massage changes the pressure inside the blood vessels, as well as changing the nerve signals to the smooth muscles, and is too risky for someone with an aneurysm.

Aneurysm Precautions

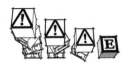 **Energy techniques only. Avoid all pressure and circulatory massage techniques.**

 Any of the following symptoms are possible indications of an aneurysm or stroke. Sudden, severe headache with no known cause, sudden confusion, trouble speaking or understanding, sudden trouble seeing in one or both eyes, dizziness, sudden trouble walking, a loss of balance or coordination. Stop or avoid massage and call emergency services immediately.

 Avoid pressure techniques until the client has healed from surgery and has the approval of their physician. ENERGY techniques are encouraged.

 Avoid the prone position during any session until the client has the approval of their physician.

 Be sure to ask about current medications and check their precautions.

 Regularly scheduled energy therapy sessions will help the client retain a semblance of normalcy and can be a significant factor in their health.

*Keep foremost in your mind
the powerful benefits of touch.*

Vasculitis

Vasculitis means the inflammation of a blood vessel. It can be due to trauma (e.g. a calf injury from a baseball). It can be a complication from another illness such as lupus. Sometimes, it is precipitated by a drug reaction. In still other cases, it occurs in conjunction with a viral illness, such as hepatitis or HIV. Pain increases whenever the blood vessel fills with fluid and can become extreme.

Vasculitis Precautions

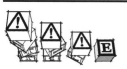 **Energy techniques only for the entire limb; avoid all pressure and circulatory massage techniques. Your full technique range is encouraged for the rest of the body.**

 Unexplained leg pain, tenderness or edema (usually in only one leg), unexplained or persistent joint pain, or sharp leg pain when the foot is bent upward are all possible signs of DVT and are considered medical emergencies. Avoid massage and have the client seek medical attention immediately.

 In cases of systemic vasculitis, consult with the treating physician before your first session with the client. ENERGY techniques are acceptable on an ongoing basis.

 Avoid pressure techniques to bruised areas for traumatic vasculitis and the regions distal to the area until all symptoms are gone.

 Anticoagulant and antithrombotic medications are common, in addition to pain medication. Be sure to ask about current medications and check their precautions.

 Remember the health benefits that relaxation brings to the client's environment through your sessions.

Deep Vein Thrombosis (DVT)

(also called thrombophlebitis)

Deep vein thrombosis is the term used to describe blood clots (thrombi) that form in the veins. These most commonly form in the legs, but can form anywhere in the body. An estimated 2 million people in the U.S. develop DVT each year. They interfere with the proper flow of blood to the heart, and sometimes the clots break loose and travel to critical organs. An embolism traveling to the lungs can result in a pulmonary embolism (PE). In fact, studies have shown that over 40 percent of the time PE is a result of deep vein thrombosis in the calf. An embolism to the brain can cause a stroke, and an embolism lodging in the heart is called a heart attack. Both can have their origins as deep vein thrombosis.

Up to half of all clients with a history of DVT will develop chronic swelling, pain and discoloration of the affected leg. The skin may be increasingly fragile due to the compromised circulation, and the client is usually encouraged to wear special elastic support stockings.

Deep Vein Thrombosis Precautions

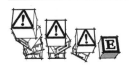 **Energy techniques only. Avoid all pressure and circulatory massage techniques.**

 Unexplained leg pain, tenderness or edema (usually in only one leg), unexplained or persistent joint pain, or sharp leg pain when the foot is bent upward are all possible signs of DVT and are considered medical emergencies. Avoid massage and have the client seek medical attention immediately.

 Chest pain, chest wall tenderness, shortness of breath, painful respiration, possibly with back or shoulder pain could all be signs of a pulmonary embolism, and are also considered a medical emergency. Avoid massage and have client seek medical attention immediately. Mere minutes may make the difference!

Deep Vein Thrombosis Precautions, cont'd.

 Avoid all pressure techniques for the entire body until the treating physician has stated that the threat of embolism has passed. Treatment may take months; ENERGY techniques can be freely utilized during this time.

 Warning: Consider the circulation of the affected leg to be compromised (and strongly consider the same for the other leg also if other cardiovascular conditions exist). Even after the physician has given approval for pressure massage, limit your techniques in these limbs to LIGHT and ENERGY techniques and be cautious about how aggressively you increase venous demands in these areas.

 Anticoagulant and antithrombotic medications are common for an extended period of time. Be sure to ask about current medications and check their precautions.

 Your knowledge about how the body normally feels and responds can be the first line of awareness for someone who may have undetected DVT. Trust your instincts and speak to your client whenever you determine something is abnormal, even if it isn't easily explained.

Varicose Veins

Veins are vessels carrying blood back to the heart. Normal veins have valves that prevent the blood from traveling away from the heart. Varicose veins have become widened such that the valves become ineffective and blood can stagnate and possibly clot. Actions that make varicose veins more likely include standing for long hours on the job, cigarette smoking, pregnancy, or chronic pressure from a leg brace or from sitting on one's legs or feet. It is estimated that 40 percent of all U.S. women will have some abnormal veins by age 50. The veins can itch or hurt with extra activity or long days.

Varicose Vein Precautions

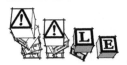 **Restrict massage to Light and Energy techniques.**

 Unexplained leg pain, tenderness or edema (usually in only one leg), unexplained or persistent joint pain, or sharp leg pain when the foot is bent upward are all possible signs of DVT and are considered a medical emergency. Avoid massage and have client seek medical attention immediately.

 Chest pain, chest wall tenderness, shortness of breath, painful respiration, possibly with back or shoulder pain could all be signs of a pulmonary embolism, and are also considered a medical emergency. Avoid massage and have client seek medical attention immediately. Mere minutes may make the difference!

 Avoid all but light pressure massage locally on visible varicose veins. Avoid vigorous massage distal to the vein to limit the extra blood flow through the area.

 Avoid vigorous massage distal to the area to limit the extra blood flow. Circulation capacity will be reduced to any area in which veins have been removed surgically, chemically or by laser.

 Be sure to ask about current medications and check their precautions.

 Varicose veins can be relieved (not cured) with a regimen of regular circulatory massage, coupled with appropriate exercise. Encourage your client to follow their physician's exercise regimen along with your therapy.

Clients find comfort
in your consistency.

Hypertension

According to recent estimates, one in four U.S. adults has high blood pressure, but because there are no symptoms, nearly one-third of these people don't know they have it. Blood pressure is defined by two numbers, *systolic pressure* (the first number) is the blood pressure measured while the heart is contracting, while *diastolic pressure* (the second number) is the blood pressure measured when the heart is at rest between beats. It measures the pressure exerted by the artery walls.

The American Heart Association currently states that normal blood pressure is rated below 120/80. If blood pressure rises for either number above 120/80 it is considered *prehypertension*, up to 140/90. If the blood pressure rises above 140/90 (either one), it is considered *Stage 1 hypertension. Stage 2 hypertension* is when systolic pressures rise to 160 or above, or diastolic pressure rises to 100 or above.

There are no symptoms for hypertension! You can feel your heart beating too fast (called tachycardia), but you cannot feel high blood *pressure*. A recent study showed that almost two thirds of those taking medicine to control high blood pressure had *stopped taking it* within three years! It is difficult to continually justify a medicine that doesn't make you feel better yet has a good chance of making you feel worse from the side effects.

Prehypertension Precautions

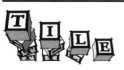 **Tolerance, Incremental, Light and Energy techniques are all encouraged.**

 If the client has developed any of the following warning symptoms, stop or avoid massage and seek emergency medical attention immediately: Chest discomfort; pain or discomfort in one or both arms, the back, neck, jaw or stomach; labored breathing; breaking out in a cold sweat; nausea or lightheadedness. Stop the massage and assist them in seeking immediate medical attention.

 Prehypertension is clearly a warning by the medical profession that healthier habits need to be adopted. Provide guidance and encouragement for your client in addition to regular massage sessions.

Stage 1 Hypertension Precautions

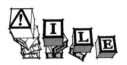 **Restrict massage to Incremental, Light and Energy techniques.**

 If the client has developed any of the following warning symptoms, stop or avoid massage and seek emergency medical attention immediately: Chest discomfort; pain or discomfort in one or both arms, the back, neck, jaw or stomach; labored breathing; breaking out in a cold sweat; nausea or lightheadedness. Stop the massage and assist them in seeking immediate medical attention.

 Avoid deep abdominal massage: There is an increased chance of returning too much blood, as well as the possibility of sympathetic or parasympathetic rebounding from nerve stimulation.

 Reduce the duration and intensity of circulatory massage to guard against overworking the cardiovascular system.

 Consistent massage sessions can improve the body's ability to control blood pressure. Explain this to your client for increased awareness about the benefits of massage, as well as the possible need to have their physician moderate their medication dosages.

Stage 2 Hypertension Precautions

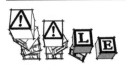 **Restrict massage to Light and Energy techniques within the client's circulatory system limits.**

 If the client has developed any of the following warning symptoms, stop or avoid massage and seek emergency medical attention immediately: Chest discomfort; pain or discomfort in one or both arms, the back, neck, jaw or stomach; labored breathing; breaking out in a cold sweat; nausea or lightheadedness. Stop the massage and assist them in seeking immediate medical attention.

Stage 2 Hypertension Precautions, cont'd.

 Avoid deep abdominal massage: There is an increased chance of returning too much blood, as well as the possibility of sympathetic or parasympathetic rebounding from nerve stimulation.

 Limit your massage to LIGHT or ENERGY massage techniques. The cardiovascular system is fragile, regardless of the medication.

 Reduce the duration and intensity of circulatory massage to guard against overworking the cardiovascular system.

 Statistically, it is likely that your client isn't taking the medication consistently, if at all. Be certain your massage is light enough to be handled if the client has uncontrolled hypertension.

 Clients with hypertension frequently have a number of ongoing prescriptions. Be sure to ask about all current medications and take enough time to check each of their precautions.

 Subtle techniques, performed with elegance and the proper attitude can have astonishing effects upon your client's health.

Remember that with massage,
you are the expert.
You are uniquely qualified
to decide what is appropriate
with your techniques.
Be firm with your decisions,
secure in the knowledge
that your client's health
is your primary goal.

Heart Diseases

Since 1900, cardiovascular disease (CVD) has been the No. 1 killer in the United States every year but 1918. Nearly 2,600 Americans die of CVD each day, an average of one death every 34 seconds.

Specific heart conditions are listed below, with varying degrees of severity. Unless it specifically says that the condition (like mitral valve prolapse) poses no concern, the following precautions should be strictly adhered to. It is always best to speak directly to the client's cardiovascular physician to be certain of the precautions. These precautions may seem excessive, and one may adapt an attitude of *"my client(s) aren't that bad."* Unfortunately, the position of *"no pain, no problem"* is exactly what makes cardiovascular disease so insidious and dangerous. Consider the consequences of being wrong, and be the cautious guardian of your client's health.

Bacterial Endocarditis
(also called infective endocarditis)

Bacterial endocarditis is an infection of the heart's inner lining and/or the heart valves. Immediate and aggressive treatment is critical, and massage is prohibited.

Heart Attack
(also called myocardial infarction)

A heart attack occurs when the blood supply to part of the heart muscle itself (the *myocardium*) is severely reduced or stopped. The reduction or stoppage happens when one or more of the coronary arteries supplying blood to the heart muscle is blocked. Immediate and aggressive treatment is critical, and massage is prohibited.

Pericarditis
Pericarditis is inflammation of the pericardium, the membrane that surrounds the heart. This squeezes the heart and restricts its action, causing severe pain. This is usually treated with antibiotics and heavy sedation in a hospital setting. Massage is prohibited.

Sudden Cardiac Death

(also called sudden arrest, cardiac arrest)

Sudden cardiac death is results from an abrupt loss of heart function. The victim may or may not have diagnosed heart disease. It occurs within minutes after symptoms appear.

Ventricular Fibrillation

Ventricular fibrillation is a condition in which the heart's lower chambers contract in a rapid, unsynchronized way, pumping little or no blood. Collapse and sudden cardiac death will follow in minutes unless medical help is provided immediately. A *defibrillator* machine is used to interrupt ventricular fibrillation and allow the heart to resume beating properly.

Acute Heart Disease Precautions

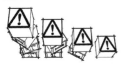 **Client is in critical condition. Avoid all therapy until approved by their physician.**

Angina Pectoris

(also called myocardial ischemia)

Angina is a sign that someone is at increased risk of heart attack, cardiac arrest and sudden cardiac death. Angina pectoris is the medical term for chest pain or discomfort due to coronary heart disease. Angina occurs when the heart muscle doesn't get as much blood or oxygen as it needs. See the precautions listed below for specifics.

Cardiomyopathy

(also called hypertrophic obstructive cardiomyopathy (HOCM), asymmetric septal hypertrophy (ASH), idiopathic hypertrophic subaortic stenosis)

Cardiomyopathy is a serious disease in which the heart muscle becomes inflamed and doesn't work as well as it should. There may be multiple causes including viral and bacterial infections. It is called hypertrophic cardiomyopathy when the muscle mass of the left ventricle enlarges and obstructs the blood flow. See the precautions listed below for specifics.

Congestive Heart Failure (CHF)

(also called diastolic failure, hypertensive heart disease, left-sided heart failure, left-ventricular heart failure (LV), right-sided heart failure, right-ventricular heart failure (RV), systolic failure)

Heart failure can involve the heart's left side, right side or both sides. The atrium receives blood into the heart, and the ventricle pumps it where it needs to go. Heart failure occurs when any of these chambers lose their ability to keep up with the amount of blood flow. As the heart's ability to pump decreases, blood flow slows down, causing fluid to build up in tissues throughout the body (edema). This excess fluid or congestion explains the term congestive heart failure. See the precautions listed below for specifics.

Cor Pulmonale

Cor pulmonale is a form of heart disease secondary to chronic obstructive pulmonary disease (COPD). The congestion from the lungs causes increased pressure in the heart, leading to a condition similar to congestive heart failure.

Coronary Heart Disease (CHD)

(also called coronary artery disease, ischemic heart disease, and silent ischemia)

These are heart problems caused by narrowed heart arteries. When arteries are narrowed, less blood and oxygen reaches the heart muscle. This can ultimately lead to heart attack. See the precautions listed below for specifics.

Left Ventricular Hypertrophy (LVH)

(also called aortic regurgitation, enlarged heart)

The muscle of the left ventricle of the heart gets larger due to aortic regurgitation, which means the valve from the left ventricle doesn't close properly, and blood can leak backward through it. This means the left ventricle must pump more blood than normal, and will gradually get bigger because of the extra workload. See the precautions listed below for specifics.

Mitral Valve Prolapse
(also called heart murmur, click-murmur syndrome, Barlow's syndrome, balloon mitral valve, floppy valve syndrome)

When the heart pumps, the mitral valve flaps don't close smoothly or evenly. Instead, a flap collapses backward into the left atrium. This lets a small amount of blood leak backward through the valve. Most people with mitral valve prolapse don't have symptoms, won't have problems and won't need treatment.

Rheumatic Heart Disease
Rheumatic heart disease is a condition in which the heart valves are damaged by rheumatic fever. Heart diseases are more likely earlier in life as a result. See the precautions listed below for specifics.

Chronic Heart Disease Precautions

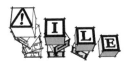 **Restrict massage to Incremental, Light and Energy techniques.**

 If the client has developed any of the following warning symptoms, stop or avoid massage and seek emergency medical attention immediately: Chest discomfort, pain or discomfort in one or both arms, the back, neck, jaw or stomach, shortness of breath, breaking out in a cold sweat, nausea or lightheadedness.

 Avoid deep tissue techniques and deep abdominal massage.

 Limit or avoid laying the client prone while performing pressure techniques. Increased pressure on the heart compounded by increasing blood flow may overload the heart.

 Warning: Your client will likely have other related conditions including hypertension. Be sure to check all conditions to understand the full range of precautions.

Chronic Heart Disease Precautions, cont'd.

 Postural hypotension can occur as a side effect of heart diseases, and may be increased with medication. Help the client to change positions and be on guard for dizziness or blacking out.

 Be sure to ask about current medications and check their precautions.

 With an understanding of your client's special needs and your unique healing abilities, you can be an invaluable asset to the improvement of their health.

Cerebrovascular Accident (CVA)

(also called stroke, transient ischemic attack, TIA)

A stroke occurs when a blood vessel that carries oxygen and nutrients to the brain ruptures (*hemorrhages*) or is blocked by a blood clot (called ische*mia*). When that happens, part of the brain cannot get the oxygen it needs and starts to die. Each year about 700,000 people experience a new or recurrent stroke. It is currently considered the third leading cause of death in the U.S.

Once a person has had a stroke, the part or side of the body affected may not function properly. Movement, sensation and healing may all be inhibited.

Acute Cerebrovascular Accident Precautions

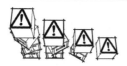 **Client is in critical condition. Avoid all therapy until approved by their physician.**

Cerebrovascular Accident, Rehabilitative Precautions

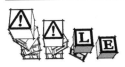 **Restrict massage to Light and Energy techniques.**

 Any of the following symptoms are possible indications of a stroke: Sudden, severe headache with no known cause, sudden numbness or weakness of the face, arm or leg, especially on one side of the body, sudden confusion, trouble speaking or understanding, sudden trouble seeing in one or both eyes, sudden trouble walking, with dizziness, loss of balance or coordination. Stop or avoid massage and call emergency services immediately.

 Avoid pressure techniques until the client has the approval of their physician after a stroke. LIGHT and ENERGY techniques are both acceptable once the client begins rehabilitation therapy. There may be widespread loss of sensation and function on the affected side, however, so be especially cautious with pressure and stretch techniques.

 Warning: Get detailed information about the client's loss of movement and sensation. Don't be shy; as a healthcare provider it is critical you get adequate information to avoid injuring them.

 Following a stroke the client will be on anticoagulant or other similar medications. Check all medications and their precautions.

 The brain has a significant ability to reroute pathways to improve function, and massage can be an important role in stimulating the nervous system for rehabilitation.

*Life is remembered
by precious moments, such as
those you give your clients.*

Cardiovascular Medications

Antianemia Medications

This group of medications stimulates red and white blood cell formation.

 If the client has recently developed any of the following, avoid massage and call the physician immediately: An unexplained skin rash, increased difficulty breathing, ringing in the ears, sudden severe headache, recent muscle weakness, unusual bleeding or bruising or swelling of the lips, tongue, or face. (This is a massage-specific list; refer to the documentation that was included with the medication for a complete list of side effects.)

 These medications are administered either intravenously or by injection. Injected medication is a subcutaneous depot, and regional massage is contraindicated within 24 hours of the injection. Confirm time restriction with physician before resuming massage to that area.

 Side Effects: Dizziness, aching muscles and fatigue all can occur with this class of medication. Limit the duration and intensity of the session if reported, and have the client contact the physician.

 Postural hypotension can occur as a side effect of this class of medication. Help the client to change positions and be on guard for dizziness or blacking out.

 Antianemia medications include: darbepoetin (Aranesp), epoetin (Epogen, Procrit), filgrastim (Neupogen), pegfilgrastim (Neulasta), and sargramostim (Leukine, Prokine).

---

*You may be the only person who
treats them with compassion.
You are truly special
in their life.*

Alpha Blockers

Alpha adrenergic blockers work specifically on peripheral arteries and veins rather than those in and around the heart. They inhibit the sympathetic nervous system, so the nervous system will be slow to respond to internal changes.

 If the client has recently developed any of the following, avoid massage and call the physician immediately: An unexplained skin rash, increased difficulty breathing, ringing in the ears, sudden severe headache, recent muscle weakness, unusual bleeding or bruising or swelling of the lips, tongue, or face. (This is a massage-specific list; refer to the documentation that was included with the medication for a complete list of side effects.)

 Avoid all heat therapies or use with extreme caution (including hot stone massage, heat pads, saunas, steam rooms, etc), as the client's ability to control their body temperature is compromised.

 Limit or avoid laying the client prone during pressure massage. Increased pressure compounded by increasing blood flow may overload the heart.

 Avoid deep tissue techniques and deep abdominal massage. Reduce and closely monitor pressure intensity and duration to avoid damaging tissue.

 Warning: Begin massage cautiously, and use your own sense of appropriate pressure. Avoid relying upon the client to determine their limits. The client is likely to have a reduced perception of pressure and pain as a result of this medication.

 Side Effects: This class of medication can create breathing difficulties, angina, and abnormal heart rate. A reduction in the normal oxygen intake and carbon dioxide elimination makes body tissues more fragile.

 Postural hypotension can occur as a side effect of this class of medication. Help the client to change positions and be on guard for dizziness or blacking out.

 Alpha blocker medications include: <u>alfuzosin</u> (UroXatral) <u>doxazosin</u> (Cardura), <u>guanadrel</u> (Hylorel), <u>guanethidine</u> (Ismelin), <u>methyldopa</u> (Aldomet, Dopamet, Hyodopa), <u>phenoxybenzamine</u> (Dibenzyline), <u>phentolamine</u> (Regitine), <u>prazosin</u> (Minipress, Minizide), <u>tamsulosin</u> (Flomax), and <u>terazosin</u> (Hytrin).

Alpha-2 Agonists

A special group of antihypertensive medications, alpha-2 agonists work by controlling nerve impulses along certain nerve pathways. They relax blood vessels so that blood passes through them more easily, which lowers blood pressure.

 If the client has recently developed any of the following, avoid massage and call the physician immediately: An unexplained skin rash, increased difficulty breathing, ringing in the ears, sudden severe headache, recent muscle weakness, unusual bleeding or bruising or swelling of the lips, tongue, or face. (This is a massage-specific list; refer to the documentation that was included with the medication for a complete list of side effects.)

 Limit or avoid laying the client prone during pressure massage. Increased pressure compounded by increasing blood flow may overload the heart.

 Avoid deep tissue techniques and deep abdominal massage. Reduce and closely monitor pressure intensity and duration to avoid damaging tissue.

 Side Effects: This class of medication can create breathing difficulties, angina and an abnormal heart rate. A reduction in the normal oxygen intake and carbon dioxide elimination makes body tissues more fragile.

 Postural hypotension can occur as a side effect of this class of medication and is more likely when combined with pressure techniques. Help the client to change positions and be on guard for dizziness or blacking out.

 Alpha-2 agonist medications include: clonidine (Catapres), guanfacine (Tenex), and hydralazine (Apresoline).

*Elegance lies in doing the
little things consistently well.*

Angiotensin-Converting Enzyme (ACE) Inhibitors

ACE inhibitors block the conversion of angiotensin I to angiotensin II, thereby reducing constriction and helping to relieve hypertension. By dilating the blood vessels leading directly from the heart, ACE inhibitors reduce the work of the failing heart in congestive heart failure.

 If the client has recently developed any of the following, avoid massage and call the physician immediately: An unexplained skin rash, increased difficulty breathing, ringing in the ears, sudden severe headache, recent muscle weakness, unusual bleeding or bruising or swelling of the lips, tongue, or face. (This is a massage-specific list; refer to the documentation that was included with the medication for a complete list of side effects.)

 Limit or avoid laying the client prone during pressure massage. Increased pressure compounded by increasing blood flow may overload the heart.

 Avoid deep tissue techniques and deep abdominal massage. Reduce and closely monitor pressure intensity and duration to avoid damaging tissue.

 Warning: Long term use of ACE inhibitors reduces white blood cell counts. Postponing the session is recommended if the therapist is unwell. The client's immune system is compromised by this medication.

 Side Effects: This class of medication can create breathing difficulties, angina, unusual bruising, excessive tiredness and an abnormal heart rate.

 Side Effects: Peripheral edema is common, along with numbness and tingling in hands and feet, cold extremities and joint pain. Recognize the client's limits in reducing their edema and have conservative goals for each session.

 Postural hypotension can occur as a side effect of this class of medication and is more likely when combined with pressure techniques. Help the client to change positions and be on guard for dizziness or blacking out.

 ACE inhibitor medications include: <u>benazepril</u> (Lotensin), <u>captopril</u> (Capoten), <u>enalapril</u> (Vasotec), <u>fosinopril</u> (Monopril), <u>lisinopril</u> (Prinivil, Zestril), <u>moexipril</u> (Univasc), <u>perindopril</u> (Aceon), <u>quinapril</u> (Accupril), <u>ramipril</u> (Altace), and <u>trandolapril</u> (Mavik).

Angiotensin-2 Receptor Blockers (ARBs)

By occupying angiotensin II receptor sites within the blood vessels, ARBs effectively relax blood vessels, reduce blood pressure and the overall workload of the heart. They also reduce the effects of sympathetic stimulation on the blood vessels.

 If the client has recently developed any of the following, avoid massage and call the physician immediately: An unexplained skin rash, increased difficulty breathing, ringing in the ears, sudden severe headache, recent muscle weakness, unusual bleeding or bruising or swelling of the lips, tongue, or face. (This is a massage-specific list; refer to the documentation that was included with the medication for a complete list of side effects.)

 Limit or avoid laying the client prone during pressure massage. Increased pressure compounded by increasing blood flow may overload the heart.

 Avoid deep tissue techniques and deep abdominal massage. Reduce and closely monitor pressure intensity and duration to avoid damaging tissue.

 Side Effects: This class of medication can create breathing difficulties, angina, unusual bruising, excessive tiredness and an abnormal heart rate.

 Side Effects: Peripheral edema is common, along with numbness and tingling in hands and feet, cold extremities and joint pain. Recognize the client's limits in reducing their edema and have conservative goals for each session.

 Angiotensin-2 receptor blocker medications include: candesartan (Atacand), eprosartan (Teveten), irbesartan (Avapro), losartan (Cozaar, Hyzaar), olmesartan (Benicar), telmisartan (Micardis), and valsartan (Diovan).

Antiarrhythmic Medications

Antiarrhythmic drugs work by making your heart more resistant to abnormal rhythms, encouraging a consistent heartbeat.

 If the client has recently developed any of the following, avoid massage and call the physician immediately: An unexplained skin rash, increased difficulty breathing, ringing in the ears, sudden severe headache, recent muscle weakness, unusual bleeding or bruising or swelling of the lips, tongue, or face. (This is a massage-specific list; refer to the documentation that was included with the medication for a complete list of side effects.)

 Side Effects: Headaches, muscle weakness, lightheadedness, nausea, and diarrhea all can occur with this class of medication. Take these into consideration as they may limit your ability to achieve your client's massage goals.

 Postural hypotension can occur as a side effect of this class of medication and is more likely when combined with pressure techniques. Help the client to change positions and be on guard for dizziness or blacking out.

 Antiarrhythmic medications include: <u>cibenzoline</u>, <u>disopyramide</u> (Norpace, Rythmodan), <u>dofetilide</u> (Tikosyn), <u>encainide</u>, <u>flecainide</u> (Tambocor), <u>lidocaine</u> (LidoPen, Xylocaine), <u>mexiletine</u> (Mexitil), <u>moricizine</u> (Ethmozine), <u>phenytoin</u> (Dilantin), <u>procainamide</u> (Procan, Promine, Pronestyl), <u>propafenone</u> (Rhythmol), <u>quinidine</u> (Cardioquin, Novoquinidin, Quinaglute, Quinalan, Quinidex, Quinora), and <u>tocainide</u> (Tonocard).

Your work in reducing your client's stress can be a deciding factor in their quality of life.

Anticoagulants and Antithrombotics

This group includes medications to inhibit how platelets stick together (antithrombotics) and reduce blood clotting (anticoagulants). They do not dissolve clots that have already formed. They are used in many circulatory disorders including heart attacks, surgery, pulmonary diseases, strokes, phlebitis and deep vein thrombosis.

 If the client has recently developed any of the following, avoid massage and call the physician immediately: Swollen or painful joints, unexplained skin rash, increased difficulty breathing, ringing in the ears, sudden severe headache, recent muscle weakness, unusual bleeding or bruising or swelling of the lips, tongue, or face. (This is a massage-specific list; refer to the documentation that was included with the medication for a complete list of side effects.)

 Limit or avoid laying the client prone during pressure massage. Increased pressure compounded by increasing blood flow may overload the heart.

 Avoid deep tissue techniques and deep abdominal massage. Reduce and closely monitor pressure intensity and duration to avoid damaging tissue.

 Side Effects: This class of medication can create breathing difficulties, angina, and abnormal heart rate. A reduction in the normal oxygen intake and carbon dioxide elimination makes body tissues more fragile.

 Postural hypotension can occur as a side effect of this class of medication. Help the client to change positions and be on guard for dizziness or blacking out.

 Antithrombotic medications include: <u>aspirin</u> (see aspirin), <u>clopidogrel</u> (Plavix), <u>dipyridamole</u> (Aggrenox, Dipimol, Dipridacot, Novodipiradol, Persantine, Pyridamole), <u>fondaparinux</u> (Arixtra), and <u>ticlopidine</u> (Ticlid).

 Anticoagulant medications include: <u>anisindione</u> (Miradon), <u>warfarin</u> (Coumadin, Panwarfarin, Sofarin, Warfilone) and <u>heparin</u> (Fragmin, Hepalean, Liquaemin, Lovenox, Uniparin).

Beta Blockers

Beta adrenergic blockers bind with the sites that would be stimulated by sympathetic neurotransmitters like adrenaline and norepinephrine in response to stress. By blocking these sites the medication slows the heart contraction rate and improves its rhythm. These drugs are also used in vascular headaches such as migraines because they have a secondary effect of reducing blood vessel constriction.

 If the client has recently developed any of the following, avoid massage and call the physician immediately: An unexplained skin rash, increased difficulty breathing, ringing in the ears, sudden severe headache, recent muscle weakness, unusual bleeding or bruising or swelling of the lips, tongue, or face. (This is a massage-specific list; refer to the documentation that was included with the medication for a complete list of side effects.)

 Avoid all heat therapies or use with extreme caution (including hot stone massage, heat pads, saunas, steam rooms, etc), as the client's ability to control their body temperature is compromised.

 Limit or avoid laying the client prone during pressure massage. Increased pressure compounded by increasing blood flow may overload the heart.

 Avoid deep tissue techniques and deep abdominal massage. Reduce and closely monitor pressure intensity and duration to avoid damaging tissue.

 Side Effects: This class of medication can create breathing difficulties, angina, and an abnormal heart rate.

 Side Effects: Peripheral edema is common, along with numbness and tingling in hands and feet, cold extremities and joint pain. Recognize the client's limits in reducing their edema and have conservative goals for each session.

 Postural hypotension can occur as a side effect of this class of medication and is more likely when combined with pressure techniques. Help the client to change positions and be on guard for dizziness or blacking out.

Beta Blocker Medication Precautions, cont'd.

 Beta blocker medications include: <u>acebutolol</u> (Monitan, Rhotral, Sectral), <u>atenolol</u> (Tenormin, Tenolin), <u>betaxolol</u> (Betoptic, Kerl-one), <u>bisoprolol</u> (Monocor, Zebeta), <u>carteolol</u> (Cartrol), <u>esmolol</u> (Brevibloc), <u>metoprolol</u> (Betaloc, Lopressor, Toprol), <u>nadolol</u> (Corgard), <u>penbutolol</u> (Levatol), <u>pindolol</u> (Visken), <u>propranolol</u> (Betachron, Detensol, Inderal, InnoPran, Novopranol), <u>sotalol</u> (Betapace, Sorine, Sotacor) and <u>timolol</u> (Betimol, Blocadren).

Calcium Channel Blockers

The expansion and contraction of the heart and smooth muscles of the blood vessels are dependent on the movement of calcium into muscle cells. Calcium channel blockers interfere with the uptake of calcium, which then helps to relax and dilate blood vessels and reduce resistance.

Calcium channel blockers also interfere with the uptake of calcium in the heart muscle, slowing the contraction of the heart and making the contractions less intense.

 If the client has recently developed any of the following, avoid massage and call the physician immediately: An unexplained skin rash, increased difficulty breathing, ringing in the ears, sudden severe headache, recent muscle weakness, unusual bleeding or bruising or swelling of the lips, tongue, or face. (This is a massage-specific list; refer to the documentation that was included with the medication for a complete list of side effects.)

 Limit or avoid laying the client prone during pressure massage. Increased pressure compounded by increasing blood flow may overload the heart.

 Warning: Long term use of calcium channel blockers reduces white blood cell counts. Postponing the session is recommended if the therapist is unwell. The client's immune system is compromised by this medication.

Calcium Channel Blocker Precautions, cont'd.

 Side Effects: This class of medication can create breathing difficulties, angina, and abnormal heart rate. A reduction in the normal oxygen intake and carbon dioxide elimination makes body tissues more fragile.

 Postural hypotension can occur as a side effect of this class of medication and is more likely when combined with pressure techniques. Help the client to change positions and be on guard for dizziness or blacking out.

 Calcium channel blocker medications include: amlodipine (Lotrel, Norvasc), bepridil (Bepadin, Vascor), diltiazem (Cardizem, Cartia, Taztia, Tiamate, Tiazac), diazoxide (Hyperstat, Proglycem), felodipine (Plendil, Renedil), flunarizine (Sibelium), isradipine (Dyna-Circ), nicardipine (Cardene), nifedipine (Adalat, Afeditab, Nifedical, Procardia), nisoldipine (Sular), nitroprusside (Nipride, Nitropress), and verapamil (Calan, Covera, Isoptin, Verelan).

Cholesterol Lowering Medications

(also called antihyperlipidemics, lipid lowering drugs, LLDs)

These medications all act to lower the *low density lipoproteins* (LDLs), *triglycerides* and *cholesterols*.

 If the client has recently developed any of the following, avoid massage and call the physician immediately: An unexplained skin rash, increased difficulty breathing, ringing in the ears, sudden severe headache, recent muscle weakness, unusual bleeding or bruising or swelling of the lips, tongue, or face. (This is a massage-specific list; refer to the documentation that was included with the medication for a complete list of side effects.)

 If the client has not had a bowel movement in several days, avoid massage and call the physician immediately. Bowel obstruction is a severe side effect of this class of medication.

Cholesterol Lowering Medication Precautions, cont'd.

 Side Effects: Aching muscles, nausea, constipation, diarrhea, and fatigue all can occur with this class of medication. Take these into consideration as they may limit your ability to achieve your client's massage goals.

 Postural hypotension can occur as a side effect of this class of medication and is more likely when combined with pressure techniques. Help the client to change positions and be on guard for dizziness or blacking out.

 Cholesterol lowering medications include: <u>atorvastatin</u> (Lipitor), <u>cholestyramine resin</u> (Cholybar, LoCholest, Prevalite, Questran), <u>clofibrate</u> (Atromid-S), <u>colesevelam</u> (Welchol), <u>colestipol</u> (Colestid), <u>ezetimibe</u> (Zetia), <u>fenofibrate</u> (Lofibra, Tricor), <u>fluvastatin</u> (Lescol), <u>gemfibrozil</u> (Lopid), <u>lovastatin</u> (Altocor, Mevacor, Mevinolin), <u>nicotinic acid</u> (Niacin, Niacor, Niaspan, Nicolar, Slo-Niacin), <u>pravastatin</u> (Eptastatin, Pravachol), <u>rosuvastatin</u> (Crestor), and <u>simvastatin</u> (Epistatin, Synvinolin, Zocor).

Cardiac Glycosides

These medications work by slowing the heart rate yet increasing the strength of each muscle contraction, thereby making the heart circulate blood more efficiently.

 If the client has recently developed any of the following, avoid massage and call the physician immediately: An unexplained skin rash, increased difficulty breathing, ringing in the ears, sudden severe headache, recent muscle weakness, unusual bleeding or bruising or swelling of the lips, tongue, or face. (This is a massage-specific list; refer to the documentation that was included with the medication for a complete list of side effects.)

 Limit or avoid laying the client prone during pressure massage. Increased pressure compounded by increasing blood flow may overload the heart.

Cardiac Glycoside Precautions, cont'd.

 Avoid deep tissue techniques and deep abdominal massage. Reduce and closely monitor pressure intensity and duration to avoid damaging tissue.

 Warning: A good percentage of clients taking these medications experience toxicity. Be alert to complaints of gastrointestinal irritation, confusion, visual disturbances, and abnormalities in heart function. These symptoms are a warning to avoid massage and seek immediate medical attention.

 Side Effects: This class of medication can create breathing difficulties, angina and an abnormal heart rate. A reduction in the normal oxygen intake and carbon dioxide elimination makes body tissues more fragile.

 Cardiac glycoside medications include: <u>digitalis</u>, <u>digitoxin</u> (Crysto-digin), and <u>digoxin</u> (Digitek, Lanoxicaps, Lanoxin). Cardiac glyco-side-like herbs include <u>foxglove</u>, <u>lily of the valley</u>, and <u>milkweed</u>.

Combined Alpha and Beta Blockers

Medications in this drug class block both alpha and beta receptors in the body to lower blood pressure.

 If the client has recently developed any of the following, avoid massage and call the physician immediately: An unexplained skin rash, increased difficulty breathing, ringing in the ears, sudden severe headache, recent muscle weakness, unusual bleeding or bruising or swelling of the lips, tongue, or face. (This is a massage-specific list; refer to the documentation that was included with the medication for a complete list of side effects.)

 Limit or avoid laying the client prone during pressure massage. Increased pressure compounded by increasing blood flow may overload the heart.

Combined Alpha and Beta Blocker Medication Precautions, cont'd.

 Avoid deep tissue techniques and deep abdominal massage. Reduce and closely monitor pressure intensity and duration to avoid damaging tissue.

 Side Effects: This class of medication can create breathing difficulties, angina and an abnormal heart rate. A reduction in the normal oxygen intake and carbon dioxide elimination makes body tissues more fragile.

 Postural hypotension can occur as a side effect of this class of medication. Help the client to change positions and be on guard for dizziness or blacking out.

 Combined alpha and beta blocker medications include: <u>carvedilol</u> (Coreg), and <u>labetalol</u> (Ibidomide, Normodyne, Presolol, Trandate).

Diuretics

Elimination of more fluid through the kidneys results in a reduced blood volume and subsequent drop in blood pressure.

 If the client has recently developed any of the following, avoid massage and call the physician immediately: An unexplained skin rash, increased difficulty breathing, ringing in the ears, sudden severe headache, recent muscle weakness, unusual bleeding or bruising or swelling of the lips, tongue, or face. (This is a massage-specific list; refer to the documentation that was included with the medication for a complete list of side effects.)

 Limit or avoid laying the client prone during pressure massage. Increased pressure compounded by increasing blood flow may overload the heart.

 Avoid deep tissue techniques and deep abdominal massage. Peripheral edema is common due to the body's circulatory challenges. Recognize the client's limits in reducing their edema and have conservative goals for each session.

Diuretic Precautions, cont'd.

 Side Effects: Aching or cramping muscles, nausea, constipation, diarrhea and fatigue all can occur with this class of medication. Take these into consideration as they may limit your ability to achieve your client's massage goals.

 Postural hypotension can occur as a side effect of this class of medication and is more likely when combined with pressure techniques. Help the client to change positions and be on guard for dizziness or blacking out.

 Thiazide diuretics include: <u>bendroflumethiazide</u> (Naturetin), <u>chlorothiazide</u> (Diurigen, Diuril), <u>chlorthalidone</u> (Hygroton, Thalitone, Uridon), <u>hydrochlorothiazide</u> (Diuchlor, Esidrix, Ezide, HCTZ, Hydro-chlor, Hydro-D, HydroDIURIL, Microzide, Neo-Codema, Oretic, Urozide), <u>hydroflumethiazide</u> (Diucardin, Saluron), <u>indapamide</u> (Lozol), <u>methyclothiazide</u> (Aquatensen, Duretic, Enduron), <u>metolazone</u> (Diulo, Mykrox, Zaroxolyn), <u>polythiazide</u> (Renese), <u>quinethazone</u> (Hydromox), <u>torsemide</u> (Demadex), and <u>trichlormethiazide</u> (Metahydrin, Naqua, Trichlorex).

 Potassium sparing diuretics include: <u>amiloride</u> (Midamor), <u>eplerenone</u> (Inspra), <u>spironolactone</u> (Aldactone, Novospiroton), and <u>triamterene</u> (Dyrenium).

 Loop diuretics include: <u>bumetanide</u> (Bumex), <u>ethacrynic acid</u> (Edecrin), and <u>furosemide</u> (Furoside, Lasix, Myrosemide, Novosemide, Uritol).

 Combination diuretics include: <u>amiloride</u> with <u>hydrochlorothiazide</u> (Moduretic), <u>atenolol</u> with <u>chlorthalidone</u> (Tenoretic), <u>benazepril</u> with <u>hydrochlorothiazide</u> (Lotensin HCT), <u>bisoprolol</u> with <u>hydrochlorothiazide</u> (Ziac), <u>captopril</u> with <u>hydrochlorothiazide</u> (Capozide), <u>enalapril</u> with <u>hydrochlorothiazide</u> (Vaseretic), <u>irbesartan</u> with <u>hydrochlorothiazide</u> (Avalide), <u>lisinopril</u> with <u>hydrochlorothiazide</u> (Prinzide, Zestoretic), <u>metoprolol</u> with <u>hydrochlorothiazide</u> (Lopressor HCT), <u>nadolol</u> with <u>bendroflumethiazide</u> (Corzide), <u>pindolol</u> with <u>hydrochlorothiazide</u> (Viskazide), <u>propranolol</u> with <u>hydrochlorothiazide</u> (Inderide LA), <u>spironolactone</u> with <u>hydrochlorothiazide</u> (Aldactazide) <u>timolol</u> with <u>hydrochlorothiazide</u> (Timolide), and <u>triamterene</u> with <u>hydrochlorothiazide</u> (Dyazide, Maxzide).

Nitrates

Even though they can be prescribed for chest pain, nitrates (also called anti-angina drugs) are not for pain relief. They dilate the veins bringing blood to the heart as well as the arteries in the heart itself. This process increases its oxygen supply, which in turn decreases the heart muscle constriction.

 If the client has recently developed any of the following, avoid massage and call the physician immediately: An unexplained skin rash, increased difficulty breathing, ringing in the ears, sudden severe headache, recent muscle weakness, unusual bleeding or bruising or swelling of the lips, tongue, or face. (This is a massage-specific list; refer to the documentation that was included with the medication for a complete list of side effects.)

 During the massage if the client experiences blurred vision, dry mouth, chest pain or fainting, stop the massage and call the doctor or emergency assistance immediately.

 Avoid regional massage to prevent an increase in circulation and absorption. Transdermal skin patches carefully administer medicine for up to 24 hours. Areas where ointments have been applied should be avoided for at least eight hours.

 Postural hypotension can occur as a side effect of this class of medication and is more likely when combined with pressure techniques. Help the client to change positions and be on guard for dizziness or blacking out.

 Nitrate medications include: erythrityl tetranitrate (Cardilate), isosorbide dinitrate (Dilatrate SR, Isordil, Isordil Tembids, Isordil Titradose, Sorbitrate), isosorbide mononitrate (Imdur, Ismo, Isotrate ER, Monoket), nitroglycerin (Deponit, Minitran, Nitro-Time, Nitrolingual, Nitrodisc, Nitroglyn, Nitrol, Nitrong, NitroQuick, Nitrostat, Transderm-Nitro), and pentaerythritol tetranitrate (Duotrate, Pentylan, Peritrate).

Thrombolytics

Thrombolytic agents are injected slowly to dissolve dangerous clots rapidly. They are given under close supervision in hospitals, and are usually reserved for life-threatening pulmonary embolisms (blood clots in the lung) or strokes since they have a greater risk of causing serious bleeding.

 Ask the physician for prior approval on the day you wish to give massage before attempting any pressure techniques.

 Avoid all pressure massage and utilize ENERGY techniques exclusively. Severe internal bleeding is a common concern when administering thrombolytics.

 Medications include: alteplase (Activase, Alteplase), anistreplase (Eminase), reteplase (Retavase), streptokinase (Streptase), tenecteplase (TNKase), and urokinase (Abbokinase).

Impressive health improvement
can be accomplished
when one focuses on performing
subtle techniques with elegance.

*Your healing energy
goes beyond your techniques
and skills. Accept the limitations
imposed by your client's
medications and conditions,
and know that your
presence alone is beneficial.*

Chapter 5

Lymph and Immune Systems

Edema

Approximately 10 percent of the fluid that enters the body tissues from the capillaries is routed back to the heart through the lymph system. A buildup of this fluid is called *edema*. Skin takes on a puffy, tight look and feel with edema. It can be throughout the body (systemic) or localized. One of the most powerful benefits of circulatory massage is the stimulation it provides the lymph system in eliminating fluid retention.

The presence of edema is a clear warning for the therapist. Determine what is causing the edema and how impaired the system is before proceeding. Some specifics are listed below, but in all cases proceed with the assumption that the client's lymphatic system is backed up and unable to handle a significant increase in fluid.

Pitting edema is the most severe form of edema. By pressing a thumb or finger firmly against the tissue for a few seconds, a dent may be produced. When the finger is withdrawn the dent may persist for seconds to as much as several minutes. All pressure techniques are to be avoided with pitting edema.

If the edema is due to an injury, determine what phase of healing they are in and follow those precautions (see sprains and strains).

Edema Precautions

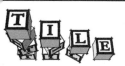 **Tolerance, Incremental, Light and Energy techniques are all encouraged. Edema is a clear warning, however, to proceed cautiously with all circulatory massage techniques.**

Edema Precautions, cont'd.

 Liver disease, kidney disease, deep vein thrombosis and advanced heart disease are all examples of conditions that produce systemic edema. Call physician before performing any pressure techniques with systemic edema. ENERGY techniques are recommended.

 Avoid all pressure techniques with pitting edema. ENERGY techniques are recommended.

 Be sure to ask about current medications and check their precautions.

 Impressive health improvement can be accomplished when one focuses on performing subtle techniques with elegance.

Lymphedema

Lymphedema is the buildup of fluid from scarring or removal of a portion of the lymph system. When surgery is performed to remove cancerous breast tissue, some or all of the lymph nodes and tissue are removed as well. Chemotherapy and radiation cancer therapy both scar the lymph tissue. These are a few examples of trauma that can eventually create lymphedema.

Special air-filled sleeves are used to gently pressure fluids toward the heart to treat lymphedema. Moving the lymph too quickly or aggressively can cause irritation, leading to a potentially life threatening increase in fluids.

Lymphedema Precautions

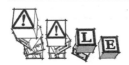 **Restrict massage to Light and Energy techniques.**

 Get the approval of the client's physician for all but the most gentle of LIGHT massage techniques. ENERGY techniques are encouraged.

Lymphedema Precautions, cont'd.

 Warning: Be cautious with the duration of massage as well as the pressure to any area. The length of your massage session must be short enough so the client has energy to spare.

 Avoid all heat therapies (including hot stone massage, heat pads, saunas, steam rooms, etc), as symptoms are exacerbated by heat.

 Be sure to ask about current medications and check their precautions.

 Sometimes the most powerful impression you make on a client is simply your compassionate presence.

Lymphadenitis and Lymphangitis

Lymphadenitis and lymphangitis are infections of the lymph nodes (also called *lymph glands*) and lymph channels, respectively. It commonly results from an acute streptococcal or staphylococcal infection of the skin (called *cellulitis*), or from an abscess in the skin or soft tissues. If the bacteria spreads to the bloodstream, it can cause a life-threatening condition called *septicemia* (blood poisoning).

With lymphadenitis, lymph nodes may be swollen, tender, and hard, and the skin over a node may be reddened and hot. With lymphangitis, you may see red streaks from infected area to the armpit or groin, with throbbing pain and a fever anywhere between 100 to 104 degrees F.

Lymphadenitis and Lymphangitis Precautions

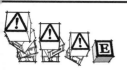 **Energy techniques only. Avoid all pressure and circulatory massage techniques.**

 Lymphadenitis and lymphangitis often becomes serious within hours. Avoid massage and seek immediate medical attention.

Lymphadenitis and Lymphangitis Precautions, cont'd.

 Avoid pressure techniques during the acute stage. ENERGY techniques are encouraged.

 When the client has the approval of their physician, begin with LIGHT techniques. Build toward more aggressive techniques over a series of sessions as their other conditions allow.

 The client's medications will likely have increased or changed after treatment for this condition. Be sure to check for any new precautions.

 Clients appreciate your knowledge of the body and will be grateful for your conservative approach.

Fibromyalgia Syndrome (FMS) and Chronic Fatigue Syndrome (CFS)

(also called myalgic encephalomyelitis)

Fibromyalgia syndrome and chronic fatigue syndrome are both characterized by scattered musculoskeletal pain (involving the muscles and bone structure), tenderness in specific areas, generalized long-term fatigue and a feeling of being tired after sleeping. FMS and CFS were originally considered unrelated conditions, however current research trends indicate that they are linked, and in fact may be the same.

Despite aggressive research and clinical studies, the causes of FMS and CFS are still unknown. Clearly one culprit cannot be to blame. The nervous system appears to run in high gear, becoming ever more sensitive to physical, mental and chemical stresses. This causes nervous system fatigue more quickly than normal, which trains the body to be more alert and sensitive to stimuli next time. Malnutrition, high toxin levels, and increased stresses are all high on the list of suspects. More research is revealing that many medications prescribed for pain and inflammation actually cause FMS symptoms if taken long-term. The Epstein-Barr virus has been blamed for chronic fatigue syndrome, but there hasn't been conclusive research to prove this.

Fibromyalgia Syndrome and Chronic Fatigue Syndrome Precautions

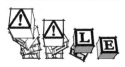 **Restrict massage to Light and Energy techniques.**

 Since symptoms vary day to day with these conditions, be sure to get specific information about their recent stress levels and symptoms, and alter your session based on this information. Avoid pressure techniques if the client is suffering from an acute systemic infection such as the flu.

 Avoid deep tissue techniques and aggressive massage. Limit full body massage to LIGHT and ENERGY techniques. Limit trigger point therapies to one to three nodes per session to avoid toxin or nerve stimulation overload.

 Be sure to ask about current medications and closely check their precautions.

 Focus on that which can provide stress relief and relaxation, rather than aggressive techniques that will likely overwhelm their system. Guard their fragile health; you have the potential to heal not only their physical body, but their emotional self as well.

Mononucleosis

(also called the kissing disease, MONO)

Infectious mononucleosis is initially an infection of the salivary glands, progressively spreading into the lymph system. It is almost universally associated with the Epstein-Barr virus (EBV). The CDC states that in the United States, as many as 95 percent of adults between 35 and 40 years of age have been infected. Transmission of EBV requires intimate contact with the saliva of an infected person; it is unlikely that salivary spray will infect someone. The incubation period, or the time from infection to appearance of symptoms, ranges from 4 to 6 weeks. Persons with infectious mononucleosis (even without symptoms) may be able to spread the infection to others for a period of weeks.

Mono causes inflammation of the liver (hepatitis) in about 1 out of every 10 people.

Mononucleosis Precautions

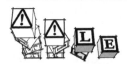 **Restrict massage to Light and Energy techniques.**

 Look for the characteristic triad: Fever, inflammation of the throat (*pharyngitis*), and swollen lymph nodes (*lymphadenopathy*), lasting from 1 to 4 weeks. Avoid all massage and contact until the client has been declared non-infectious.

 Mono may be misdiagnosed as strep throat and treated with antibiotics. The vast majority of adolescents and adults with mono who receive ampicillin-like antibiotics develop a red raised rash over a good portion of the body. Have the client contact their physician immediately.

 Avoid deep tissue techniques and aggressive massage. Guard against taxing the recuperating lymph system during this stage by limiting your massage to LIGHT and ENERGY techniques. Recovery from mono after the infectious stage can be lengthy, often as long as four months.

 Warning: The spleen becomes swollen and traumatized during mononucleosis, so protect it by avoiding all percussive techniques for 6 months after they have recovered from the infection.

 Short-term steroids and NSAIDs may be prescribed, as well as antivirals (rarely). Once the client has recovered and been approved for massage, check all their current medications review those precautions.

 An invigorating massage may seem to the client to be the "wake-up call" they need. Help your client understand the need for caution, and they will appreciate you standing guard over their health.

HIV Infection and AIDS

Acquired Immunodeficiency Syndrome (AIDS) is a chronic, progressive, life-threatening condition caused by the Human Immunodeficiency Virus (HIV). By damaging or destroying the immune system cells, HIV interferes with the body's ability to effectively fight off disease. The term AIDS applies to the most advanced stages of HIV infection.

According to the U.S. National Institutes for Health, as many as 950,000 Americans may be infected with HIV, one-quarter of whom are unaware of their infection.

There are no clear symptoms for HIV. Although a person newly infected with the virus can pass it along to others, symptoms may not appear for almost a decade. Early signs include swollen lymph nodes, fever and diarrhea, but can often be attributed to other conditions. Until recently, HIV could only be diagnosed by a long, emotionally traumatic series of tests. Now, reliable tests are available that reveal results in as little as 20 minutes, and one is even available as a home test.

HIV and AIDS Precautions

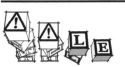 **Restrict massage to Light and Energy techniques.**

 Ask before each session if the client has any new symptoms. Be on guard for things that may signal a drop in their immunity (like a cold, flu or increased fatigue) and postpone pressure techniques if suspicious. ENERGY massage is always encouraged (following the guidelines below).

 Clients with AIDS may have a complicated set of conditions. Consulting with their physician before their first session is recommended to gain complete understanding of the appropriate precautions.

 Postponing the session is recommended if the therapist is unwell, as the client's immune system is compromised.

HIV and AIDS Precautions, cont'd.

 Warning: Be cautious with the duration of massage as well as the pressure to any area. The length of your massage session must be short enough so the client has energy to spare.

 Warning: HIV is spread through the exchange of body fluids containing lymphocytes, specifically blood, semen and vaginal secretions. The virus can live in fluids indefinitely and only dies when the fluid dries. Avoid unprotected contact with these fluids.

 Warning: Someone infected with HIV is more likely to develop certain cancers, especially Kaposi's sarcoma, cervical cancer and lymphoma. Follow the precautions listed in the chapter on Cancer if your client has been diagnosed. Signs of Kaposi's sarcoma in light-skinned people are round brown, reddish, or purple raised blotches or nodules that develop on the skin or in the mouth. In dark-skinned people, the spots are more pigmented.

 Note: Sweat, saliva and sputum has been researched and found not to transmit HIV. Clients who are asymptomatic are encouraged to receive any and all forms of massage.

 Ongoing medications to treat the lymphatic system are common. Be sure to ask about all current medications, recent treatments including chemotherapy and check their precautions.

 Your compassionate interest in your client's health, fueled by your knowledge of HIV and AIDS, is a rare and priceless gift. It can be most rewarding for the therapist as well.

*Find your strength
in the Golden rule.*

Lymph and Immune System Medications

Non-Nucleoside Reverse Transcriptase Inhibitors (NNRTIs)

NNRTIs are used to treat HIV and AIDS. They prevent healthy T-cells in the body from becoming infected with HIV by binding to the enzyme called *reverse transcriptase* (which is used to convert RNA into DNA).

 If the client has recently developed any of the following, avoid massage and call the physician immediately: An unexplained skin rash, increased difficulty breathing, ringing in the ears, sudden severe headache, recent muscle weakness, unusual bleeding or bruising or swelling of the lips, tongue, or face. (This is a massage-specific list; refer to the documentation that was included with the medication for a complete list of side effects.)

 Warning: Begin massage cautiously, and use your own sense of appropriate pressure. Avoid relying upon the client to determine their limits. The client is likely to have a reduced perception of pressure and pain as a result of this medication.

 Side Effects: Mild to moderate rashes, peripheral edema and neuropathy, headaches, cold extremities, yellowed skin, muscle and joint pain, nausea, and/or vomiting all can occur with this class of medication. Take these into consideration as they may limit your ability to achieve your client's massage goals. If any of these symptoms persist or are severe, avoid massage and have the client call their doctor.

 Postural hypotension can occur as a side effect of this class of medication. Help the client to change positions and be on guard for dizziness or blacking out.

 Non-nucleoside reverse transcriptase inhibitor medications include delavirdine (DLV, Rescriptor), efavirenz (EFV, Sustiva), emtricit-abine (Emtriva), and nevirapine (NVP, Viramune).

Nucleoside/Nucleotide Reverse Transcriptase Inhibitors (NRTIs)

(also called nucleoside analogs, nucleotide analogues, "nukes", RT inhibitors)

NRTIs were the first antiretroviral drugs to be developed. When HIV infects a cell in a person's body, it copies it's own genetic code into the cell's DNA. They prevent healthy T-cells in the body from becoming infected with HIV by inhibiting the enzyme called *reverse transcriptase* (which is used to convert RNA into DNA).

While nucleotide analogues are technically different from nucleoside analogues, they act very much the same way and are combined here for reference purposes.

 If the client has recently developed any of the following, avoid massage and call the physician immediately: An unexplained skin rash, increased difficulty breathing, ringing in the ears, sudden severe headache, recent muscle weakness, unusual bleeding or bruising or swelling of the lips, tongue, or face. (This is a massage-specific list; refer to the documentation that was included with the medication for a complete list of side effects.)

 Warning: Begin massage cautiously, and use your own sense of appropriate pressure. Avoid relying upon the client to determine their limits. The client is likely to have a reduced perception of pressure and pain as a result of this medication.

 Side Effects: Peripheral edema and neuropathy, headaches, yellowed skin, cold extremities, muscle and joint pain, nausea, and/or vomiting all can occur with this class of medication. Take these into consideration as they may limit your ability to achieve your client's massage goals. If any of these symptoms persist or are severe, avoid massage and have the client call their doctor.

 Postural hypotension can occur as a side effect of this class of medication. Help the client to change positions and be on guard for dizziness or blacking out.

Nucleoside/Nucleotide Reverse Transcriptase Inhibitors Precautions, cont'd.

 Nucleoside/nucleotide reverse transcriptase inhibitor medications include: <u>abacavir</u> (Ziagen, ABC), <u>abacavir</u> <u>with</u> <u>lamivudine</u> (Epzicom), <u>abacavir</u> <u>with</u> <u>zidovudine</u> <u>and</u> <u>lamivudine</u> (Trizivir), <u>alovudine</u>, <u>amdoxovir</u> (DAPD), <u>didanosine</u> (ddI, Videx, Videx EC), <u>elvucitabine</u>, <u>emtricitabine</u> (Emtriva, FTC), <u>lamivudine</u> (3TC, Epivir), <u>stavudine</u> (d4T, Zerit), <u>tenofovir DF</u> (BisPOC, PMPA, TDF, Viread), <u>tenofovir DF</u> with <u>emtricitabine</u> (Truvada), <u>zalcitabine</u> (ddC, Hivid), <u>zidovudine</u> (AZT, Retrovir, ZDV), and <u>zidovudine</u> <u>with</u> <u>lamivudine</u> (Combivir).

Protease Inhibitors (PI)

PIs interrupt HIV replication at a later stage in its life cycle by interfering with an enzyme known as *HIV protease*. This causes HIV particles in your body to become structurally disorganized and noninfectious.

When NRTIs and protease inhibitors are used in combination, it is referred to as highly active antiretroviral therapy, or HAART.

 If the client has recently developed any of the following, avoid massage and call the physician immediately: An unexplained skin rash, increased difficulty breathing, ringing in the ears, sudden severe headache, recent muscle weakness, unusual bleeding or bruising or swelling of the lips, tongue, or face. (This is a massage-specific list; refer to the documentation that was included with the medication for a complete list of side effects.)

 Warning: Begin massage cautiously, and use your own sense of appropriate pressure. Avoid relying upon the client to determine their limits. The client is likely to have a reduced perception of pressure and pain as a result of this medication.

Protease Inhibitor Precautions, cont'd.

 Side Effects: Peripheral edema and neuropathy, headaches, yellowed skin, cold extremities, muscle and joint pain, nausea, and/or vomiting all can occur with this class of medication. Take these into consideration as they may limit your ability to achieve your client's massage goals. If any of these symptoms persist or are severe, avoid massage and have the client call their doctor.

 Postural hypotension is a common side effect of this class of medication. Help the client to change positions and be on guard for dizziness or blacking out.

 Protease inhibitor medications include: amprenavir (Agenerase, APV), atazanavir (ATZ, Reyataz), fosamprenavir (FPV, Lexiva), indinavir (Crixivan, IDV), lopinavir (Kaletra, LPV), nelfinavir (NFV, Viracept), ritonavir (Norvir, RTV), saquinavir (Fortovase, Invirase, SQV), and tipranavir (TPV).

Fusion Inhibitors

(also called entry inhibitors)

Recently developed for the treatment of HIV infections that have become resistant to the long-standing anti-HIV drugs, fusion inhibitors block the HIV from entering the T-cells.

 If the client has recently developed any of the following, avoid massage and call the physician immediately: An unexplained skin rash, increased difficulty breathing, ringing in the ears, sudden severe headache, recent muscle weakness, unusual bleeding or bruising or swelling of the lips, tongue, or face. (This is a massage-specific list; refer to the documentation that was included with the medication for a complete list of side effects.)

Fusion Inhibitor Precautions, cont'd.

 Side Effects: Peripheral edema and neuropathy, headaches, yellowed skin, cold extremities, muscle and joint pain, nausea, and/or vomiting all can occur with this class of medication. Take these into consideration as they may limit your ability to achieve your client's massage goals. If any of these symptoms persist or are severe, avoid massage and have the client call their doctor.

 Postural hypotension is a common side effect of this class of medication. Help the client to change positions and be on guard for dizziness or blacking out.

 Fusion inhibitor medications include: enfuvirtide (ENF, Fuzeon), T-1249.

Immunosuppressants

This class of medication is primarily used to prevent rejection of kidney, liver, heart, and other organ transplants as well as to prevent rejection problems in bone marrow. The transplanted organ is considered "foreign" by the immune system and will be attacked and rejected unless these medications are administered. It can again become "foreign" years later, requiring additional medication. These medications work by inhibiting the body's ability respond to infection and foreign matter. Immunosuppressant drugs are also used for conditions such as severe eczema, psoriasis, rheumatoid arthritis or acne.

 If the client has recently developed any of the following, avoid massage and call the physician immediately: Fever, yellowing of the skin, unexplained skin rash, increased difficulty breathing, ringing in the ears, sudden severe headache, recent muscle weakness, unusual bleeding or bruising or swelling of the lips, tongue, or face. (This is a massage-specific list; refer to the documentation that was included with the medication for a complete list of side effects.)

Immunosuppressant Medication Precautions, cont'd.

 Postponing the session is recommended if the therapist is unwell. The client's immune system is compromised from this medication.

 Avoid all heat therapies or use with extreme caution (including hot stone massage, heat pads, etc), as normal heat dissipation is compromised and burns may occur.

 Side Effects: Muscle stiffness, bone or joint pain, increased bruising, vomiting and diarrhea are all common with this class of medication. Take these into consideration as they may limit your ability to achieve your client's massage goals. If any of these symptoms are severe or persistent, have the client contact their physician.

 Postural hypotension is a common side effect of this class of medication. Help the client to change positions and be on guard for dizziness or blacking out.

 Topical immunosuppressant medications include: anthralin, coal tar, calcipotriene (Dovonex), psoralen, salicylic acid, and tazarotene (Tazorac).

 Systemic immunosuppressant medications include: acitretin (Neotigason, Soriatane), adapalene (Differin), alefacept (Amevive), alitretinoin (Panretin), azathioprine (Azasan, Imuran), bexarotene (Targretin), cyclosporine (Gengraf, Neoral, Sandimmune), efalizumab (Raptiva), fenretinide, hydroxyurea (Hydrea), isotretinoin (Accutane, Amnesteem, Claravis, Sotret), methotrexate (Amethopterin, Folex, Mexate, Rheumatrex, Trexall), mycophenolate (CellCept), sirolimus (Rapamune) sulfasalazine (Azulfidine), tacrolimus (FK 506, Prograf), tazarotene (Tazorac), thioguanine (6-TG, Lanvis), and tretinoin (Retin A, Renova).

Chapter 6

Integumentary System

Standard/Universal Precautions

(Adapted from the Center for Disease Control publication, *Universal Precautions for Prevention of Transmission of HIV and Other Bloodborne Infections.*)

Standard/Universal Precautions are designed to reduce the risk of transmission of bloodborne pathogens to health care providers as well as reduce the risk of transmitting microorganisms from one client to another. Standard/Universal Precautions apply to contact with blood, all body fluids, secretions and excretions (except sweat), nonintact skin, and mucous membranes.

These practices should be followed for all clients since it is not always possible to recognize an infection by visual inspection.

Handwashing
Hands should be washed after touching blood, body fluids, secretions, excretions, and contaminated items, whether or not gloves are worn. Hands should be washed immediately after gloves are removed, and when otherwise indicated to avoid transfer of microorganisms to the therapist, other clients or environments. It may be necessary to wash hands between tasks and procedures on the same client to prevent cross-contamination of different body sites.

Handwashing is critical between clients, and is recommended before any other activity is performed. Soap is naturally antimicrobial, and special soap is not necessary. A waterless microbial hand cleanser is an acceptable alternative when facilities for handwashing are not available.

Gloves

Nonsterile gloves should be worn when touching blood, body fluids, secretions, excretions, and contaminated items. Gloves should be changed between tasks and procedures on the same client after contact with material that may contain a high concentration of microorganisms. Gloves should be removed promptly after use, before touching noncontaminated items and environmental surfaces, and hands should be washed to avoid transfer of microorganisms to other persons or environments.

Mask and Face Protection

A mask and eye protection (goggles or glasses with solid side shields) or a face shield should be worn to protect mucous membranes of the eyes, nose, and mouth during procedures and activities that are likely to generate splashes or sprays of blood, body fluids, secretions, and excretions.

Gowns

A gown should be worn to protect skin and to prevent soiling of clothing during procedures and activities that are likely to generate splashes or sprays of blood, body fluids, secretions, or excretions. A soiled gown should be removed promptly, and hands should be washed to avoid transfer of microorganisms to other persons or environments.

Cleanup of Body Fluids

A freshly prepared solution of one part bleach to nine parts water should be used to clean any surface contaminated with body fluids. Extra solution should be discarded daily (not stored) and new solution prepared as needed.

Skin Lesions on Therapist

Since different massage techniques utilize different portions of the therapist's body, gloves may not be adequate protection in preventing the transfer of infectious microorganisms. Inspect all skin that may touch the client in the course of performing your techniques (including elbows, forearms, feet and ankles) and refrain from using that body part if the skin is not intact or if there is a possibility of infection.

Visual Inspection

Never touch an area of skin that you have not seen that day. You must visually inspect any skin that your hand or skin will be touching. This includes massage techniques while gloved, as you can spread infection to other areas of the body even though your skin is protected. Many diseases and drugs inhibit the client's sensation, and it is not enough to rely upon the client's description and feelings to tell you if the skin is safe for massage.

Massaging through linens or clothing doesn't require visual inspection, although verbally questioning the client about inflammation or other conditions is still necessary.

*When it comes to the skin,
your client regards
you as the expert.
Use this authority
to encourage them to seek
appropriate care without delay
whenever either of you
have a concern.*

Bacterial Skin Infections

Specific conditions are listed on the following pages with the description of the condition, but certain precautions should be taken for all bacterial skin infections:

Bacterial Skin Infection Precautions

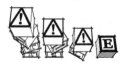 **Avoid all touch directly on the infected area. Energy techniques only. Your full technique range is encouraged for the rest of the body.**

 If lymph nodes are swollen, tender, hard, and hot, or if there are visible red streaks on the skin pointing towards the armpit or groin, with throbbing pain and/or fever, stop or avoid massage and seek immediate medical attention. Lymphadenitis and lymphangitis may spread within hours.

 Avoid any area of skin you suspect may be infected along with a generous margin for safety. Keep that area of the body covered with bandages or the client's clothing to limit contamination.

 Warning: Touching the skin under linens or clothing is acceptable as long as you have visually inspected the skin that day. Never touch an area of skin that you have not seen.

 Follow the Standard Precautions detailed at the beginning of this chapter for all equipment and linen that may have been in contact with a suspected infection.

 The various antibiotic classes each use different methods to eliminate bacteria. Check these precautions and any other medications the client is currently taking.

 Clients appreciate your knowledge of the body and will be grateful for your conservative approach.

Acne

The pores of your skin contain oil glands that lubricate your hair and skin. Sometimes a pore may become clogged with too much oil, dead skin cells or bacteria. Specific acne lesions are as follows:

Whiteheads result when a pore is completely blocked, trapping sebum (oil), bacteria, and dead skin cells, causing a white appearance on the surface.

Blackheads result when a pore is only partially blocked, allowing some of the trapped sebum, bacteria, and dead skin cells to slowly drain to the surface. The black color is a reaction of the skin's own pigment (melanin), reacting with the oxygen in the air.

Papules are small, red, solid bumps with no head.

A *pustule* (*zit*) is similar to a whitehead, but is inflamed, and appears as a red circle with a white or yellow center.

As opposed to the lesions mentioned above, *nodules* are hard bumps under the skin's surface that can be quite painful and can last a long time.

An acne *cyst* can appear similar to a nodule, but is pus-filled and has as diameter of 5mm or more.

 Note: Although acne is not contagious, it is an infection with localized acute inflammation and may become irritated with massage.

Boils

A boil is a bacterial skin infection involving the entire hair follicle and the adjacent subcutaneous tissue. A cluster of boils connected under the surface is called a *carbuncle*.

 Symptoms: A boil begins as a tender, red nodule, ultimately becoming filled with pus and rupturing.

Cellulitis

(also called erysipelas)

Cellulitis is a skin infection that sometimes accompanies damage to the skin, poor circulation, or diabetes. Streptococcal or staphylococcal bacteria enter the skin through a cut, puncture, ulcer, or sore, producing enzymes that break down the skin cells. Lymphadenitis and lymphangitis (infection of the lymph nodes and lymph channels) can occur as a complication and requires immediate medical attention.

 Symptoms: One or both lower limbs show large areas of redness, swelling, tenderness and increased warmth.

Folliculitis

Folliculitis is a group of skin conditions in which hair follicles become infected, most commonly by bacteria.

 Symptoms: Beginning as a tender red spot, folliculitis often transforms into a pustule.

Impetigo

(also called school sores)

Impetigo is an aggressively contagious bacterial skin infection. It most often occurs on exposed areas such as the hands and face.

 Symptoms: Lesions include pustules and round, crusted oozing patches which progressively increase in size.

Necrotizing Fasciitis

(also called flesh eating disease)

Necrotizing fasciitis is a very serious bacterial infection of the skin and soft tissues. It begins as an open wound becomes infected with a particularly aggressive bacteria. The bacteria multiply and release toxins and enzymes that result in thrombosis. The resulting loss of blood supply kills the tissue.

 Symptoms: Lesions begin as a swollen, purplish rash, with large dark marks turning into blisters. There can be severe pain, but other conditions such as diabetes may inhibit sensation. If left untreated, the tissue blackens and dies (*necrosis*).

Fungal Skin Infections

(also called dermatophytosis, mycosis)

Fungal skin infections are caused by mold-like fungi called dermatophytes that live on skin proteins (*keratin*) on the surface of the skin.

Fungal skin infections are contagious. It can be passed by direct skin-to-skin contact or by contact with contaminated items such as the outside of massage bottles or unwashed sheets. You can also catch it from pets that carry the fungus, especially cats.

Tinea corporis, also called *ringworm*, is a fungal infection usually originating on the torso and spreading to a much larger area. If it is found on the scalp it is called *tinea capitis*. *Tinea cruris*, also called *jock itch* or *ringworm of the groin*, is an infection of the groin area occurring almost exclusively in adult men. *Tinea pedis*, also called *athlete's foot,* is a fungal infection of the foot.

Fungal Skin Infection Precautions

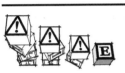 **Avoid all touch directly on the infected area. Energy techniques only. Your full technique range is encouraged for the rest of the body.**

 Secondary bacterial infections can occur if the skin is broken from itching. If lymph nodes are swollen, tender, hard, and hot, or if there are visible red streaks on the skin pointing towards the armpit or groin, with throbbing pain and/or fever, stop or avoid massage and seek immediate medical attention. Lymphadenitis and lymphangitis may spread within hours.

 Avoid any area of skin you suspect may be infected, along with a generous margin for safety. If the client shows swelling of lymph nodes and/or fever, stop or avoid massage and have client consult with their physician.

 Symptoms: Lesions include itchy, red, raised, scaly patches that may blister and ooze. The patches often have sharply-defined edges. They are often redder around the outside with normal skin tone in the center, which may look like a ring.

 Follow the Standard Precautions detailed at the beginning of this chapter for all equipment and linen that may have been in contact with a suspected infection.

 Antifungal medications are available over-the-counter as well as on a prescription basis. Check other current medications also for additional precautions.

 Treating this infection typically requires persistence as well as patience. Encourage the client to follow through for success.

Parasitic Skin Infections

Parasites on the skin are usually small insects or worms that burrow into the skin to live there and/or lay their eggs. The two most common are scabies and lice.

Scabies

Scabies is caused by a tiny mite that is often hard to detect. It causes an allergic reaction that manifests as severe itching. Mites can live in bedding for up to 24 hours or more, and newly infected persons can be contagious for 6 to 8 weeks before symptoms occur.

Scabies Precautions

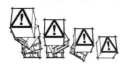 **Avoid all therapy until approved by their physician.**

 Avoid all contact and massage with clients infected with scabies for one week after treatment has begun or the physician has cleared the client for contact.

 Warning: The skin may remain irritated for weeks following treatment. Be cautious about oils and pressure to avoid further irritation.

 Symptoms: Lesions begin weeks after initial infestation, causing severe itching on warmer sites such as skin folds, where clothing is tight, between the fingers, under the nails, or on the elbows or wrists. Symptoms are worse at night. Hives, tiny bites, or pimples appear, and in more advanced cases, the skin may be crusty or scaly.

 Scabicide drugs cause severe itching, often mimicking a second scabies infestation.

 This infection can be humiliating to the client, so remember to lead with compassion.

Lice

Lice are tiny insects that can infest the skin anywhere on the body. This infection is characterized by intense itching, which is often worse at night. Lice are highly contagious, spreading from person-to-person by close body contact, shared clothes, linens or other items such as hats or brushes.

Lice, or their eggs (called nits), can usually be seen on the hair, behind the ears, and on the neck. In some cases, lice and eggs can be found in the seams of clothing.

Lice Precautions

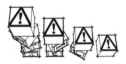 **Avoid all therapy until approved by their physician.**

 Avoid all contact and massage with clients infected with lice until the treatment is complete or the physician has cleared the client for contact.

 After massage has been cleared: Follow the Standard Precautions detailed at the beginning of this chapter for all equipment and linen that may have been infected with lice.

 Medications (other than special shampoos) are not necessary for lice.

 Lice infestation is only a temporary delay in your sessions with the client. Be supportive and they in turn will be grateful.

---

*Trust and loyalty blossoms
from the wellspring of
compassion.*

Viral Skin Infections

Herpes
(also called cold sores, genital herpes, shingles)

Infections around the outside of the mouth, eye or the genitalia are caused by the *Herpes Simplex* virus. Shingles is caused by the *varicella-zoster virus*, which is also called *Herpes Zoster*. This is the same virus that causes chickenpox.

An opportunistic virus, herpes lies dormant in the nerve roots that correspond to the areas of the skin originally infected. When stresses are high and the immune system is challenged, the virus seizes the opportunity to erupt at the skin level. Wherever it erupts it causes extremely painful, thin-topped pimple clusters that rupture and grow into larger skin erosions and ulcerations. These stay inside the skin areas (called *dermatomes*) controlled by the infected nerve root. A small percentage of eruptions cause *postherpetic neuralgia* (PHN), a persistent pain that can last for a month or longer after the skin has healed.

Herpes is extremely contagious by touch from the moment the skin becomes hypersensitive to the end of the skin's final healing stage. While it is dormant the area is not contagious. The virus does not travel inside the nerves to other areas; spreading to other areas occurs on the skin surface only.

Herpes Infection Precautions

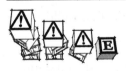 **Avoid all touch directly on the lesions. Energy techniques only. Your full technique range is encouraged for the rest of the body.**

 Serious skin infections and those endangering the eye should be treated by a physician.

 Avoid any area of skin you suspect may be infected along with a generous margin for safety. Keep that area of the body covered with bandages or the client's clothing to limit contamination.

Herpes Precautions, cont'd.

 Avoid any movements that would cause stretching of the skin around the lesion, as the infected areas are extremely painful. Also consider avoiding positions that would put pressure on the area.

 Warning: Touching the skin under linens or clothing is acceptable as long as you have visually inspected the skin that day. Never touch an area of skin that you have not seen.

 Follow the Standard Precautions detailed at the beginning of this chapter for all equipment and linen that may have been in contact with a suspected infection.

 Anticonvulsants, pain medications, and topical pain relievers are all common to control the pain, and antivirals may be prescribed to minimize the duration and spread of the infection. Check each of their current medications for additional precautions.

 Even as common as this infection is (the **WHO** states that one third of the world's population is infected with the herpes simplex virus), clients are often still embarrassed by the social stigma. Take all necessary precautions, and then change topics and focus on your massage. Your client will appreciate your tact and professionalism.

Warts

Warts are caused by a virus, which generally invades the skin through small or invisible cuts and abrasions. They can appear anywhere on the skin. Those on the sole of the foot are called *plantar warts*. They are often mistaken for *corns* or *calluses*, which are layers of dead skin that build up to protect an area subjected to repeated stress.

Plantar warts tend to be hard and flat, with a rough surface and well-defined boundaries. Plantar warts vary in color from gray to brown with a center that appears as one or more pinpoints of black. When they appear on other parts of the body warts are generally raised and lumpy.

Wart Precautions

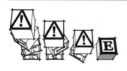

Avoid all touch directly on the wart. Energy techniques only. Your full technique range is encouraged for the rest of the body.

 If you suspect that there may be some abnormality, recommend that they consult a dermatologist without delay.

 Avoid massage directly on the wart. Surrounding skin is non-contagious and massage is recommended.

 There are many self treatments available. These can damage the surrounding tissue as well. Consider any area treated as still infected and possibly inflamed unless it was performed by a physician.

 This is one of the least threatening conditions the client will ever have; keep this in perspective whenever the subject comes up to avoid embarrassment or discomfort.

Conjunctivitis

(also called pink eye)

Conjunctivitis is an inflammation of the conjunctiva, the clear membrane that covers the white part of the eye and lines the inner surface of the eyelids. It is a fairly common, temporary condition and usually causes no permanent danger to the eye or vision. There are four major causes:

Viral Conjunctivitis
Viral conjunctivitis usually affects only one eye and causes excessive eye watering and a light discharge.

Bacterial Conjunctivitis
Bacterial conjunctivitis affects both eyes and causes a heavy, sometimes greenish discharge.

Allergic Conjunctivitis

Allergic conjunctivitis affects both eyes and causes itching and redness in the eyes and sometimes the nose, as well as excessive tearing.

Giant Papillary Conjunctivitis (GPC)

Giant papillary conjunctivitis usually affects both eyes and causes excess tears, contact lens intolerance, itching, a heavy discharge, and red bumps on the underside of the eyelids.

Conjunctivitis Precautions

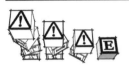 **Avoid all touch techniques on the client's face. Your full technique range is encouraged for the rest of the body.**

 Any infection of the eye can be dangerous and should be treated by a physician.

 Warning: Infectious conjunctivitis is highly contagious. Avoid contact with any portion of the client's face or any linen that has touched their face. Use the standard precautions detailed in this chapter for proper hygiene and safety.

 Warning: The client may be unable to use the face cradle due to the pressure on the area surrounding the eye. Ask if a seated or side posture would be more comfortable before attempting to place them in a prone position.

 Local drops are usually the only medications prescribed for conjunctivitis. Ask in any case to be sure you have a complete list, and before you begin, ask if they wish to have their drops ready during the session.

 This temporary condition may be extremely uncomfortable and temporarily disfiguring. Take necessary precautions and then focus elsewhere to ease the client's mind as well as their body.

Eczema and Dermatitis

Eczema is a general term encompassing a group of inflammatory skin conditions known as dermatitis. Although the exact causes are unknown, eczema appears to be an abnormal response of the body's immune system. It is not infectious and therefore not contagious. The National Institutes of Health estimates that 15 million people in the U.S. have some form of eczema.

Atopic Dermatitis
Signs and symptoms of this common form of eczema include itchy, thickened, scaly skin, most often in the folds of the elbows or backs of the knees. It is also common on the face, hands and feet. When this type occurs in infants it is called *infantile eczema*.

Contact Dermatitis
This type of eczema occurs after exposure to an allergen such as poison ivy or cosmetics such as eye makeup, or an irritant such as soap or detergent. Signs and symptoms include redness and itching, and blisters and weeping sores may form in severe cases.

Neurodermatitis
This type occurs because of repeated scratching due to pruritis (*itching*). Chronic scratching can cause patches of thickened, brownish skin. These patches have definite margins that are thick and leather-like (*lichenified*). This type of dermatitis is also known as *lichen simplex chronicus*.

Seborrheic Dermatitis
This type can appear as a stubborn, itchy *dandruff.* Dandruff is usually due to mild seborrheic dermatitis of the scalp. It also appears as greasy, scaling areas at the sides of the nose, eyebrows, behind the ears or over the breastbone. In infants, seborrheic dermatitis is called *cradle cap* — a crusty, scaly skin on a baby's scalp.

Stasis Dermatitis

This type often is associated with swelling of the lower legs from venous insufficiency and varicose veins. Stasis dermatitis may cause the skin at the ankles and shins to become discolored (red or brown), thick and itchy. Decubitus ulcers (*bed sores*) also may develop.

Eczema and Dermatitis Precautions

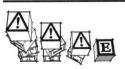 **Avoid all pressure and circulatory massage techniques to affected area(s). Energy techniques only. Your full technique range is encouraged for the rest of the body.**

 If you suspect that there may be some abnormality, recommend that they consult a dermatologist without delay.

 Avoiding local areas of eczema is recommended as the massage lubricants and pressure may further irritate the area. If the cause is well known and the client has a full awareness of the potential reactions then massage may be warranted. Have the client check with the treating physician to be sure in these cases.

 Avoid the local area and keep it covered with bandages or the client's clothing to limit contamination. Open wounds such as cracks or ulcerations are vulnerable to infection.

 Topical and oral medications may be prescribed for this condition. The client may also be self-medicating. Check each of their current medications for additional precautions.

 Discussing possible physical and chemical irritants (and how to eliminate them) can have a significant effect on the clients' ability to manage this condition.

Psoriasis

Researchers believe that with psoriasis, the immune system sends faulty signals that speed up the growth cycle in skin cells. This is called an autoimmune response. Think about cleaning the walls of your house with steel wool; the intent is healthy, but the overaggressive nature damages the surface. The more signals that come in for healing or repair, the more aggressive the cleaning becomes.

Certain people carry genes that make them more likely to develop psoriasis, but not everyone with these genes develops psoriasis. Instead, a "trigger" makes the psoriasis appear in those who have these genes. Emotional stress, chemical or physical skin irritation, infections, and certain medications can all act as triggers.

Psoriasis produces red, irritating skin patches with loose, whitish scales. In up to 15 percent of the cases it also damages the joints much like rheumatoid arthritis (see psoriatic arthritis).

Psoriasis Precautions

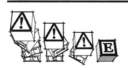 **Avoid all pressure and circulatory massage techniques to affected area(s). Energy techniques only. Your full technique range is encouraged for the rest of the body.**

 Have the client consult their physician if there has been any dramatic change in symptoms, or if the client has a persistent fever and severe fatigue.

 Avoid pressure massage on acutely inflamed joints or lesions.

 Any pressure massage on the skin lesions stimulates the growth and cleaning response and will likely aggravate the condition. If you and the client both agree that massage is warranted, preapprove any lubricant with the client and test for irritation on a small area of skin. Using linen as an alternate to lubricants may be preferred.

Psoriasis Precautions, cont'd.

 Medications vary frequently with clients as they build resistance. Immunosuppressants, anti-inflammatory and pain medications are common and ever changing. Ask before each visit what topical and oral medications are currently being used.

 Physical irritation can flare local lesions, yet the stress-relieving benefits of massage are also undeniable. Find the unique balance with your client and help them flourish!

Systemic Sclerosis

(also called scleroderma)

Scleroderma is a rare, chronic autoimmune disease that causes *fibrosis* (scar tissue) to be formed in the skin and/or internal organs due to a production of excess collagen. The fibrosis eventually causes the involved skin or organs to harden. There is decreased blood supply, which makes them very sensitive to cold temperatures (Raynaud's syndrome), and *calcinosis* is common (calcium lumps under the skin.) The cause is unknown.

Systemic Sclerosis Precautions

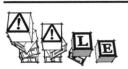 **Restrict massage to Light and Energy techniques.**

 Before your first session including pressure techniques, consult with the physician to discuss the proper precautions for this client.

 Avoid pressure techniques designed to activate the healing response because of the body's excess collagen production. Scleroderma produces progressively fragile, atrophic skin. LIGHT and ENERGY techniques are recommended to increase circulation.

Systemic Sclerosis Precautions, cont'd.

 Check all other conditions the client reports to gain a complete understanding of the necessary precautions.

 NSAIDs, steroids and circulatory medicines are all common and ongoing. Be sure to ask about current medications and check their precautions.

 Teach your client gentle massage techniques they can use to increase circulation and they'll be grateful for life!

Skin Trauma

Abrasion

An abrasion is any friction trauma that destroys tissue. Most abrasions are shallow scrapes that do not extend into the dermis and do not bleed. While there is often little or no blood loss from an abrasion, there can be a great deal of pain because of the exposed nerve endings.

 Avoid local massage as abrasions are vulnerable to infection.

Bites and Stings

Some normally minor insect bites may cause life-threatening anaphylaxis in sensitive people. Any dramatic or increasing swelling should be treated as a serious problem; avoid massage and seek immediate medical attention.

 If local lymph nodes are tender, swollen and hot (lymphadenitis), or if you see red streaks radiating from the bite or sting (lymphangitis), avoid massage and seek immediate medical attention. Contact the physician before regional massage to ensure that any possible infection is under control.

 Avoid massage directly over the bite or sting.

Burns and Scalds

Burns can be caused by contact with heat, flame, chemicals, electricity, or radiation. A burn occurs when the temperature at skin level cannot dissipate fast enough through blood supply and radiating into the air. Tissue damage begins at the skin's surface and penetrates deeper as the burn progresses through three degrees of severity.

First-Degree Burns

First-degree burns (including sunburn) only damage the epidermis. They cause redness and possibly swelling and pain, and typically within a few days.

Second-Degree Burns

Second-degree burns affect both the epidermis and the dermis, causing redness, pain, swelling and blisters. The skin typically heals in a few weeks without scarring.

Third-Degree Burns

Third-degree burns affect the epidermis, dermis and tissues beneath the skin. Blood and nerve supply is destroyed, which inhibits healing. Third-degree burns usually result in extensive scarring and take up to 12 months to heal completely.

A *skin graft* is healthy skin transplanted from one area of the body (called the *source area* or *donor site*) to the damaged area (called the *recipient area*). The source sites most commonly used for skin grafts are the inner thigh, leg, buttocks, upper arm, and forearm. Since there are no functioning sweat or oil glands in a skin graft it is necessary to keep the area oiled.

Burn Precautions

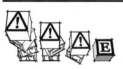 **Avoid all pressure and circulatory massage techniques to the burned area(s). Energy techniques only. Your full technique range is encouraged for the rest of the body.**

Burn Precautions, cont'd.

 Contact the client's physician before any massage over skin grafts. The increased circulation is undoubtedly beneficial, yet care is needed to ensure that the skin is able to endure pressure massage.

 Avoid all heat therapies on burned areas, as well as any lubricant that may produce a heat sensation.

 Avoid local massage over all burns until fully healed.

 Warning: Healing second and third degree burns are very vulnerable to infection and can be extremely painful. Have the client keep all burns covered. When performing massage in adjacent areas, avoid techniques that would pull or stretch the burned tissue.

 NSAIDs, steroids, and antibiotics are all common prescription medications and may be ongoing. Be sure to ask about current medications and check their precautions.

 The pain from burns can be excruciating; calming massage wherever appropriate will reduce their stress and build the body's healing ability.

Contusion (Bruise)

A contusion is a bruise caused by a blow to the muscle, tendon or ligament; caused when blood pools around the injury and discolors the skin.

 Avoid local massage to all visible acute bruises, as well as those that are invisible but tender, as blood clotting may be present.

Crust (Scab)

An area on the surface of the skin containing dried body fluid (*exudate*).

 Avoid local massage as the tissues beneath scabs are vulnerable to infection.

Excoriation

Excoriation refers to a hollow, crusted area caused by scratching or picking at a skin lesion.

 Avoid local massage as the lesion may be vulnerable to infection.

Erosion

The term erosion refers to a loss of epidermal tissue. The basement membrane remains intact, protecting the body from a systemic infection.

 Avoid local massage over erosions to prevent further trauma and possible infection.

Fissures, Ulcers, and Lacerations

An ulcer is a lesion where epidermal tissue and at least part of the dermal tissue is lost. This makes the body vulnerable to a systemic infection. A *decubitus ulcer* (*bed sore*) is caused by a loss of blood supply due to persistent pressure on a body part (e.g. a wheelchair-bound or bedridden person). A fissure is a linear ulcer. A laceration is any torn, ragged, mangled, or stabbed wound.

 If local lymph nodes are tender, swollen and hot (lymphadenitis), or if you see red streaks radiating from the area (lymphangitis), avoid massage and seek immediate medical attention.

 Avoid local massage as well as a generous margin for safety. All open wounds are vulnerable to infection.

With your thoughts and energy,
reinforce the fact that
beauty transcends the skin.

Frostbite

Frostbite is a form of localized tissue destruction from freezing where ice crystals form in the skin and possibly deeper tissues. It occurs once skin temperatures fall below 32° F.

The frostbitten body part becomes pale, cold, hard, and insensitive to touch or deep pressure. The skin becomes hypersensitive to temperature, and even the slightest exposure to temperature changes can result in a severe inflammatory reaction and ulceration.

Frostbite may be classified by three stages according to the severity or depth of the injury: First degree frostbite is called *erythema,* which when thawed becomes reddened, painful and hypersensitive. Second degree frostbite is called *vesication.* The damage is deeper and blistering occurs. *Necrosis* is the third and most severe form of frostbite, where deep tissues and blood supply are destroyed and amputation may be necessary.

 Tissues suspected of frostbite should be thawed with warm (not hot) water. Do not rub or create friction on the skin, and do not use direct heat such as heated air or a heat pad. Separate each finger or body part with sterile dressings, and only thaw the skin if it can be kept warm. Refreezing the tissue will cause more extensive damage.

 Avoid all heat, ice and cold therapies on all frostbitten areas, as well as any lubricant that may produce a heat sensation.

 Reduce your local massage duration to guard against overwhelming the tissues. After tissue has healed, only LIGHT and ENERGY techniques should be used locally due to the fragile tissue.

Puncture

A puncture wound is any hole extending past the epidermis.

 If local lymph nodes are tender, swollen and hot (lymphadenitis), or if you see red streaks radiating from the puncture wound (lymphangitis), avoid massage and seek immediate medical attention.

 If the wound is deep, hasn't bled, or if there is a fever, avoid massage and seek immediate medical attention to rule out the possibility of tetanus.

 Avoid the local area and any tender areas surrounding the puncture.

Scar and Keloid

When an injury occurs, the body forms a special collagen 'glue' known as *granulation scar tissue*. It takes up to 12 months for a scar to mature. Mature scar tissue has a tensile strength that is only 30 percent as strong as normal skin. Scars are permanent and never revert to the original local tissue.

Excessive scar tissue is classified as either a keloid or a *hypertrophic scar* and can be painful and chronically itchy. There is a genetic predisposition for the formation of keloids.

 Avoid deep tissue techniques directly over scars. Reduce and closely monitor pressure intensity and duration to avoid damaging the scar tissue.

 Releasing the adhesions that form in the tissues surrounding the scar can greatly increase mobility and function.

Benign Skin Lesions

The usual precautions about neoplasms and massage do not apply in benign neoplasms of the skin. They are extremely slow growing, non-contagious and relatively harmless. Most are painless, although they may become irritated more easily than the surrounding tissue.

Angiomas

Strawberry hemangiomas (also called a *strawberry mark, vascular nevus* or *capillary hemangioma*) consist of small, closely packed blood vessels. They may be present at birth or develop in the first several weeks of life. They usually grow rapidly, remain a fixed size, and then subside. 95 percent of strawberry hemangiomas disappear by the time the child is 9 years old, although there may be some permanent discoloration or puckering of the skin where a strawberry hemangioma existed.

Cavernous hemangiomas are similar to strawberry hemangiomas but are deeper. They may appear as a red-blue spongy mass of tissue filled with blood. Some of these lesions disappear on their own, usually as a child approaches school age. Others become permanent marks with possible darkening from melanin infiltration.

A *port-wine stain* is a flat hemangioma made of dilated capillaries. The most common location is the face. The size varies from very small lesions, to lesions covering over half the surface of the body.

Salmon patches (stork bites) are small, pink, flat spots. They are extremely common, appearing on 30 to 50 percent of newborns. They are small blood vessels (capillaries) that are visible through the skin. Patches on the face often fade as the infant grows. Salmon patches on the back of the neck may not fade but are usually not noticeable as the hair grows.

Dermatofibroma

This benign neoplasm is the most prevalent of all painful skin tumors. It can be asymptomatic, but frequently produces some level of pain and itching. Dermatofibromas typically arise slowly and most often occur as a solitary nodule on an extremity with a wide range of coloring from flesh to any darker or lighter pigment.

Lipoma

This neoplasm is formed of *adipocytes* (fat cells), and is a nodule that does not discolor the skin's surface and moves slightly when pressed. There may be one or many, but they do not spread and pose no health concern.

Mole

Also called a *nevus*, a mole is a benign neoplasm formed of melanocytes that looks like a pigmented macule, papule or nodule. This means it can be flat or elevated, but typically not larger than a pencil eraser. They can be present at birth or develop at any age. Any new skin lesion should be evaluated by a physician.

Seborrheic keratosis

Seborrheic keratoses are the most common benign tumors in older individuals. Located on the face, chest, shoulders, back, or other areas, they are elevated with brown, black, yellow or other hues, with a rough or wart-like texture and a waxy surface. They look as if they were "pasted" onto the skin. They can itch, grow, and become cosmetically unattractive but pose no health threat.

Skin tag

This is a soft, small, flesh-colored benign neoplasm that appears to hang from a stalk (*pedunculated*). Skin tags are primarily found where a person sweats. They are harmless, but may bleed profusely if torn or cut.

Benign Skin Lesion Precautions

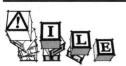 **Avoid deep pressure on the lesion(s). Your full technique range is encouraged for the rest of the body.**

 If you suspect that there may be some abnormality, clearly state to the client that your experience is in recognizing "normal" tissue, and that the spot in question does not fit the normal pattern. Do not offer any names, as you may be misleading and unnecessarily traumatizing your client. Recommend (as firmly as you feel it is necessary) that they consult a dermatologist without delay and report the findings to you.

 Avoid local pressure techniques after surgery until the client has healed and has the approval of their physician. ENERGY techniques are encouraged, and all techniques are encouraged in the surrounding tissues.

 Avoid deep massage directly on the lesion. All techniques are encouraged in the surrounding tissues.

 No specific medications are prescribed for benign neoplasms. As always, check the client's current medications for specific precautions.

 These conditions are far more aesthetically uncomfortable than physically threatening. Help the client recognize that the value of the human body is far greater than the surface blemishes.

Malignant Skin Lesions

A thorough discussion of cancer as it relates to the massage profession is discussed in the chapter entitled Cancer. Please refer to that chapter for additional precautions.

Listed below are the most commonly seen skin malignancies. The descriptions are designed to be used as an indicator of what may occur with each condition. It is beyond the scope of any massage therapist to even hint that a suspected lesion is cancerous.

Basal Cell Carcinoma (BCC)

Basal cell carcinoma is the most common malignancy in humans. It typically occurs in areas of chronic sun exposure. BCC is usually slow growing and rarely metastasizes. Early detection and treatment is important, however, to prevent further tissue destruction and to minimize the scar.

BCC appears as one or more pearly, waxy papules with central depression, erosion or ulcerations and a raised, distinct border. Small spider veins (called *telangiectasia*) are commonly seen, and the lesion may bleed easily.

Kaposi's Sarcoma (KS)

Kaposi's sarcoma currently is the most common AIDS-associated malignancy. They appear as brown, pink, red, or purple nodules or raised lesions, and may be less distinctive in dark-skinned individuals.

Squamous Cell Carcinoma (SCC)

Squamous cell carcinoma is the second most common form of skin cancer and frequently arises on sun-exposed skin as people age. SCC begins as a red papule or plaque with a scaly, crusted surface. It grows to a nodular size, with the bulk of the lesion below the surface.

Malignant Melanoma

Melanoma is a malignancy of pigment-producing cells (melanocytes) occurring in the skin and mucous membranes. Melanomas account for only 4 percent of all skin cancers; however, they are responsible for 75 percent of all skin cancer deaths in the U.S. Early detection is essential for survival.

Melanomas are often mistaken for moles. The **ABCD** criteria for the difference between a mole and a melanoma is as follows:

Asymmetry

Melanomas are unusually shaped. Moles are typically round or oval in shape, rising distinctly from the surrounding skin.

Border Notching

The edges of a melanoma are irregular and may blend in with the surrounding normal skin. Moles have clearly defined edges.

Color Variegation

More than one color is apparent on melanomas, with black, brown, red, or white hues possible. Each mole is limited to one color, although the same body part may have moles of different shades.

Diameter

The size of a melanoma is typically greater than 6 mm across. Moles should be less than the width of a pencil eraser or your smallest fingernail (your pinkie fingernail).

Malignant Skin Lesion Precautions

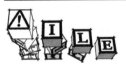 **Avoid deep pressure on the lesion(s). Your full technique range is encouraged for the rest of the body.**

 If you suspect that there may be some abnormality, clearly state to the client that your experience is in recognizing "normal" tissue, and that the spot in question does not fit the normal pattern. Do not offer any names, as you may be misleading and unnecessarily traumatizing your client. Recommend (as firmly as you feel it is necessary) that they consult a dermatologist without delay and report the findings to you.

 Avoid all pressure techniques until the client has healed from surgery and has the approval of their physician. ENERGY techniques are encouraged.

Malignant Skin Lesion Precautions, cont'd.

 If the client has undergone radiation therapy at any time in the past, or is currently undergoing therapy, refer to that section in the chapter on cancer for a complete understanding of massage precautions.

 Avoid deep massage directly on the lesion. All techniques are encouraged in the surrounding tissues.

 If the client is undergoing chemotherapy, check that section for additional precautions. Check the client's current medications for specific precautions.

 Encourage the client to get checked and treated without delay. As the expert in skin conditions, they look to you for guidance. Stress to them that early detection is the key to success.

The uncertainty you may feel when faced with a difficult or unpopular decision comes from the same place in your soul as compassion and integrity. Trust your instincts and training.

Anti-Infection Medications

Antibiotics

(also called antibacterials)

Bacteria are the oldest, simplest, and the most numerous forms of life. Bacteria are simple, one-celled organisms called *prokaryotes* (cells that do not contain a nucleus). 10,000 bacteria lined up side-by-side would only take one inch of space, and they can replicate as fast as every twenty minutes!

There are many thousands of species of bacteria, about two thousand species of which are identified. Most are harmless, and many are helpful -- even vital to our existence. For example, the bacteria that live in the roots of plants help extract nitrogen from the atmosphere to enrich the soil. Healthy bacteria that exist in our intestines are called *probiotics*. They break down food into the components we can absorb and are as necessary to proper nutrition as chewing our food. Unfortunately, antibiotics wipe out this normal flora. This is becoming increasingly obvious as a fundamental cause of long-term malnutrition and illnesses such as candida.

Most bacteria may be placed into one of three groups. *Aerobic bacteria* (like those causing staphylococcal or streptococcal infections) thrive in the presence of oxygen and require it for their continued growth and existence. Other bacteria are *anaerobic* (like those that cause gangrene, botulism, or tetanus), and cannot tolerate gaseous oxygen. The third group are the *facultative anaerobes* (like Salmonella and Escherichia Coli), which prefer growing in the presence of oxygen, but can continue to grow without it.

70 percent of the antibiotics used in the US are fed to livestock, which translates to about 25 million pounds of antibiotics. This is almost *eight times* the amount given to humans to treat disease. Only about 10 percent of that amount is actually intended to treat disease. Antibiotics provide a double benefit for the meat industry -- they reduce the spread of disease and at the same time dramatically accelerate growth. For example, antibiotics force chickens to mature fast enough to be ready for slaughter in only five to six weeks. The only way for consumers to be certain that meat and dairy has not been treated with antibiotics is to purchase those labeled antibiotic-free. Farmers in the U.S. are not required to report antibiotic use in livestock.

Ingesting antibiotics in any fashion increases the likelihood of contracting bacteria resistant to those antibiotics in the future.

Aminoglycosides

Aminoglycosides are broad-spectrum antibiotics that are often injected into veins or muscles to treat serious bacterial infections. Some aminoglycosides are also used orally to treat intestinal infections or topically to treat eye infections.

 If the client has recently developed any of the following, avoid massage and have them call their physician immediately: Unexplained joint pain or skin rash, increased difficulty breathing, ringing in the ears, sudden severe headache, recent muscle weakness, unusual bleeding or bruising or swelling of the lips, tongue, or face. (This is a massage-specific list; refer to the documentation that was included with the medication for a complete list of side effects.)

 Side Effects: Nausea and numbness or tingling of the hands or feet, drowsiness, headache and stomach cramping are side effects that can occur with antibiotics. Take these into consideration as they may limit your ability to achieve your client's massage goals.

 Aminoglycoside antibiotic medications include: amikacin (Amikin), gentamicin (Garamycin), kanamycin (Kantrex), neomycin (Mycifradin), netilmicin (Netromycin), paromomycin (Humatin), streptomycin, and tobramycin (TOBI, TobraDex, Nebcin).

Anaerobic Antibiotics

Anaerobic antibiotics eliminate bacteria that thrive without oxygen and cause internal infections.

 If the client has recently developed any of the following, avoid massage and call the physician immediately: Unexplained joint pain or skin rash, increased difficulty breathing, ringing in the ears, sudden severe headache, recent muscle weakness, unusual bleeding or bruising or swelling of the lips, tongue, or face. (This is a massage-specific list; refer to the documentation that was included with the medication for a complete list of side effects.)

Anaerobic Antibiotic Precautions, cont'd.

 Warning: Permanent peripheral neuropathy is a complication with long-term use of this class of antibiotics. Be extra cautious with pressure, as the client may not be able to accurately determine their limits.

 Side Effects: Dark brown or reddish urine, headache, nausea, mild stomach pain or cramps and diarrhea often occur as a result of this class of medication. Take these into consideration as they may limit your ability to achieve your client's massage goals.

 Anaerobic antibiotic medications include <u>metronidazole</u> (Flagyl, Protostat) and <u>paromomycin</u> (Humatin).

Cephalosporins

Cephalosporins kill bacteria by destroying the outer cell wall.

 If the client has recently developed any of the following, avoid massage and call the physician immediately: Unexplained joint pain or skin rash, increased difficulty breathing, ringing in the ears, sudden severe headache, recent muscle weakness, unusual bleeding or bruising or swelling of the lips, tongue, or face. (This is a massage-specific list; refer to the documentation that was included with the medication for a complete list of side effects.)

 Side Effects: Nausea and numbness or tingling of the hands or feet, drowsiness, headache and stomach cramping are side effects that can occur with antibiotics. Take these into consideration as they may limit your ability to achieve your client's massage goals.

 Cephalosporin antibiotic medications include: <u>cefaclor</u> (Ceclor), <u>cefadroxil</u> (Duricef, Ultraef), <u>cefamandole</u> (Mandol), <u>cefazolin</u> (Ancef, Kefzol, Zolicef), <u>cefdinir</u> (Omnicef), <u>cefditoren</u> <u>pivoxil</u> (Spectracef), <u>cefepime</u> (Maxipime), <u>cefixime</u> (Suprax), <u>cefmetazole</u> (Zefazone), <u>cefonicid</u> (Monocid), <u>cefoperazone</u> (Cefobid), <u>cefotaxime</u> (Claforan), <u>cefotetan</u> (Cefotan), <u>cefoxitin</u> (Mefoxin), <u>cefpodoxime</u> (Vantin), <u>cefprozil</u> (Cefzil), <u>ceftazidime</u> (Ceptaz, Fortaz, Tazicef, Tazidime), <u>ceftibuten</u> (Cedax), <u>ceftizoxime</u> (Cefizox), <u>ceftriaxone</u> (Rocephin), <u>cefuroxime</u> (Ceftin), <u>cephalexin</u> (Biocef, Cefanex, Ceporex, Keflex, Keftab, Novolexin), <u>cephradine</u> (Anspor, Velosef), and <u>loracarbef</u> (Lorabid).

Macrolides

Macrolides are narrow-spectrum antibiotics that alter the chemical activity inside the bacteria, preventing the production of proteins needed by the bacteria to survive.

 If the client has recently developed any of the following, avoid massage and call the physician immediately: Unexplained joint pain or skin rash, increased difficulty breathing, ringing in the ears, sudden severe headache, recent muscle weakness, unusual bleeding or bruising or swelling of the lips, tongue, or face. (This is a massage-specific list; refer to the documentation that was included with the medication for a complete list of side effects.)

 Side Effects: Nausea and numbness or tingling of the hands or feet, drowsiness, headache and stomach cramping are side effects that can occur with antibiotics. Take these into consideration as they may limit your ability to achieve your client's massage goals.

 Macrolide antibiotic medications include: azithromycin (Zithromax), clarithromycin (Biaxin), dirithromycin (Dynabac), erythromycin (Diomycin, EryPed, Erythrocin, Ilosone, Ilotycin), telithromycin (Aventis, Ketek), and troleandomycin (TAO).

Oxazolidinones

These medications are used to treat susceptible serious bacterial infections such as skin infections, hospital and community acquired pneumonia, and other resistant infections.

 If the client has recently developed any of the following, avoid massage and call the physician immediately: Unexplained joint pain or skin rash, increased difficulty breathing, ringing in the ears, sudden severe headache, recent muscle weakness, unusual bleeding or bruising or swelling of the lips, tongue, or face. (This is a massage-specific list; refer to the documentation that was included with the medication for a complete list of side effects.)

 Side Effects: Nausea and numbness or tingling of the hands or feet, drowsiness, headache and stomach cramping are side effects that can occur with antibiotics. Take these into consideration as they may limit your ability to achieve your client's massage goals.

 Oxazolidinone antibiotic medications include linezolid (Zyvox).

Penicillins

Penicillins kill bacteria by destroying the outer cell wall.

 If the client has recently developed any of the following, avoid massage and call the physician immediately: Unexplained joint pain or skin rash, increased difficulty breathing, ringing in the ears, sudden severe headache, recent muscle weakness, unusual bleeding or bruising or swelling of the lips, tongue, or face. (This is a massage-specific list; refer to the documentation that was included with the medication for a complete list of side effects.)

 Side Effects: Nausea and numbness or tingling of the hands or feet, drowsiness, headache and stomach cramping are side effects that can occur with antibiotics. Take these into consideration as they may limit your ability to achieve your client's massage goals.

 Penicillin antibiotic medications include: <u>amoxicillin</u> (Amoxil, Bio-mox, Polymox, Trimox, Wymox), <u>amoxicillin</u> <u>with</u> <u>clavulanate</u> (Augmentin), <u>ampicillin</u> (D-Amp, Marcillin, Omnipen, Penbritin, Polycillin, Principen, Totacillin), <u>ampicillin</u> with <u>sulbactam</u> (Unasyn), <u>bacampicillin</u> (Spectrobid), <u>carbenicillin</u> (Geocillin), <u>cloxacillin</u> (Cloxapen), <u>dicloxacillin</u> (Dycill, Dynapen, Pathocil), <u>mezlocillin</u> (Mezlin), <u>nafcillin</u> (Unipen), <u>flucloxacillin</u> (Floxapen), <u>oxacillin</u> (Bactocill), <u>penicillin G</u> (Ayercillin, Bicillin, Crystapen, Crysticillin, Megacillin, Permapen, Pfizerpen, Wycillin), <u>penicillin V</u> (Beepen, Beta-pen, Ledercillin, Pen-Vee, Robicillin, Truxcillin, Novo-pen, V-Cillin, Veetids), <u>piperacillin</u> (Pipracil, Pipril), <u>piperacillin</u> <u>with</u> <u>tazobactam</u> (Zosyn), <u>ticarcillin</u> (Ticar), and <u>ticarcillin</u> with <u>clavulanate</u> (Timentin).

Quinolones

(also called fluoroquinolones)

Quinolones are broad-spectrum antibiotics that work by interfering with an enzyme that allows bacteria to reproduce, thereby halting the growth of bacteria and eventually leading to their death.

 If the client has recently developed any of the following, avoid massage and call the physician immediately: Unexplained joint pain or skin rash, increased difficulty breathing, ringing in the ears, sudden severe headache, recent muscle weakness, unusual bleeding or bruising or swelling of the lips, tongue, or face. (This is a massage-specific list; refer to the documentation that was included with the medication for a complete list of side effects.)

Quinolone Precautions, cont'd.

 Side Effects: Nausea and numbness or tingling of the hands or feet, drowsiness, headache and stomach cramping are side effects that can occur with antibiotics. Take these into consideration as they may limit your ability to achieve your client's massage goals.

 Quinolone antibiotic medications include: <u>ciprofloxacin</u> (Cipro), <u>enoxacin</u> (Penetrex), <u>gatifloxacin</u> (Tequin), <u>gemifloxacin</u> (Factive), <u>levofloxacin</u> (Levaquin), <u>lomefloxacin</u> (Maxaquin), <u>moxifloxacin</u> (Avelox), <u>norfloxacin</u> (Noroxin), <u>ofloxacin</u> (Floxin), <u>sparfloxacin</u> (Zagam), and <u>trovafloxacin</u> (Trovan).

Rifamycins

Rifamycins help slow the replication of certain bacteria.

 If the client has recently developed any of the following, avoid massage and call the physician immediately: Unexplained joint pain or skin rash, increased difficulty breathing, ringing in the ears, sudden severe headache, recent muscle weakness, unusual bleeding or bruising or swelling of the lips, tongue, or face. (This is a massage-specific list; refer to the documentation that was included with the medication for a complete list of side effects.)

 Side Effects: Nausea and numbness or tingling of the hands or feet, drowsiness, headache and stomach cramping are side effects that can occur with antibiotics. Take these into consideration as they may limit your ability to achieve your client's massage goals.

 Rifamycin antibiotic medications include: <u>rifabutin</u> (Mycobutin), <u>rifampin</u> (Rifadin, Rifamate, Rifampicin, Rifater, Rimactane), <u>rifaximin</u> (Xifaxan), and <u>rifapentine</u> (Priftin).

Sulfonamides and Related Compounds

Bacterial cells produce folic acid, a chemical necessary for their growth. Sulfonamides interfere with the enzyme that helps form folic acid, subsequently killing the bacteria.

 If the client has recently developed any of the following, avoid massage and call the physician immediately: Unexplained joint pain or skin rash, increased difficulty breathing, ringing in the ears, sudden severe headache, recent muscle weakness, unusual bleeding or bruising or swelling of the lips, tongue, or face.

Sulfonamide Precautions, cont'd.

 Side Effects: Nausea and numbness or tingling of the hands or feet, drowsiness, headache and stomach cramping are side effects that can occur with antibiotics. Take these into consideration as they may limit your ability to achieve your client's massage goals.

 Sulfonamide antibiotic medications (and related compounds) include: co-trimoxazole (Bactrim, Bethaprim, Cotrim, Septra, Sulfatrim, Trimethoprim), sulfadiazine (Azulfidine, Microsulfon, Salazopyrin), sulfamethoxazole (Gantanol), and sulfisoxazole (Gantrisin, Sulfizole, Truxazole).

Tetracyclines

Tetracyclines prevent the bacteria from producing proteins needed to survive.

 If the client has recently developed any of the following, avoid massage and call the physician immediately: Unexplained joint pain or skin rash, increased difficulty breathing, ringing in the ears, sudden severe headache, recent muscle weakness, unusual bleeding or bruising or swelling of the lips, tongue, or face. (This is a massage-specific list; refer to the documentation that was included with the medication for a complete list of side effects.)

 Side Effects: Nausea and numbness or tingling of the hands or feet, drowsiness, headache and stomach cramping are side effects that can occur with antibiotics. Take these into consideration as they may limit your ability to achieve your client's massage goals.

 Tetracycline antibiotic medications include: demeclocycline (Declomycin), doxycycline (Adoxa, Doryx, Doxy, Doxycin, Monodox, Periostat, Vibramycin), minocycline (Dynacin, Minocin, Vectrin), oxytetracycline (Terramycin), and tetracycline (Achromycin, Brodspec, Panmycin, Robitet, Sumycin, Tetracap, Wesmycin).

Miscellaneous Antibiotics

As we learn more about bacteria and their growth patterns, specific antibiotics can be designed for specific conditions. Drugs that do not fit other categories are listed here.

 If the client has recently developed any of the following, avoid massage and call the physician immediately: Unexplained joint pain or skin rash, increased difficulty breathing, ringing in the ears, sudden severe headache, recent muscle weakness, unusual bleeding or bruising or swelling of the lips, tongue, or face. (This is a massage-specific list; refer to the documentation that was included with the medication for a complete list of side effects.)

 Side Effects: Nausea and numbness or tingling of the hands or feet, drowsiness, headache and stomach cramping are side effects that can occur with antibiotics. Take these into consideration as they may limit your ability to achieve your client's massage goals.

 Miscellaneous antibiotic medications include: aztreonam (Azactam), chloramphenicol, clindamycin (Benzaclin, Cleocin, Dalacin), cycloserine (Seromycin), daptomycin (Cubicin), fosfomycin (Monurol), furazolidone (Furoxone), imipenem with cilastatin (Primaxin), lincomycin (Lincocin), meropenem (Merrem), mupirocin (Bactroban), neomycin (Myciguent), nitrofurantoin (Furadantin, Macrobid, Macrodantin), trimethoprim (Primsol, Proloprim, Trimpex), and vancomycin (Vancocin, Vancoled).

*Client limitations are
an opportunity for you to
utilize your resourcefulness.*

Antifungals

Antifungals work by exploiting differences between mammalian and fungal cells to kill off the fungal organism without significantly harming the host.

There are three main classes of commonly used antifungal drugs: *Polyenes*, *imidazoles* and *triazoles*. Polyenes interact with ergosterol in the fungal cell wall, causing the cell's contents to leak out and the cell to die. Imidazoles block the synthesis of ergosterol in fungal cells, inhibiting cell growth. Triazoles also act by blocking ergosterol synthesis, inhibiting fungal cell growth.

 If the client has recently developed any of the following, avoid massage and call the physician immediately: An unexplained skin rash or itching, sudden severe headache, recent muscle weakness, increased difficulty breathing, ringing in the ears, unusual bleeding or bruising or swelling of the lips, tongue, or face. (This is a massage-specific list; refer to the documentation that was included with the medication for a complete list of side effects.)

 Side Effects: Headaches may occur as a result of this class of medication. Take this into consideration as it may limit your ability to achieve your client's massage goals.

 Postural hypotension can occur as a side effect of oral antifungals. Help the client to change positions and be on guard for dizziness or blacking out.

 Polyene antifungal medications include <u>amphotericin</u> and <u>nystatin</u> (Mycostatin, Nilstat, Nystex).

 Imidazole antifungal medications include: <u>ketoconazole</u> (Nizoral) and <u>clotrimazole</u> (Cruex, Desenex, Fungoid, Lotrimin, Lotrisone, Mycelex).

 Triazole antifungal medications include <u>fluconazole</u> (Diflucan) and <u>itraconazole</u> (Sporanox).

 Miscellaneous antifungal medications include <u>terbinafine</u> (Lamisil), <u>flucytosine</u> (Ancobon), and <u>griseofulvin</u> (Fulvicin, Grifulvin, Gris-PEG, Grisactin).

Scabicides and Pediculicides

Scabies infections (infestation with mites) and pediculosis infections (infestation with lice) are treated with these medication creams.

 If the client has recently developed any of the following, avoid massage and call the physician immediately: Joint or muscle pain, headache, fever, painful and tender glands in neck, armpits, or groin, or swelling of the face, hands, arms, feet, or legs. (This is a massage-specific list; refer to the documentation that was included with the medication for a complete list of side effects.)

 Side Effects: Severe itching with irritation is common with this medication. Take this into consideration as it may limit your massage techniques.

 Scabicide and pediculicide medications include: crotamiton (Eurax), ivermectin (Mectizan, Stromectol), lindane (Gamma Benzene, Kwell, Scabene), and permethrin (Acticin, Elimite, Nix).

Antiparasitics

(also called antihelminthics)

Antiparasitics are used to treat *roundworm*, hookworm, *pinworm*, *whipworm*, *tapeworm* and other worm infections.

 If the client has recently developed any of the following, avoid massage and call the physician immediately: An unexplained skin rash, increased difficulty breathing, ringing in the ears, sudden severe headache, recent muscle weakness, unusual bleeding or bruising or swelling of the lips, tongue, or face. (This is a massage-specific list; refer to the documentation that was included with the medication for a complete list of side effects.)

 Side Effects: Diarrhea and stomach pain may result from this medication. Take these into consideration as they may limit your ability to achieve your client's massage goals.

 Antiparasitic medications include: mebendazole (Vermox), niclosamide (Niclocide), nitazoxanide (Alinia), and tinidazole (Tindamax).

Antivirals

Unlike bacteria, viruses aren't complete organisms. They are DNA and RNA strands that become introduced to the host cell and have different properties and mechanisms of infection than bacteria do. Rather than killing the viruses, anti-viral drugs block steps in the process through which viruses reproduce.

 If the client has recently developed any of the following, avoid massage and call the physician immediately: An unexplained skin rash, increased difficulty breathing, ringing in the ears, sudden severe headache, recent muscle weakness, unusual bleeding or bruising or swelling of the lips, tongue, or face. (This is a massage-specific list; refer to the documentation that was included with the medication for a complete list of side effects.)

 Side Effects: Headaches, dizziness, lower extremity swelling and nausea are side effects that may occur as a result of this class of medication. Take these into consideration as they may limit your ability to achieve your client's massage goals.

 Postural hypotension can occur as a side effect of oral medications in this class. Help the client to change positions and be on guard for dizziness or blacking out.

 Antiviral medications include: acyclovir (Avirax, Zovirax), adefovir dipivoxil (Hepsera), amantidine (Antadine, Endantadine, Symadine, Symmetrel), docosanol (Abreva), famciclovir (Famvir), foscarnet (Foscavir), ganciclovir (Cytovene), penciclovir (Denavir), oseltamivir (Tamiflu), ribavirin (Tribavirin, Virazid, Virazole), rimantadine (Flumadine), valacyclovir (Valtrex), and zanamivir (Relenza).

Guard against emotionally overwhelming your client with your passion for massage.

*The nervous system is the
instrument by which you create
a harmonious symphony
for your client's benefit.*

Chapter 7

Nervous System

Peripheral Neuropathy

Peripheral neuropathy describes damage to the nerves as they exit the brain and spinal cord and extend through the body. It is a general term rather than a specific disease, and can refer to virtually any nerve condition that does not come directly from the brain or spinal cord (which is called the central nervous system, or CNS).

It may be caused by diseases of the nerves or as the result of systemic illnesses. Diabetes, for example, is one of the most common causes of peripheral neuropathy. It can be from a loss of blood supply, as in Raynaud's syndrome. Other causes include mechanical pressure such as nerve entrapment from a vertebral subluxation or other bones (e.g. carpal tunnel syndrome) or other tissues.

Although the causes of peripheral neuropathy are diverse, they produce common symptoms including weakness, numbness, abnormal sensations such as burning, tickling, pricking or tingling (called paresthesia) and/or pain in the affected body part. It can be area-specific (e.g. just the thumb may be numb in cervical nerve entrapment), throughout the body part (like the whole-hand tingling of carpal tunnel syndrome), or systemic (as a complication of diabetes).

Peripheral Neuropathy Precautions

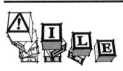 **Restrict massage to Incremental, Light and Energy techniques, and avoid relying upon the client to determine their limits.**

Peripheral Neuropathy Precautions, cont'd.

 Encourage the client to seek care from a neurological physician like a chiropractor and/or neurologist to discover the best treatments. Your understanding about their body can have significant influence in motivating them towards a solution.

 Warning: Pressure massage and/or lubricants may be irritating rather than soothing in certain cases. Discuss your therapy approach prior to working with the client to reveal specifics about their condition.

 Warning: Begin massage cautiously, and use your own sense of appropriate pressure. Avoid relying upon the client to determine their limits. The client is likely to have a reduced perception of pressure and pain. When the nerve supply is compromised, the pain threshold can be reached without warning.

 Some medications can cause peripheral neuropathy, which can compound the problem. Research the client's current medications for additional precautions.

 Your flexibility in touch therapy techniques makes you uniquely qualified to improve your client's quality of life. Client limitations are an opportunity for you to utilize your resourcefulness.

Complex Regional Pain Syndrome (CRPS)

(also called Causalgia, reflex sympathetic dystrophy syndrome, RSDS)

Complex regional pain syndrome is a chronic pain condition that is believed to be the result of dysfunction in the autonomic nervous system. Dramatic changes in the color and temperature of the skin over the affected limb or body part, intense burning pain, skin sensitivity, sweating, and swelling are all typical symptoms. There is no single cause, and the exact mechanism is as yet unknown. Typically, the onset of CRPS follows an injury to tissue, although in about 30 percent of the cases there is no apparent trigger. The intensity of the original trauma has no relationship to the severity of CRPS, and the condition spreads to other limbs in 70 percent of those afflicted.

Some experts believe there are three stages associated with CRPS, marked by progressive changes in the skin, muscles, joints, ligaments, and bones of the affected area. It is not an infectious condition and therefore not contagious. It is emotionally and physically traumatic and disfiguring, lasting often for years, but it is not fatal.

Stage One

Stage one is thought to last from 1 to 3 months and is characterized by severe burning pain, muscle spasms, joint stiffness, and alterations in the blood vessels that cause the skin to change color and temperature.

Stage Two

Stage two lasts from 3 to 6 months and is characterized by intensifying pain, swelling, decreased hair growth, cracked, brittle, grooved, or spotty nails, softened bones, stiff joints, and weak muscle tone.

Stage Three

In stage three the changes in the skin and bone become irreversible. Pain becomes unyielding and may involve the entire limb or affected area. There may be marked muscle loss (*atrophy*), severely limited mobility, and involuntary contractions of the muscles and tendons that flex the joints. Limbs may become contorted.

Various treatment combinations in addition to medication include the following: Injection of an anesthetic (called sympathetic nerve-blocking medication) blocks pain fibers in the affected nerves is designed to relieve pain. A TENS unit (called *Transcutaneous Electrical Nerve Stimulation*) applies electrical impulses to pressure nerve endings which "crowd out" pain signals and provide relief. In rare cases, surgically cutting the nerves in the affected area may be necessary to provide relief (called *surgical sympathectomy*). This permanent treatment is controversial as it frequently destroys the sensations and function of the surrounding tissue.

Complex Regional Pain Syndrome Precautions

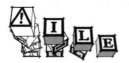 **Restrict massage to Incremental, Light and Energy techniques.**

 Communication with the client's physician and other members of their healthcare team is essential with CRPS. The nature of the treatment regime makes this a complex case. The physician must be kept informed about your therapies and observations to make appropriate changes in treatment.

 Avoid deep tissue massage techniques. Local and regional osteoporosis occurs with CRPS. There are no visible signs to determine if a client has bone loss. Use LIGHT and ENERGY techniques only for those with a history of osteoporosis, and be especially careful with pressure on the torso.

 Warning: Limit your sessions to calming and soothing techniques. Those techniques that stimulate a sympathetic response will only antagonize the nervous system.

 Many different classes of medication are used to treat CRPS, including topical analgesics, antiseizure drugs, antidepressants, corticosteroids, and narcotics. No single drug or combination of drugs has produced consistent long-lasting improvement in symptoms, so be alert for changes in their medication.

 Your special knowledge about the body can assist the client in working through the physical aspects of this condition; your unique healing energy can help them heal mentally and emotionally.

The art of massage lies in discovering and delivering exactly what your client needs.

Headaches

A headache happens when pain-sensitive nerve fibers (called *nociceptors*) are triggered in the network of nerves that extends over the scalp, face, and along the surface and the base of the brain. 90 percent of all headaches are triggered by stress or tension. Other types of headache have different triggers and are not as easily treated.

Headaches have been separated into four main categories by their general cause: Inflammatory headaches, muscle contraction headaches, traction headaches, and vascular headaches. Each category is detailed below.

Inflammatory Headaches
Inflammatory headaches are caused by irritation or infection of the arteries or nerves in the head, sinuses or neck. Pain is usually mild to moderate and can be periodic or continuous depending on its cause.

Muscle Contraction Headaches
Muscle contraction headaches are caused by sustained tension in the muscles of the face and/or neck. The pain is usually mild to moderate and feels like pressure is being applied to the head or neck. Tension headaches fall under this category.

Tension Headaches
Tension headaches are a subgroup of muscle contraction headaches and account for more than 75 percent of all headaches. They are typically a steady ache rather than a throbbing one and affect both sides of the head. They can occur frequently, even daily in some cases.

Traction Headaches
Traction headaches happen when nerve fibers are pulled, stretched, or displaced (e.g., squinting to compensate for poor eyesight). Brain tumors can cause traction headaches as they press against pain-sensitive blood vessels. Traction headaches typically feel as if a strong pressure is being applied to the head.

Vascular Headaches

Vascular headaches are caused by abnormal blood flow changes in the brain. Vascular headaches are characterized by intense, throbbing pain on one or both sides of the head. The three sub-categories of vascular headaches include *migraine headaches*, *cluster headaches*, and *sinus headaches*.

Migraine Headaches

Migraines are a specific subgroup of vascular headaches and afflict 25 to 30 million people in the United States alone. About 20 percent are *classic* migraines, in which an *aura* (a painless visual disturbance) occurs before the head pain begins. The other 80 percent are *common* migraines without an aura. More than half of the time migraines hurt on only one side of the head. Regardless of whether they are unilateral or bilateral, they can be debilitating, excruciating, and often last days with nausea, vomiting and an extreme sensitivity to light.

Cluster Headaches

These headaches strike in groups or clusters over several weeks. The pain centers around one eye and is extremely severe but brief, lasting no more than an hour or two. The National Headache Foundation reports studies that show most cluster headaches can be stopped by inhaling 100 percent oxygen.

Sinus Headaches

A 2001 study by the American Academy of Neurology found that 97 percent of self-described sinus headaches were actually migraine attacks. The absence of upper respiratory symptoms is the biggest clue. Tension headaches can also be felt in the area of the sinuses. A physician should be consulted for proper diagnosis and treatment.

Headache Precautions

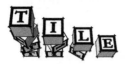 **Tolerance, Incremental, Light and Energy techniques are all encouraged.**

Headache Precautions, cont'd.

 Some types of headache are signals of more serious disorders and call for prompt medical care. Avoid massage if you suspect a headache fits one or more of these descriptions:

➢ A sudden, severe headache of a type not experienced before,

➢ A persistent headache or repetitive headaches following a blow to the head,

➢ A severe headache associated with a stiff neck,

➢ Recurring headaches in children,

➢ A headache associated with fever or convulsions,

➢ A persistent headache in a person who was previously headache free,

➢ A headache accompanied by confusion or loss of consciousness,

➢ A headache triggered by exertion, coughing, bending or sexual activity.

 Warning: Discuss your intentions with the client before working on their head and neck. Give them clear support to signal if they feel the technique is aggravating their headache. This will encourage the client to experiment with solutions while feeling safe and in control.

 Many medications can produce headaches as a side effect. Be sure to eliminate this as a possibility, and if their medication does have headaches listed as a side effect, have them consult with their physician.

 Antiemetic and antipsychotic medications are frequently prescribed for the treatment of migraines, as well as any combination of other pain and anti-inflammatory medication. Ask about current medications and check their precautions.

 Virtually all headaches respond well to massage. Your stress-reducing massage techniques may be a key in keeping them at bay.

Trigeminal Neuralgia (TN)

(also called tic douloureux)

Trigeminal neuralgia is a condition that affects the *trigeminal nerve* (the 5th cranial nerve). The trigeminal nerve is responsible for touch, pain, pressure, and temperature sensations of the face, jaw, gums, forehead, and around the eyes. Rarely affecting anyone younger than 50, it can be caused by an unusual aneurysm, vascular compression or tumor along the path of the nerve, but usually there is no definitive explanation for the disorder.

Trigeminal neuralgia is characterized by a sudden, severe, electric shock-like or stabbing pain typically felt on one side of the face. The attacks of pain, which generally last several seconds and may be repeated one after the other, may be triggered by talking, brushing teeth, rubbing the face, shaving, chewing, or swallowing. It is not fatal, but can cause significant anxiety in anticipation of an impending attack.

Trigeminal Neuralgia Precautions

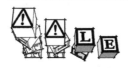 **Restrict massage to Light and Energy techniques for the face and skull. Your full technique range is encouraged for the rest of the body.**

 Encourage the client to seek care from a neurological physician like a chiropractor and/or neurologist to discover the best treatments. Your understanding about their body can have significant influence in motivating them towards a solution.

 Avoid heat and cold therapies to the head and neck unless specifically requested by the client as they are also likely antagonists.

 Warning: Pressure on the face is a common trigger for TN. Clients will likely wish to have you avoid the entire head area. Respect their desires and assist them in finding a safe position for their head, as face cradles may also be antagonistic.

 Anticonvulsants are used either intermittently or as a regular dosage in the treatment of TN. Check these and any other medication the client is currently taking for massage precautions.

Trigeminal Neuralgia Precautions, cont'd.

 Pain from TN is one of the most excruciating sensations of all. Reduce their anxiety by discussing with your client each area you intend to massage before beginning the session.

Bell's Palsy

Bell's palsy is a form of facial paralysis resulting from damage to the 7th cranial nerve (the *facial nerve*). This nerve disorder afflicts approximately 40,000 Americans each year. It can strike almost anyone at any age; however, it disproportionately attacks pregnant women and people who have diabetes, influenza, a cold, or some other upper respiratory ailment.

In addition to one-sided facial paralysis with possible inability to close the eye, symptoms of Bell's palsy may include pain, tearing, drooling, hypersensitivity to sound in the affected ear, and impairment of taste. Most people begin to get significantly better within two weeks, and about 80 percent recover completely within three months.

Bell's Palsy Precautions

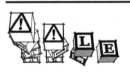 **Restrict massage to Light and Energy techniques for the face and skull. Your full technique range is encouraged for the rest of the body.**

 Immediate medical response can make a difference in the severity of this condition and how quickly the client recovers. Avoid massage and strongly encourage the client to seek medical attention if this condition is suspected.

 Contact the physician before your first session to confirm that any infection is under control and no other precautions exist.

 Avoid all heat and cold therapies to the affected tissues. Normal sensation is compromised.

Bell's Palsy Precautions, cont'd.

 Avoid deep tissue techniques to the affected tissues. Reduce and closely monitor pressure intensity and duration to avoid damaging tissue. LIGHT and ENERGY techniques are encouraged to limit muscle and tissue atrophy.

 This condition is commonly treated with antivirals and corticosteroids. Be sure to ask about current medications and check their precautions.

 Facial paralysis is emotionally traumatic. Focus on nurturing and supportive techniques during the recovery period to assist their growth through this process. Utilizing a full-body approach will remind them that their condition is but a small and temporary part of their life.

Spinal Cord Injury (SCI)

The spine is made up of 24 movable segments (called *vertebrae*). 98 percent of the nerve supply that controls body sensation and function comes through the spinal cord and exits between these vertebrae. Spinal cord injury may stem from a sudden, traumatic blow to the spine that fractures, dislocates, crushes or compresses one or more vertebrae. It may also result from a gunshot or knife wound that penetrates and cuts the spinal cord.

Spinal cord injuries are classified as partial or complete, depending on how much of the cord width is damaged. With a partial spinal cord injury, the spinal cord is able to convey some messages and retain some sensation and possibly some motor function below the affected area. A complete injury is defined by complete loss of motor function and sensation below the area of injury. However, even in a complete injury, the spinal cord is almost never completely cut in half. Portions of the nervous system may be in shock for an extended period of time without actually being destroyed. A persistent therapy regime can awaken these nerves and improve body function and sensation long after the acute stage of the illness has passed.

In general, injuries that are higher in the spinal cord produce more paralysis than those that occur lower. Respiratory tract, urinary tract and intestinal troubles are likely complications for all SCI, as is lower body osteoporosis and atrophy of the paralyzed tissues.

Spinal Cord Injury Precautions

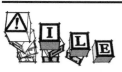 **Restrict massage to Incremental, Light and Energy techniques in the affected area(s). Your full technique range is encouraged for the rest of the body.**

 Avoid all pressure massage until the acute stage has passed, the injury is stable and the extent of the damage is known. Contact the physician for approval and guidance in the client's specific needs.

 Avoid all heat and cold therapies to the affected tissues. Normal sensation is compromised.

 Avoid deep tissue techniques to the affected tissues. Reduce and closely monitor pressure intensity and duration to avoid damaging tissue. LIGHT and ENERGY techniques are encouraged to limit muscle and tissue atrophy. Light mobility and stretching techniques are recommended within the client's limits.

 Warning: Cardiovascular diseases, osteoporosis, and tissue atrophy are likely the longer the client has paralysis. Adjust your massage techniques to take into account the loss of mobility, tissue endurance and impaired healing capacity.

 Warning: A lack of mobility makes pressure ulcers (bed sores) likely. These are highly vulnerable to infection. Avoid the area directly adjacent to the lesion and avoid breathing on the wound.

 Inhaled steroids are commonly used in the acute stage of SCI, followed by ongoing medications to control pain and muscle spasticity, as well as medications that can improve bladder control, bowel control, sexual functioning, etc. Keep up to date on each of the client's medications and their specific massage precautions.

 Trust in your skills and perceptions about what is appropriate in helping those with spinal cord injuries. You can be of valuable assistance in their quality of life.

Traumatic Brain Injury (TBI)

A traumatic brain injury is any sudden, physical damage to the brain. The term does not apply to brain injuries that are hereditary, congenital or degenerative, or brain injuries induced by birth trauma, toxins, diseases or infections.

Concussions (also called *closed head injuries*) are a type of brain injury resulting in confusion and possibly short-term loss of consciousness. The brain may be bruised, but the skull remains intact. The bruising of the brain tissue is called a contusion. *Shaken baby syndrome* is a severe form of traumatic brain injury in which the skull violently jolted. Other causes of TBI include skull fractures and open head injuries that penetrate the skull and brain tissue.

Symptoms of a TBI may include headache, nausea, confusion or other cognitive problems, a change in personality, depression, irritability, and other emotional and behavioral problems. Some people may have seizures as a result of a TBI or they may slip into a coma.

The injured person will have restrictions in physical activities for a time, depending upon the severity of the trauma. A second trauma to the bruised brain tissue can be catastrophic and life-threatening. Long-term disabilities resulting from traumatic brain injuries fall into three categories:

Cognition
Cognitive disabilities include losses in comprehension, concentration, judgment, memory, mood, and/or reasoning.

Movement abilities
Disability in movement includes a loss of muscle strength, coordination, and/or balance. It could also include the physical loss of speech to varying degrees.

Sensation
Losses in sensation may include tactile sensation and/or special senses like taste or vision.

Traumatic Brain Injury Precautions

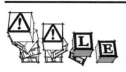 **Restrict massage to Light and Energy techniques in general. More intense massage may be appropriate on an individual basis.**

 If the client has recently suffered a TBI, consult the physician for approval before your first session with the client. Massage is appropriate once their physician has lifted all restrictions against physical activity.

 Warning signs for a TBI include confusion, severe headache or stiff neck, fever, vomiting, unusual sleepiness or unequal pupils. If any of these symptoms are present, stop or avoid massage and call for emergency medical help immediately.

 Ask about any residual disabilities to consider in designing a session for a client with TBI.

 Be sure to ask about current medications and check their precautions.

 Sadly, a sharp mind is often 'trapped" inside a body less responsive than it used to be. Your patience with their lessened abilities will be well appreciated by your client.

Sometimes the most powerful impression you make on a client is simply your compassionate presence.

Epilepsy Disorder

(also called seizure disorder)

Seizures are usually divided into two classes based on how much of the brain is involved at the onset of the seizure. In *partial seizures*, only part of the brain is involved, and the entire brain is involved with *generalized seizures*. The most severe form is known as *status epilepticus*, where a loss of consciousness may continue for 30 minutes or longer.

Symptoms vary and can include any combination of muscle rigidity, convulsions, atonicity, or other dramatic movements. They may last only a minute or so with limited conscious, or may be longer lasting with full loss of consciousness. Following any seizure the person will be disoriented and emotional for a period of time.

Epilepsy Disorder Precautions

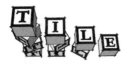 **Tolerance, Incremental, Light and Energy techniques are all encouraged.**

 Do not attempt to restrain anyone having a seizure. It will cause harm to that individual. Call emergency services as soon as a seizure begins. If possible, roll the person on their side to help keep the airway open. If the client is on the table at the onset of a seizure, help them to the floor if possible and move the table and other items away. *Place nothing inside the mouth* (especially not your priceless fingers), as it is likely there will be more trauma resulting from the object than the protection it was intended to provide.

 No massage in any fashion during or immediately after a seizure, regardless of its duration or intensity. Avoid all massage until the client has been treated and released by their physician.

 Benzodiazepines, anticonvulsants and barbiturates may all be utilized in the management of seizure disorders. Be sure to ask about these and all other medications and check their precautions.

 A normal lifestyle is recommended for persons with seizure disorders, and the full range of massage techniques can be utilized as well whenever seizures are absent. Be supportive in your client's ability to achieve their full health potential.

Depression

In real life, depression does not always fall into neat categories. It is sometimes hard to know when depression crosses the line from a difficult life situation to being a depressive illness. As such, many times a person suffering from depression remains undiagnosed and untreated. It is estimated that over 18 million American adults suffer from a depressive illness each year.

Depression strikes in several forms. When a psychiatrist makes a diagnosis of a patient's depressive illness, he or she may use a number of terms to describe it. These labels confuse many people who don't understand that they can overlap. People with depressive illness may also receive more than one diagnosis since the illness is often linked with other problems, such as alcoholism or other substance abuses, eating disorders, or anxiety disorders. In an estimated 10 to 15 percent of major depressive episodes, the cause is an underlying factor such as a particular medication or a medical condition.

Atypical Depression
This type of depression is very common in women. The feeling of depression will get better for a period and then worsen again. The symptoms of oversleeping, overeating, hypersensitivity to rejection and intermittent panic attacks, are characteristic of atypical depression. This type of depression usually begins in adolescence and, if untreated, will often continue throughout life.

Bipolar Depression
(also known as bipolar disorder, manic-depression, and manic-depressive illness)

In bipolar depression, the lows alternate with terrible highs in an often bewildering oscillation. Scientists now believe this up-and-down mood roller coaster is the product of an imbalance in brain chemistry, which can be treated successfully 80 percent of the time with medication.

Dysthymia
While many people have single or infrequent episodes of severe depression, some suffer with recurrent or long-lasting depression. For these people, who almost always seem to have symptoms of a mild form of the illness, the diagnosis is dysthymia or *minor depression*.

Major Depression

(also known as major depressive disorder, unipolar depression)

When you hear the term *clinical depression,* it merely means the depression is severe enough to require treatment. When a person is badly depressed during a single severe period, he or she can be said to have had an episode of clinical depression. More severe symptoms mark the period as an episode of major depression.

The more severe or the depression, the more it is likely to affect its sufferer's life. Loss of enjoyment in activities that used to provide pleasure, along with loss of motivation to perform routine daily habits, are two patterns of behavior that factor into the diagnosis of clinical depression.

Postpartum Depression (PPD)

Postpartum depression is thought to be a form of major depression. Most women suffer from a down feeling the first few days after giving birth. About 10 percent of new mothers develop postpartum depression, experiencing symptoms that are severe and disabling. Postpartum depression can occur at any time within the first six months after giving birth. If left untreated, it can last up to a year or longer. It often arises from a combination of dramatic hormonal changes in addition to emotional and lifestyle stresses.

Premenstrual Dysphoric Disorder (PMDD)

This condition is experienced by approximately 4 percent of menstruating women. Different from premenstrual syndrome (PMS), women who suffer from premenstrual dysphoric disorder have more severe symptoms of deep depression or irritability for the week or two prior to or during menses.

Psychotic Depression

Approximately 15 percent of people who suffer from major depression also show symptoms of psychotic depression. These symptoms include hearing voices inside one's head, having visions of people or things that are not actually, and delusional thinking. People who suffer from this extreme form of major depression are in need of immediate attention.

Seasonal Affective Disorder (SAD)

SAD is a mood disorder associated with depression episodes and related to seasonal light variations. People sometimes react emotionally to changes in the amount of daylight available. With less sunlight in the winter, some individuals become depressed, sad and irritable. When spring arrives with more daylight hours, they feel better and their mood improves.

Depression Precautions

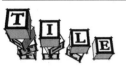 **Tolerance, Incremental, Light and Energy techniques are all encouraged.**

 Listen attentively to the client's conversation. Statements such as, *"I can't go on," "Nothing matters any more,"* or even *"I'm thinking of ending it all,"* are remarks that should always be taken seriously. Contact their physician as well as a close family member without delay. Share the responsibility of ensuring that the client gets the help these statements are asking for.

 Clients can respond enthusiastically to the antidepressive benefits of massage and may desire to reduce or eliminate their medications. Strongly recommend that they consult the physician that prescribed the medication before changing dosages, as there are often specific chemical needs to be addressed.

 Physical stress adds to a person's depression, just as mental and chemical stressors do. Aggressive techniques requiring a healing response from the client may add to their fatigue. Comforting massage techniques, on the other hand, are well known to have antidepressive benefits.

 Medications designed to treat depression can have a wide range of side effects. Check each of their current medications for precautions.

 People who feel depressed don't want answers or solutions. They want a safe place to express their fears and anxieties, to be themselves. They do not necessarily want to be alone. They want someone to listen, to trust, and to care without trying to fix them or make light of their concerns. Control your urge to make a comment, add to a story or offer advice. Don't analyze, compare, criticize or cheer them up. Just listen.

Anxiety Disorders and Panic Disorders

An estimated 19 million adult Americans suffer from anxiety or panic disorders. They can develop from a complex set of factors, including genetics, brain chemistry, personality, and life events. They range from isolated incidents to lifelong challenges, from feelings of uneasiness to immobilizing bouts of terror. They have a common set of precautions for the therapist and are individually explained below.

Generalized Anxiety Disorder (GAD)

Generalized anxiety disorder is a condition characterized by chronic anxiety, exaggerated worry and tension. It is diagnosed when someone spends at least six months worrying excessively about a number of everyday problems. Their worries are accompanied by physical symptoms, especially fatigue, headaches, muscle tension and body aches.

Obsessive-Compulsive Disorder (OCD)

Obsessions are thoughts, images, or impulses that occur over and over again and feel beyond control. *Compulsions* are acts the person performs over and over again, often according to certain "rules" to try to make their obsessions go away. The most common form of OCD involves contamination. The thought of germs, disease or the mere presence of dirt evokes a sense of threat and inspires incredible motivation to eliminate these contaminants. The next most common form of OCD involves checking door locks, light switches, faucets, stoves or items that might pose a risk to either one's well-being, or the well-being of others. It is not uncommon for persons with OCD to wash, clean or check items up to 100 times in a row. Hoarding, ordering, thought avoidance and *hypochondriasis* (chronic and abnormal anxiety about imaginary symptoms) are all additional forms of OCD.

Discuss each part of your session in detail with your client prior to beginning the session, and encourage their participation in designing a regime with which they can feel confident. Avoiding lubricants, retaining clothing, shortening sessions and providing breaks may all be helpful to the client.

Panic Disorder

People with panic disorder experience white-knuckled, heart-pounding terror that strikes suddenly and without warning. Many live in persistent worry about when the next bout will occur. Multiple symptoms include a pounding heart, chest pains, lightheadedness or dizziness, nausea, shortness of breath, shaking or trembling, choking, and a fear of dying or going crazy. This diagnosis is considered when multiple attacks occur within four weeks, or one or more attacks followed by at least a month of persistent fear of having another attack.

Phobias

Phobias are irrational fears that lead people to altogether avoid specific things or situations that trigger intense anxiety. Agoraphobia, for example, is the fear of being in any situation that might trigger a panic attack and from which escape might be difficult. *Social phobia* (also called *social anxiety disorder*) can be characterized as an intense fear of situations, usually social or performance situations, where embarrassment may occur. Physical symptoms can include heart palpitations, faintness, blushing and profuse sweating. Psychological counseling is typically necessary to differentiate phobias from other anxiety disorders.

Posttraumatic Stress Disorder (PTSD)

(also called Acute Stress Disorder)

Posttraumatic stress disorder was first used as a diagnosis for military personnel, but has been expanded to explain exposure to traumas such as a serious accident, a natural disaster, or criminal assault. To be diagnosed, symptoms must be present for more than one month and be accompanied by a dropoff in the ability to socialize, work, or participate in other areas of daily functioning. The symptoms associated with PTSD include "reliving" the traumatic event in flashbacks and nightmares, avoidance behaviors such as avoiding places or circumstances related to the trauma, emotional numbing, and physiological challenges such difficulty sleeping, irritability or poor concentration.

Anxiety and Panic Disorder Precautions

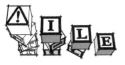

Restrict massage to Incremental, Light and Energy techniques.

Anxiety and Panic Disorder Precautions, cont'd.

 A consultation with the client's psychotherapist or counselor may be beneficial in creating a feeling of safety and assurance for your client. A team approach can greatly benefit both your therapies.

 Avoid any technique that may possibly be perceived as aggressive or intense. Even though your intent is pure, some techniques may threaten a client's feeling of safety.

 Warning: Take time before the first session with your client to "walk them through" the process, including choices in disrobing, body areas to address or avoid, and clear verbal signals for mental or physical discomfort. Discussing all actions in advance will enhance the client's feeling of control and security. Repeating this for subsequent sessions may seem redundant but can build needed confidence in the client.

 Medications designed to treat anxiety and panic disorders have a wide range of side effects. Check each of their current medications for precautions.

 You may very well be the portal by which the client finds the path for healing. Be vigilant in your nurturing through your actions as well as your thoughts.

Dementia

Dementia is caused by many conditions. Some can be reversed, while others are permanent. The two most common forms of permanent dementia are Alzheimer's disease and multi-infarct dementia.

Reversible dementia can be caused by a high fever, dehydration, vitamin deficiency and poor nutrition, bad reactions to medicines, problems with the thyroid gland, or a minor head injury. Refer to the specific condition causing dementia for precautions.

Alzheimer's Disease (AD)

AD is named after Dr. Alois Alzheimer, a German doctor who discovered the condition in 1906. It is a progressively deteriorating mental condition in which there is a loss of nerve cells in areas of the brain that are vital to thought, memory, and language. There are insufficient levels of certain chemicals in the brain (including *acetylcholine*) that carry complex messages back and forth between nerve cells.

Mild forgetfulness is typical during the earliest stages of Alzheimer's disease. Anxiety and depression are also common. The next stage is usually marked by poor concentration, trouble with speech and language, and aimless wandering. Many people who have Alzheimer's disease deny the significance of their symptoms. As the disease advances, they may need help with daily activities, such as food preparation and bathing. In the final stages, they can become incapacitated and disoriented to the point of not knowing their own name and not recognizing loved ones.

There is currently no cure for AD. Treatment is mainly aimed at alleviating or improving symptoms of the disease. The lifespan of an Alzheimer's disease victim is generally reduced, although a person may live anywhere from 3 to 20 years after diagnosis.

Multi-Infarct Dementia (MID)

(also called vascular dementia)

MID is a progressively debilitating condition which occurs when blood clots block small blood vessels and destroy brain tissue. CADASIL (Cerebral Autosomal Dominant Arteriopathy with Subcortical Infarcts and Leukoencephalopathy) is an inherited form of MID.

Symptoms include confusion, migraine-like headaches, problems with recent memory, wandering or getting lost in familiar places, loss of bladder or bowel control (*incontinence*), emotional problems such as laughing or crying inappropriately, difficulty following instructions, and problems handling money.

Currently the treatment focuses on reducing the high blood pressure and incidence of blood clots. There is no reversal of the damage that has occurred. It is stubbornly progressive and permanent.

Dementia Precautions

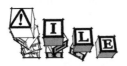 **Restrict massage to Incremental, Light and Energy techniques.**

 Be sure to gather a complete health history from a competent individual well in advance of your session. Clients with dementia invariably have other health concerns and each should be investigated for specific precautions.

 Plan ahead for a session with a client with dementia. Have the caregiver write a short note explaining to the client what they are going for and when the caregiver will return, including the phone number where they can be reached. This can be beneficial should the client become disoriented. In advanced cases, have a caregiver in attendance for additional support and comfort.

 Avoid any technique that may possibly be perceived as aggressive or intense. Restrict your massage techniques to those that are light, comforting and stress-reducing. Be alert for non-verbal cues to guide your massage, rather than verbal guidance from the client. Even though your intent is pure, some techniques may threaten a client's feeling of safety.

 Prior to your session, gather a complete list of the client's medications and research all precautions with the client's caregiver, as you may not be able to question the client as the session progresses.

 Medications that reduce blood pressure, clotting and cholesterol are all commonly used for both **AD** and **MID**. Cholinesterase inhibitors and N-methyl-D-aspartate antagonists are used specifically for AD. Be sure to ask about all other medications and check their precautions.

 Not only does a diagnosis of dementia have an enormous effect on the person with the disease, but the progressive nature of the disease also places a tremendous strain on the person's family, friends and especially the primary caretaker. Stress-reducing massage for these people will be especially well received.

Parkinson's Disease (PD)

Parkinson's disease is a chronic neurological condition named after Dr. James Parkinson, who first identified and described the syndrome in 1817. The disease progresses slowly, affecting a small area of cells in the mid-brain known as the *substantia nigra*. Degeneration of these cells causes a reduction in the chemical called *dopamine*. When approximately 80 percent of the dopamine-producing cells are damaged, the symptoms of Parkinson disease appear. Although there is no cure to date, the disease is not fatal. Treatment focuses on medically replacing dopamine and using drugs to help dopamine last longer in the brain.

The classic symptom of Parkinson's disease is a tremor in one hand or arm when the body is at rest (called a *resting tremor*). Other common symptoms include slow movement (*bradykinesia*), rigid limbs, a shuffling gait, and a stooped posture. People with PD often show reduced facial expressions and speak in a soft voice.

Parkinson's Disease Precautions

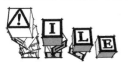 **Restrict massage to Incremental, Light and Energy techniques.**

 Massage may have significant benefits in improving the quality of life for those with PD. It is best to coordinate your sessions with the other members of the client's healthcare team. Discuss your massage therapy with the client's physician as it may have an effect on their medication, especially anti-depression medicine.

 Avoid deep tissue techniques because of the fragile condition of the bones due to osteoporosis. Reduce and closely monitor pressure intensity and duration to avoid damaging soft tissues. LIGHT and ENERGY techniques are encouraged. LIGHT mobility and stretching techniques are also recommended within the client's limits.

 Warning: Trunk muscles (especially flexors) become progressively stiff and inflexible. Recognize your client's movement limitations, and be extra cautious about stretching techniques.

Parkinson's Disease Precautions, cont'd.

 Plan for extra time and assistance in changing positions as the client with PD may be unable to get on or off the table without your help.

 Be sure to ask about current medications and check their precautions. COMT inhibitors, dopamine agonists and other anti-Parkinson's medications are common.

 Depression is as much a factor in PD as muscle rigidity. Your professional skills can provide a unique way to nurture the client and soothe both their mental and physical distress.

Amyotrophic Lateral Sclerosis (ALS)

(also called Lou Gherig's disease)

ALS is a nervous system disease of unknown origin that causes degeneration throughout the brain and spinal cord. Over 90 percent of those afflicted have no family history of ALS. A common first symptom is a painless weakening of a hand, foot, arm or leg, followed by difficulty in speaking, swallowing and walking. It inevitably progresses, causing atrophy and paralysis of the muscles of the limbs and torso. The ability to breathe unaided deteriorates. In most cases, mental faculties are not affected, and ALS is not infectious or contagious. About 20 percent of people with ALS live five years or more, and 5 percent will live 20 years. To date there is no cure.

Amyotrophic Lateral Sclerosis Precautions

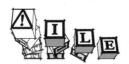 **Restrict massage to Incremental, Light and Energy techniques.**

 Massage may have significant benefits in improving the quality of life for those with ALS. It is best to coordinate your sessions with the other members of the client's healthcare team.

Amyotrophic Lateral Sclerosis Precautions, cont'd.

 Postponing the session is recommended if the therapist is unwell. The client's respiratory system is compromised and an infection can have disastrous consequences.

 Avoid deep tissue techniques. Reduce and closely monitor pressure intensity and duration to avoid damaging tissue. LIGHT and ENERGY techniques are encouraged.

 Light mobility and stretching techniques are recommended within the client's limits to limit muscle and tissue atrophy. Remember that the normal therapeutic responses to massage are absent in the client's muscular system.

 Heat therapies are encouraged within the client's limits.

 At this time, <u>riluzole</u> (Rilutek) is the only drug that has been approved by the FDA for treatment of ALS. COMT inhibitors, dopamine agonists and other anti-Parkinson's medications are commonly prescribed. Be sure to ask about current medications and check their precautions.

 Guard against emotionally overwhelming your client with your actions, your unconscious emotional exuberance or your words. Keep in mind that the most appropriate, compassionate action in some cases may be simply being present and in touch with them.

Multiple Sclerosis (MS)

MS is a chronic, unpredictable neurological disease that affects the central nervous system. It is suspected that the body's immune system attacks the insulating sheath *(myelin sheath)* in the brain. The scar tissue *(sclerosis)* that forms allows adjacent nerves to "short circuit" and stop functioning. Think of the wires leading to and from a light bulb. If the insulation separating the electrical wires is destroyed, they would "short circuit" together, re-routing the electrical signal before it reached the bulb. The light bulb would be permanently off. Since MS is not specific to any one area of the brain, virtually all nerve functions (like the light bulb) are at risk of being permanently shut off.

Symptoms for multiple sclerosis can include almost anything arising from nerve loss. Organ dysfunction, difficulty moving limbs, and numbness or pain are all possible symptoms. Unfortunately, once the diagnosis of MS has been made, both clients and their medical physicians tend to stop looking for solutions to new symptoms. Subluxations, for example, resulting in nerve dysfunction may remain undiscovered and untreated.

MS is not contagious, not directly inherited, and is not considered a fatal disease. There is no cure for MS yet, but drugs can help slow the course and/or symptoms in some people. Many afflicted with this condition experience long periods of remission where there is no worsening. Minimizing stress is a factor encouraging these remissions, and appropriate massage can play an important role in stress management.

Multiple Sclerosis Precautions

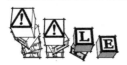 **Restrict massage to Light and Energy techniques.**

 Massage may have significant benefits in improving the quality of life for those with MS. It is best to coordinate your sessions with the other members of the client's healthcare team. If the client has recently suffered a setback, consult the physician for approval before pressure massage in the affected areas.

 Postponing the session is recommended if the therapist is unwell. The client's immune system is challenged and an infection can have disastrous consequences during the acute stage of this condition.

 Avoid all heat therapies (including hot stone massage, heat pads, saunas, steam rooms, etc), as symptoms are exacerbated by heat.

 Warning: Care must be taken not to overstimulate the client, which can result in painful muscle spasms. Limit your massage to LIGHT and ENERGY techniques, and limit the duration of each session.

 A wide array of medications are possible due to the variable pattern of symptoms. Be sure to ask about current medications and check their precautions.

Multiple Sclerosis Precautions, cont'd.

 Teaching MS clients to save energy curbs fatigue and helps ward off deterioration, says a recent research study from the University of Minnesota. Clients have limited energy to spend on their health; be a mentor and counsel them to rest frequently before they run out of energy. Encourage them to work with a variety of healthcare practitioners to maintain their health.

Cerebral Palsy (CP)

Cerebral palsy is a term used to describe a group of chronic disorders impairing muscle control. It appears in the first few years of life and generally does not worsen over time. The disorders are caused by developmental problems or damage to portions of the brain that disrupt the ability to control movement and posture.

Cerebral palsy is caused by an injury to the brain before, during, or shortly after birth, including severe loss of oxygen before or during birth, an infection causing meningitis, or labor trauma. About 10 to 20 percent of children who have cerebral palsy acquire the disorder after birth, through infection or head injury.

Some massage therapists, the most well-known of which is Maier Schneider, have had success with cerebral palsy clients. There are four types of cerebral palsy: Spastic, athetoid, ataxic, and mixed. They are described in more detail below, but they all share similar precautions.

Spastic Cerebral Palsy
Spastic cerebral palsy is the most common type of cerebral palsy, accounting for nearly 80 percent of all CP cases. Symptoms include one or more tight muscle groups limiting movement. The remaining mobility is stiff and jerky (*spastic*) with limited control.

Athetoid Cerebral Palsy
About 10 percent of those with cerebral palsy have athetoid CP, which includes involuntary, purposeless movements, especially in the face, arms, and trunk. These involuntary movements often interfere with speaking, feeding,

reaching, grasping, and other skills requiring coordinated movements. This condition often produces low muscle tone including problems maintaining posture for sitting and walking.

Ataxic Cerebral Palsy

Ataxic cerebral palsy produces involuntary, uncontrolled movements and poor coordination resulting in an unsteady walk with a wide based gait. This rare form of cerebral palsy also affects their sense of balance and depth perception.

Mixed Cerebral Palsy

About 10 percent of those with cerebral palsy have what is known as a mixed-type. These people have both the tight muscle tone of spastic cerebral palsy, and the involuntary movements of athetoid cerebral palsy.

Cerebral Palsy Precautions

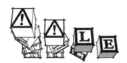 **Restrict massage to Light and Energy techniques.**

 Massage may have significant benefits in improving the quality of life for those with CP. It is best to coordinate your sessions with the other members of the client's healthcare team.

 The client may have difficulty communicating their goals and limitations. Discuss verbal and nonverbal signals as well as physical goals and limitations with the client and/or guardian before your first session.

 Warning: Care must be taken not to overwhelm the client. Limit your massage to LIGHT and ENERGY techniques, and limit the duration of each session.

 Although there is no medical cure for CP, drugs can be used to control seizures and muscle spasms. Ask about any medications and check their precautions.

 Compassionate touch is welcome with most anyone; with someone struggling with CP it can be powerfully unique and gratifying. It is your healing energy not just your technique that they cherish.

Guillain-Barré Syndrome (GBS)

(also called acute inflammatory demyelinating polyneuropathy, acute idio-pathic polyneuritis, Landry's ascending paralysis)

Guillain-Barré (ghee-yan bah-ray) Syndrome, is an autoimmune disorder in which the body's immune system attacks the insulating sheath *(myelin sheath)* of the peripheral nervous system. GBS is the most common cause of rapidly acquired paralysis in the United States today, affecting one to two people in every 100,000. The cause is not known, however, it frequently follows a significant immune suppression such as a viral infection.

GBS begins with weakness and/or abnormal sensations of the legs and arms. It often progresses into paralysis of the legs, arms, chest and/or face. The condition usually reaches the point of greatest weakness or paralysis within days or weeks after the first symptoms occur. The recovery period may be as little as a few weeks or as long as a few years. Most recover fully but about 30 percent have some permanent weakness.

With supportive hospital care GBS is rarely fatal. Treatment includes medication combined with a process called *plasmapheresis*. In autoimmune conditions, the body's immune system mistakenly turns against itself, attacking its own tissues, in part by producing substances known as *autoantibodies*.

Plasmapheresis is a process in which autoantibody-filled plasma is filtered from the blood. It unfortunately filters out supportive antibodies also, which leaves the client extremely vulnerable to other diseases and infections.

Guillain-Barré Syndrome Precautions

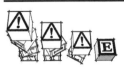 **Energy techniques only. Avoid all pressure and circulatory massage techniques.**

 Talk with the physician and rehabilitation team before attempting any therapy other than ENERGY techniques.

Guillain-Barré Syndrome Precautions, cont'd.

 Postponing the session is recommended if the therapist is unwell. The client's immune system is compromised, especially if they are on medication and/or plasmapheresis.

 Avoid all pressure techniques during the acute stage of this condition. Limit your massage to ENERGY techniques. With the physician's approval, you may gently move the client's limbs to help keep the muscles flexible and limit atrophy.

 As the client begins to recover limb control, more active rehabilitation can begin. Limit initial sessions to LIGHT and ENERGY techniques with short duration to avoid further stimulating the immune response.

 Medications will change as the client progresses through this condition. Be sure to ask about current medications and check their precautions.

 Remember that although their body is essentially attacking itself and you are extremely limited in your active responses, your compassionate presence alone can be uplifting and energizing.

Encephalitis and Meningitis

Meningitis is an inflammation of the membranes that cover the brain and spinal cord (*meninges*). The inflammation is usually caused by bacteria or viruses. Many of the bacteria or viruses that can cause meningitis are fairly common and are associated with other everyday illnesses. *Encephalitis* means "inflammation of the brain" and is also caused by bacterial or viral infection.

Common symptoms include high fever, headache, and stiff neck. These symptoms can develop over several hours, or they may develop over a couple of days. Other symptoms can include nausea, vomiting, sensitivity to light, confusion, and sleepiness.

Encephalitis and Meningitis Precautions

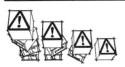 **Client is in critical condition. Avoid all therapy until approved by their physician.**

 Meningitis and encephalitis are medical emergencies and all forms of massage are to be avoided. Even ENERGY techniques such as cranial-sacral therapy affect the cerebrospinal fluid and can worsen the condition.

Encephalitis and Meningitis, Rehabilitative Precautions

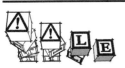 **After the client has recovered completely and has been given approval by their physician for massage, Light and Energy techniques are encouraged.**

 There may be specific precautions after a client has been successfully treated. Contact the physician to determine appropriate techniques before your session.

 Postponing the session is recommended if the therapist is unwell. The client's immune system has been compromised and an infection can have disastrous consequences.

 Warning: Care must be taken not to overwhelm the client. Limit your massage to LIGHT and ENERGY techniques as the client rehabilitates, and limit the duration of each session.

 Focus your massage techniques on gentle and relaxation techniques. Guard their recovering strength by reducing the duration of each session if necessary.

 The client may be on continuing medication after the condition has been treated; check all medications for specific precautions.

 The client will especially appreciate your help and expertise in regaining their health once this condition has passed.

Hydrocephalus

Hydrocephalus is strictly translated as "water on the brain," referring to the *cerebrospinal fluid* (CSF). Increased pressure from the CSF can be a result of developmental problems, infections producing encephalitis or meningitis, or traumatic episodes. Often the cause is unknown. Spinal taps may be performed during the diagnostic phase. A *shunt* is often surgically implanted to normalize the amount of cerebrospinal fluid being produced with the amount being reabsorbed.

Hydrocephalus Precautions

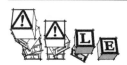 **Restrict massage to Light and Energy techniques.**

 Call physician before your first session to confirm that the condition is stable and can accommodate massage.

 Warning: Children with hydrocephalus have to be handled with extreme care to avoid trauma to the skull or spine. LIGHT and ENERGY techniques are recommended to soothe the client.

 In adults with hydrocephalus, the therapy goals are to gently reduce muscle spasticity and help limit the loss of mobility. LIGHT techniques and gentle movements without stretching can be effective.

 Be sure to ask about current medications and check their precautions.

 Although limited, your massage can provide the emotional release that no other therapy can offer.

Glaucoma

Glaucoma is a group of eye diseases that gradually steals sight, often without warning or symptoms. *Primary open angle glaucoma* (POAG) is the most common form, affecting about three million Americans. It occurs when the drainage system in the eye becomes clogged and pressure builds. It was once thought that high intraocular pressure (IOP) was the exclusive cause of *optic nerve* damage. The optic nerve is also known as the 2nd cranial nerve, a grouping of over a million nerve endings attached to the back of the eye. Although IOP is clearly a risk factor, we now know that other factors must also be involved as even people with "normal" pressure (called *normal tension glaucoma*) can experience vision loss from glaucoma.

Glaucoma can occur as the result of an eye injury, inflammation, tumor or a disease such as diabetes. It can also be caused by certain drugs such as steroids. Both cataracts and glaucoma can be a natural part of the aging process, and the two are not associated. Vision loss is caused by damage to the optic nerve, and the damage is irreversible.

Glaucoma Precautions

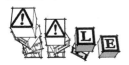 **Restrict massage to Light and Energy techniques.**

 If the client has developed sudden, severe headaches or tremors of the hands or feet, avoid massage and have them call their doctor. These are serious drug side effects requiring immediate medical attention. (This is a massage-specific list; refer to the documentation that was included with the medication for a complete list of side effects.)

 Warning: The client may be unable to use the face cradle due to the pressure on the area surrounding the eye. Ask if a seated or side posture would be preferred before attempting to place them in a prone position.

 Glaucoma is treated with miotics, sympathomimetics, and prostaglandin analogues. Research their specific medicine in this text, and be sure to check their other medications also for a complete set of precautions.

 Unfortunately, massage has little to offer in the treatment of glaucoma. Your help in removing stress and pressure in the rest of the body will be most appreciated.

Nervous System Medications

Selective Serotonin Reuptake Inhibitors (SSRIs)

These medications are mood elevators used to treat depression. They act by blocking the breakdown of serotonin so that more is available for the brain to use. Depression can be caused by low serotonin levels.

 If the client has recently developed any of the following, avoid massage and call the physician immediately: Jaw, neck, and back muscle spasms, unexplained skin rash or itchy skin, increased difficulty breathing, ringing in the ears, sudden severe headache, recent muscle weakness, unusual bleeding or bruising or swelling of the lips, tongue, or face. (This is a massage-specific list; refer to the documentation that was included with the medication for a complete list of side effects.)

 Side Effects: Headaches, muscle pain or weakness, tremors, constipation, diarrhea and drowsiness all can occur with this class of medication. Take these into consideration as they may limit your ability to achieve your client's massage goals.

 Selective serotonin reuptake inhibitor medications include: citalopram (Celexa), escitalopram (Lexapro), fluoxetine (Prozac, Sarafem), fluvoxamine (Luvox), paroxetine (Paxil), and sertraline (Zoloft).

Monoamine Oxidase (MAO) Inhibitors

These drugs are used in the treatment of panic disorder, social phobia, and obsessive-compulsive disorder (OCD). They may also be used in the treatment of difficult recurring headaches. Anyone taking a MAO inhibitor must avoid wine, beer, and cheeses that contain the amino acid *tyramine*.

 If the client has recently developed any of the following, avoid massage and call the physician immediately: Jaw, neck, and back muscle spasms, unexplained skin rash or itchy skin, increased difficulty breathing, ringing in the ears, sudden severe headache, recent muscle weakness, unusual bleeding or bruising or swelling of the lips, tongue, or face. (This is a massage-specific list; refer to the documentation that was included with the medication for a complete list of side effects.)

MAO Inhibitor Medication Precautions, cont'd.

 Avoid stretching techniques as the sensory feedback is depressed. Reduce and closely monitor pressure intensity and duration to avoid damaging tissue.

 Side Effects: Headaches, swelling of the feet or legs, muscle aches or spasm, constipation, drowsiness, tiredness, tremors, nausea and vomiting all can occur with this class of medication. Take these into consideration as they may limit your ability to achieve your client's massage goals.

 Postural hypotension can occur as a side effect of this class of medication and is more likely when combined with pressure techniques. Help the client to change positions and be on guard for dizziness or blacking out.

 Monoamine oxidase inhibitor medications include: isocarboxazid (Marplan), moclobemide (Manerix), phenelzine (Nardil) and tranylcypromine (Parnate).

Tricyclic Antidepressants (TCAs)

These medications are used to treat depression and anxiety. They may also be used to lower the frequency of migraines or for other chronic pain. Tricyclic antidepressants work by normalizing the amount of certain mood-altering chemicals in your brain.

 If the client has recently developed any of the following, avoid massage and call the physician immediately: Jaw, neck, and back muscle spasms, unexplained skin rash or itchy skin, increased difficulty breathing, ringing in the ears, sudden severe headache, recent muscle weakness, unusual bleeding or bruising or swelling of the lips, tongue, or face. (This is a massage-specific list; refer to the documentation that was included with the medication for a complete list of side effects.)

 Avoid all heat therapies or use with extreme caution (including hot stone massage, heat pads, saunas, steam rooms, etc), as the resistance to heat is compromised.

Tricyclic Antidepressant Precautions, cont'd.

 Avoid deep pressure massage and reduce the duration of massage to each area. These medications have a drying effect on the skin, making it more fragile.

 Avoid stretching techniques as the sensory feedback is depressed. Reduce and closely monitor pressure intensity and duration to avoid damaging tissue.

 Side Effects: Nausea, constipation, sleeplessness and fatigue are side effects that may occur as a result of this class of medication. Take these into consideration as they may limit your ability to achieve your client's massage goals.

 Tricyclic antidepressant medications include: <u>amitriptyline</u> (Elavil, Endep, Vanatrip), <u>amitriptyline</u> <u>with</u> <u>chlordiazepoxide</u> (Limbitrol), <u>amitriptyline</u> <u>with</u> <u>perphenazine</u> (Etrafon, Triavil), <u>amoxapine</u> (Asendin), <u>buspirone</u> (BuSpar), <u>clomipramine</u> (Anafranil), <u>desipramine</u> (Norpramin), <u>doxepin</u> (Adapin, Sinequan), <u>imipramine</u> (Tofranil), <u>nortriptyline</u> (Aventyl, Pamelor), <u>protriptyline</u> (Vivactil), and <u>trimipramine</u> (Surmontil).

Miscellaneous Antidepressants

These medications do not fall under any specific drug class. They are used to treat depression, anxiety and some forms of migraine headaches.

 If the client has recently developed any of the following, avoid massage and call the physician immediately: Jaw, neck, and back muscle spasms, unexplained skin rash or itchy skin, increased difficulty breathing, ringing in the ears, sudden severe headache, recent muscle weakness, unusual bleeding or bruising or swelling of the lips, tongue, or face. (This is a massage-specific list; refer to the documentation that was included with the medication for a complete list of side effects.)

 Avoid stretching techniques as the sensory feedback is depressed. Reduce and closely monitor pressure intensity and duration to avoid damaging tissue.

Miscellaneous Antidepressant Precautions, cont'd.

 Side Effects: Headaches, constipation, dizziness, drowsiness, tremors, nausea and vomiting all can occur with this class of medication. Take these into consideration as they may limit your ability to achieve your client's massage goals.

 Miscellaneous antidepressant medications include: <u>bupropion</u> (Wellbutrin, Zyban), <u>lithium</u> (Cibalith, Eskalith, Lithane, Lithobid, Lithonate, Lithotabs), <u>maprotiline</u> (Ludiomil), <u>mirtazapine</u> (Remeron), <u>nefazodone</u> (Serzone), <u>trazodone</u> (Desyrel), and <u>venlafaxine</u> (Effexor).

Miscellaneous Sedatives and Hypnotics

Many drugs used to treat sleep disorders are difficult to group together with other drugs based on their mechanism of action, because the exact mechanism may be unknown, or no other medication works in the same manner.

 If the client has developed severe muscle weakness, confusion, or an unexplained rash, avoid massage and have them call their doctor immediately. These drug side effects are considered very serious and require medical attention. (This is a massage-specific list; refer to the documentation that was included with the medication for a complete list of side effects.)

 Side Effects: Headaches, muscle weakness, lightheadedness, nausea, diarrhea, and stomach irritation all can occur with this class of medication. Take these into consideration as they may limit your ability to achieve your client's massage goals.

 Postural hypotension can occur as a side effect of this class of medication. Help the client to change positions and be on guard for dizziness or blacking out.

 Miscellaneous sedative and hypnotic medications include: <u>chloral hydrate</u> (Aquachloral), <u>ethchlorvynol</u> (Placidyl) <u>glutethimide</u> (Doriden), <u>zaleplon</u> (Sonata), and <u>zolpidem</u> (Ambien).

Central Nervous System Stimulants

This class of medication is primarily used for Attention Deficit Hyperactivity Disorder (ADHD) and improves concentration, allowing the child or adult to focus.

 If the client has recently developed any of the following, avoid massage and call the physician immediately: Sudden severe headache, recent muscle weakness or joint pain, muscle twitching, unexplained skin rash, increased difficulty breathing, ringing in the ears, unusual bleeding or bruising or swelling of the lips, tongue, or face. (This is a massage-specific list; refer to the documentation that was included with the medication for a complete list of side effects.)

 Heat therapies (including hot stone massage, heat pads, etc.) are not appropriate with medications that constrict the blood vessel walls. Normal heat dissipation is compromised and burns may occur.

 Cold therapies are contraindicated with medications causing vasoconstriction, as the smooth muscle may spasm and produce painful ischemia.

 Side Effects: Headaches, stomach upset and nervousness can occur with this class of medication. Take these into consideration as they may limit your ability to achieve your client's massage goals.

 CNS stimulant medications include: atomoxetine (Strattera), amphetamine with dextroamphetamine (Adderall), dexmethylphenidate (Focalin), dextroamphetamine (Dexedrine, Dextrostat), methylphenidate (Concerta, Metadate, Methylin, Ritalin), pemoline (Cylert, PemADD), phentermine (Adipex-P, Fastin, Ionamin, Zantryl), and phenylpropanolamine (PPA).

Antipsychotic Medications

This class of medication is primarily used for mental illnesses and eating disorders.

 If the client has recently developed any of the following, avoid massage and call the physician immediately: Jaw, neck, and back muscle spasms, unexplained skin rash or itchy skin, increased difficulty breathing, ringing in the ears, sudden severe headache, recent muscle weakness, unusual bleeding or bruising or swelling of the lips, tongue, or face. (This is a massage-specific list; refer to the documentation that was included with the medication for a complete list of side effects.)

 All heat therapies should be avoided (including hot stone massage, heat pads, saunas, steam rooms, etc.) as the client's ability to control their body temperature is compromised.

 Side Effects: Headaches, skin rash, swollen ankles, dry or discolored skin, anxiety, insomnia, drowsiness, lightheadedness, upset stomach, vomiting, constipation, and restlessness are common side effects of this class of medication. Take these into consideration as they may limit your ability to achieve your client's massage goals.

 Postural hypotension can occur as a side effect of this class of medication. Help the client to change positions and be on guard for dizziness or blacking out.

 Antipsychotic medications include: chlorpromazine (Thorazine), fluphenazine (Permitil, Prolixin), haloperidol (Haldol), loxapine (Loxitane), mesoridazine (Serentil), molindone (Moban), perphenazine (Trilafon), thiothixene (Navane), and trifluoperazine (Stelazine).

Atypical Antipsychotics

Atypical antipsychotics work by binding to certain receptors in the brain to help correct imbalances of certain *neurotransmitters*. (Neurotransmitters are chemicals that allow for communication between brain nerve cells.

 If the client has developed any of the following, avoid massage and have them call their doctor or emergency services immediately: Very stiff muscles, fever, tremors, excessive sweating, unusual face, mouth, tongue, or jaw movements, slow or difficult speech, or a pounding heartbeat. These drug side effects are considered very serious and require medical attention. (This is a massage-specific list; refer to the documentation that was included with the medication for a complete list of side effects.)

 All heat therapies should be avoided (including hot stone massage, heat pads, saunas, steam rooms, etc.), as the client's ability to control their body temperature is compromised.

 Side Effects: Headaches, skin rash, swollen ankles, dry or discolored skin, anxiety, insomnia, drowsiness, lightheadedness, upset stomach, vomiting, constipation, and restlessness are common side effects of this class of medication. Take these into consideration as they may limit your ability to achieve your client's massage goals.

 Postural hypotension can occur as a side effect of this class of medication. Help the client to change positions and be on guard for dizziness or blacking out.

 Atypical antipsychotic medications include: aripiprazole (Abilify), clozapine (Clozaril), olanzapine (Zyprexa, Zydis), quetiapine (Seroquel), risperidone (Risperdal) and ziprasidone (Geodon).

Cholinergic Agonists

This class of drugs stimulates the action of acetylcholine, increasing parasympathetic responses including dilating blood vessels, slowing the heart rate and relaxing body tissues. Since massage techniques also encourage these responses, focus on the purpose of the medication to determine if massage is recommended. Oral medications are more likely to be suspect than topical applications or eye drops.

Cholinergic Agonist Precautions

 If the client has developed a sudden rash, confusion, a fever, severe nausea or vomiting, shortness of breath, or very low blood pressure, stop or avoid all massage and have them call their doctor immediately. These drug side effects are considered very serious and require medical attention. (This is a massage-specific list; refer to the documentation that was included with the medication for a complete list of side effects.)

 Side Effects: Nausea, increased sweating and salivation, and urinary frequency all can occur with this class of medication. Take these into consideration as they may limit your ability to achieve your client's massage goals.

 Postural hypotension is common with this class of medication. Help the client to change positions and be on guard for dizziness or blacking out.

 Cholinergic agonist medications include: <u>acetylcholine</u> (Miochal), <u>bethanechol</u> (Duvoid, Myotonachol, Urecholine), <u>carbachol</u> (Carbastat, Carboptic, Isopto Carbachol, Miostat), and <u>pilocarpine</u> (Diocarpine, Milocarpine, Ocusert Pilo, Pilocar, Pilopine, Piloptic, Salagen).

Cholinesterase Inhibitors

Also called *anticholinesterase* medications, this class of drug inhibits the breakdown of *acetylcholine*. Patients with dementia and Alzheimer's disease have decreased levels of acetylcholine, a chemical that acts as a messenger to allow communication between nerve cells. Cholinesterase breaks down acetylcholine. Preventing the destruction of acetylcholine improves memory and cognitive function.

 If the client has developed any of the following, stop or avoid all massage and have them call their doctor immediately: Skin rash or hives, changes in vision or balance, severe diarrhea, difficulty breathing, difficulty urinating, dizziness, vomiting, nervousness, increased confusion, slow heartbeat, or palpitations, severe stomach pain, uncontrollable movements, or unexplained weight loss. (This is a massage-specific list; refer to the documentation that was included with the medication for a complete list of side effects.)

Cholinesterase Inhibitor Precautions, cont'd.

 Side Effects: Headaches, upset stomach, vomiting, diarrhea, dizziness, loss of balance, muscle aches, and fatigue are all common side effects of this class of medication. Take these into consideration as they may limit your ability to achieve your client's massage goals.

 Cholinesterase Inhibitor medications include: <u>donepezil</u> (Aricept), <u>galantamine</u> (Reminyl), <u>rivastigmine</u> (Exelon) and <u>tacrine</u> (Cognex, Tetrahydroaminoacridine, THA).

N-methyl-D-aspartate Antagonists

These medications block the amino acid *glutamate*, which is thought to be responsible for symptoms of Alzheimer's.

 If the client has developed any of the following, stop or avoid all massage and have them call their doctor immediately: Severe dizziness, hallucinations, not able to hold your urine, shortness of breath, swelling in throat or tongue, skin rash or redness, or vomiting. These drug side effects are considered very serious and require medical attention. (This is a massage-specific list; refer to the documentation that was included with the medication for a complete list of side effects.)

 Side Effects: Headaches, mild diarrhea, and dizziness are all common side effect of this medication. Take these into consideration as they may limit your ability to achieve your client's massage goals.

 Postural hypotension can occur as a side effect of this class of medication. Help the client to change positions and be on guard for dizziness or blacking out.

 N-methyl-D-aspartate antagonist medications include <u>memantine</u> (Namenda).

Anticholinergics and Antispasmodics

Anticholinergics reduce parasympathetic nerve responses. Some of these medications are used to relieve cramps or spasms of the stomach, intestines, and bladder. Others are used to prevent nausea, vomiting, and motion sickness. Still others are given before surgery help relaxation and to decrease secretions like saliva.

 If the client has developed any of the following, stop or avoid all massage and have them call their doctor immediately: Skin rash or hives, unusual warmth, dryness, and flushing of skin, severe muscle weakness, persistent dizziness, eye pain, blurred vision, unsteadiness, confusion, seizures, difficulty in breathing, fast heartbeat, fever, or slurred speech. These drug side effects are considered very serious and require medical attention. (This is a massage-specific list; refer to the documentation that was included with the medication for a complete list of side effects.)

 Side Effects: Common side effects from this class of medication include headaches, decreased sweating, constipation, drowsiness, and dry eyes. Take these into consideration as they may limit your ability to achieve your client's massage goals.

 Anticholinergic and antispasmodic medications include: aniso-tropine, atropine (Atropisol, Isopto-Atropine, Sal-Tropine), belladonna, clidinium (Quarzan), dicyclomine (Bentyl, Bentylol, Formulex, Spasmoban), flavoxate (Urispas), glycopyrrolate (Robinul), homatropine (Homapin, Levbid, Levsin), hyoscyamine (Anaspaz, A-Spas, Cystospaz, Donnamar, ED-SPAZ, Gastrosed, Levsinex, Symax SL), mepenzolate (Cantil), methantheline (Banthine), methscopolamine (Pamine), oxybutynin (Ditropan), pirenzepine (Gastrozepin), propantheline (Pro-Banthine, Propanthel), scopolamine (Buscopan, Transderm-Scop, Transderm-V) and tolterodine (Detrol).

COMT Inhibitors

Catechol O-MethylTransferase inhibitors are the newest class of medications for the treatment of Parkinson's disease. COMT inhibitors increase the availability of anti Parkinson's medications, which subsequently relieves the tremors, stiffness and movement difficulties for longer periods.

 If the client has recently developed any of the following, avoid massage and call the physician immediately: Severe back or neck spasms, unusual or uncontrolled movements, unexplained skin rash, severe headache, increased tremors, increased difficulty breathing, ringing in the ears, recent muscle weakness, unusual bleeding or bruising or swelling of the lips, tongue, or face. (This is a massage-specific list; refer to the documentation that was included with the medication for a complete list of side effects.)

 Side Effects: Back pain, abdominal pain, increased sweating, nausea, vomiting, diarrhea, weakness, anxiety, and fatigue all can occur with this class of medication. Take these into consideration as they may limit your ability to achieve your client's massage goals.

 Postural hypotension can occur as a side effect of this class of medication. Help the client to change positions and be on guard for dizziness or blacking out.

 COMT inhibitor medications include entacapone (Comtan) and tolcapone (Tasmar).

Anti-Parkinson's Medications

Current evidence shows that symptoms of Parkinson's disease are related to a lack of dopamine in the brain. *Levodopa* is a precursor that is converted to dopamine in the brain. Other medications combined with levodopa assist in its effectiveness (e.g. the monoamine oxidase inhibitor called selegiline).

 If the client has recently developed any of the following, avoid massage and call the physician immediately: Severe back or neck spasms, unusual or uncontrolled movements, unexplained skin rash, severe headache, increased tremors, increased difficulty breathing, ringing in the ears, recent muscle weakness, unusual bleeding or bruising or swelling of the lips, tongue, or face. (This is a massage-specific list; refer to the documentation that was included with the medication for a complete list of side effects.)

Anti-Parkinson's Medication Precautions, cont'd.

 Side Effects: Headaches, muscle pain, abdominal pain, increased sweating, nausea, vomiting, diarrhea, weakness, anxiety, and fatigue are all common side effects of this class of medication. Take these into consideration as they may limit your ability to achieve your client's massage goals.

 Postural hypotension can occur as a side effect of this class of medication. Help the client to change positions and be on guard for dizziness or blacking out. If dizziness does occur, have the client consult their doctor before the next session.

 Anti-Parkinson's medications include: <u>amantadine</u> (Symadine, Symmetrel), <u>apomorphine</u> <u>hydrochloride</u> (Apokyn), <u>carbidopa</u> <u>with</u> <u>levodopa</u> (Sinemet), <u>carbidopa</u> <u>with</u> <u>levodopa</u> <u>and</u> <u>entacapone</u> (Stalevo), and <u>selegiline</u> (Carbex, Eldepryl).

Antidyskinetics

Antidyskinetics are used to treat Parkinson's disease by improving muscle control and reducing stiffness, allowing for more normal body motion.

 If the client has recently developed any of the following, avoid massage and call the physician immediately: An unexplained skin rash, severe headache, increased tremors or seizures, increased difficulty breathing, ringing in the ears, recent muscle weakness, unusual bleeding or bruising or swelling of the lips, tongue, or face. (This is a massage-specific list; refer to the documentation that was included with the medication for a complete list of side effects.)

 Side Effects: Headaches, muscle cramps, nausea, vomiting, constipation, drowsiness, numbness or weakness in hands or feet and fatigue are all common side effects of this class of medication. Take these into consideration as they may limit your ability to achieve your client's massage goals.

Antidyskinetic Medication Precautions, cont'd.

 Postural hypotension can occur as a side effect of this class of medication. Help the client to change positions and be on guard for dizziness or blacking out. If dizziness does occur, have the client consult their doctor before the next session.

 Antidyskinetic medications include: benztropine (Cogentin), biperiden (Akineton), ethopropazine (Parsidol), procyclidine (Procyclid, Kemadrin), and trihexyphenidyl (Artane, Trihexane, Trihexy).

Dopamine Receptor Agonists

Dopamine receptor agonists mimic the effects of dopamine in the brain, and cause the neurons to react as if dopamine was present.

 If the client has recently developed any of the following, avoid massage and call the physician immediately: Severe back or neck spasms, unusual or uncontrolled movements, unexplained skin rash, severe headache, increased tremors, increased difficulty breathing, ringing in the ears, recent muscle weakness, unusual bleeding or bruising or swelling of the lips, tongue, or face. (This is a massage-specific list; refer to the documentation that was included with the medication for a complete list of side effects.)

 Side Effects: Headaches, muscle pain, abdominal pain, edema, increased sweating, nausea, vomiting, diarrhea, weakness, anxiety and fatigue are all common side effects of this class of medication. Take these into consideration as they may limit your ability to achieve your client's massage goals.

 Postural hypotension can occur as a side effect of this class of medication. Help the client to change positions and be on guard for dizziness or blacking out. If dizziness does occur, have the client consult their doctor before the next session.

 Dopamine receptor agonist medications include: bromocriptine (Parlodel), carbidopa (Lodosyn), pergolide (Permax), pramipexole (Mirapex), and ropinirole (Requip).

Amyotrophic Lateral Sclerosis Medications

At this time, riluzole is the only drug that has been approved by the FDA for treatment of ALS. It helps to delay the deterioration of muscle strength, limb control and respiratory function.

 Fever, difficulty breathing or shortness of breath, or yellowing of the skin or eyes are all serious side effects of the medication. Stop or avoid massage and have the client seek medical attention immediately.

 Side Effects: Back pain, stomach pain, dizziness, drowsiness, nausea and/or vomiting are all side effects of the medication. Adjust your massage goals accordingly if these symptoms are present.

 Postural hypotension can occur as a side effect of this class of medication. Help the client to change positions and be on guard for dizziness or blacking out.

 Amyotrophic lateral sclerosis medications include riluzole (Rilutek).

Ophthalmic Beta Blockers

These medications decrease the rate that the fluids flow into the eye, which reduces internal pressure.

 If the client has recently developed any of the following, avoid massage and call the physician immediately: Unusual weight gain, unexplained skin rash, increased difficulty breathing, ringing in the ears, sudden severe headache, recent muscle weakness, unusual bleeding or bruising or swelling of the lips, tongue, or face. (This is a massage-specific list; refer to the documentation that was included with the medication for a complete list of side effects.)

 Side Effects: Headaches, dizziness and drowsiness can occur with this class of medication. Take these into consideration as they may limit your ability to achieve your client's massage goals.

 Postural hypotension can occur as a side effect of this class of medication. Help the client to change positions and be on guard for dizziness or blacking out.

Ophthalmic Beta Blocker Precautions, cont'd.

 Opthalmic beta blocker medications include: <u>betaxolol</u> (Betoptic), <u>carteolol</u> (Ocupress), <u>levobunolol</u> (AKBeta, Betagan), <u>metipranolol</u> (OptiPranolol), and <u>timolol</u> (Betimol, Ocudose, Timoptic).

Carbonic Anhydrase Inhibitors

Carbonic anhydrase inhibitors are used to treat glaucoma. Acetazolamide is also used as an anticonvulsant to control certain seizures in the treatment of epilepsy.

 If the client has developed any of the following, avoid massage and have them call their doctor or emergency services immediately: Very stiff muscles, fever, tremors, excessive sweating, unusual face, mouth, tongue, or jaw movements, slow or difficult speech, or a pounding heartbeat. These drug side effects are considered very serious and require medical attention. (This is a massage-specific list; refer to the documentation that was included with the medication for a complete list of side effects.)

 Side Effects: Headaches, dizziness or drowsiness can occur with this class of medication. Take these into consideration as they may limit your ability to achieve your client's massage goals.

 Warning: These medications reduce the levels of potassium in the body, which can result in recurring muscle cramps. Be aware of this and explain to the client the need to consult with their physician if muscle cramping persists.

 Carbonic anhydrase inhibitor medications include: <u>acetazolamide</u> (AK-Zol, Diamox, Storzolamide), <u>brinzolamide</u> (Azopt), <u>dichlor-phenamide</u> (Daranide), <u>dorzolamide</u> (Trusopt), <u>methazolamide</u> (GlaucTabs, Neptazane), and <u>dorzolamide</u> with <u>timolol</u> (Cosopt).

Miotics

Miotics are topical eye medications that cause the pupil to contract. This helps to drain the fluid from the eye and decrease internal pressure.

 If the client has developed any of the following, avoid massage and have them call their doctor or emergency services immediately: Very stiff muscles, fever, tremors, excessive sweating, unusual face, mouth, tongue, or jaw movements, slow or difficult speech, nausea, vomiting or diarrhea, or a pounding heartbeat. These drug side effects are considered very serious and require medical attention. (This is a massage-specific list; refer to the documentation that was included with the medication for a complete list of side effects.)

 Side Effects: Headaches can occur with this class of medication. Take these into consideration as they may limit your ability to achieve your client's massage goals.

 Miotic medications include: <u>carbachol</u> (Carboptic, Isopto Carbachol), <u>demecarium bromide</u> (Humorsol), <u>ecothiophate iodide</u> (Phospholine Iodide), <u>physostigmine</u> (Isopto Eserine), and <u>pilocarpine</u> (Adsorbocarpine, Akarpine, Isopto Carpine, Ocusert Pilo, Pilocar, Pilopine HS, Piloptic, Pilostat).

Prostaglandin Analogues

These medications reduce the internal eye pressure for clients with glaucoma.

 If the client has recently developed any of the following, avoid massage and call the physician immediately: An unexplained skin rash, severe headache, increased difficulty breathing, ringing in the ears, recent muscle weakness, unusual bleeding or bruising or swelling of the lips, tongue, or face. (This is a massage-specific list; refer to the documentation that was included with the medication for a complete list of side effects.)

 Side Effects: Headaches, dizziness or drowsiness can occur with this class of medication. Take these into consideration as they may limit your ability to achieve your client's massage goals.

Prostaglandin Analogue Precautions, cont'd.

 Postural hypotension can occur as a side effect of this class of medication. Help the client to change positions and be on guard for dizziness or blacking out.

 Prostaglandin analogue medications include: <u>bimatoprost</u> (Lumigan), <u>latanoprost</u> (Xalatan), <u>travoprost</u> (Travatan), and <u>unoprostone</u> (Rescula).

Ocular Sympathomimetics

Ocular sympathomimetics reduce the amount of fluid formed in the eye and increase the flow of the fluid out of the eye. This lowers internal eye pressure for clients with glaucoma. They also act as decongestants and can sometimes be found in cold medicines.

 If the client has developed unusual muscle pain, unusual swelling, itching, rash or hives, or difficulty breathing or swallowing, avoid all massage and have them call their doctor immediately. These drug side effects are considered very serious and require medical attention. (This is a massage-specific list; refer to the documentation that was included with the medication for a complete list of side effects.)

 If the client complains of a full bladder and an inability to urinate, seek emergency medical attention immediately.

 Side Effects: Headaches, dizziness and drowsiness can occur with this class of medication. Take these into consideration as they may limit your ability to achieve your client's massage goals.

 Ocular sympathomimetic medications include: <u>apraclonidine</u> (Iopidine), <u>brimonidine</u> (Alphagan), and <u>dipivefrin</u> (AKPro, Propine).

Chapter 8

Respiratory System

Influenza

(also called the flu)

The flu is a respiratory infection caused by a variety of flu viruses. Symptoms begin aggressively 1 to 4 days after infection, and can include headache, severe fatigue, chills, dry cough, body aches, fever, stuffy nose and a sore throat (*pharyngitis*). Typically, the fever begins to decline on the second or third day of the illness. The flu can be spread (is contagious) before symptoms start and for 3 to 4 days afterwards.

Reye's syndrome (a condition affecting the nervous system) sometimes develops in children and teenagers who are recovering from the flu. This is extremely rare; nonetheless as a precaution it is recommended that children avoid taking aspirin for fever or pain.

Influenza Precautions

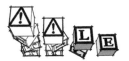 **Restrict massage to Light and Energy techniques.**

 If the client has recently developed any of the following warning symptoms, stop or avoid massage and have the client seek emergency attention: Difficulty breathing, chest or abdominal pain, sudden or severe dizziness, lethargy, confusion, or a fever with a rash.

 Avoid TOLERANCE and INCREMENTAL techniques, and limit the duration of your session to avoid overwhelming the client. Flu shots do not prevent illness. The flu vaccine actually weakens the immune system and makes someone more predisposed to this and other illnesses.

Influenza Precautions, cont'd.

 Avoid close contact with immunocompromised individuals if the therapist has received the FluMist vaccine in the last 21 days. Viral replication and shedding occurs in the upper respiratory system during this time and the virus can be spread to others. (Immunocompromised individuals include those on steroid or immunosuppressant medications, pregnant women, and those who are battling cancer, HIV, allergies, eczema, etc.)

 Warning: If the client is easily fatigued and their immunity seems to be particularly challenged, limit or avoid pressure techniques until the client's infection is past the acute stage. ENERGY techniques can be helpful.

 Antiviral medications may be prescribed, as well as many over-the-counter drugs. Clients routinely self-medicate in addition to prescription medications. Be sure to ask about current medications and check their precautions.

 In the subacute stage of influenza, LIGHT or ENERGY techniques may speed healing. Be sure to inform the client, however, that they must support the massage with good nutrition and rest, or the body will struggle and symptoms may worsen.

Common Cold

A cold is an illness caused by a virus infection located in the nose, sinuses, ears, and bronchial tubes. Colds are highly contagious and spread when droplets of fluid containing the virus are transferred by touch or are inhaled. They are the number one reason for visits to the doctor in the U.S., yet there are no antiviral medications available for the cold, and antibiotics are ineffective and should only be taken to treat bacterial complications.

Symptoms begin 1 to 3 days after becoming infected and can include a runny nose, respiratory congestion, coughing and sneezing, weakened senses of taste and smell, and a scratchy throat. Fever, headache and severe fatigue are less likely and may indicate the flu.

Common Cold Precautions

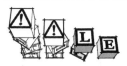 **Restrict massage to Light and Energy techniques.**

 If the client has recently developed any of the following warning symptoms, stop or avoid massage and have the client seek emergency attention: Difficulty breathing, chest or abdominal pain, sudden or severe dizziness, lethargy, confusion, or a fever with a rash.

 If you as the therapist have a cold, be extremely cautious with whom you choose to massage. Postpone massage for immunocompromised individuals, including those on steroid or immunosuppressant medications, pregnant women, and those who are battling cancer, HIV, allergies, eczema, etc.

 Limit or avoid pressure techniques if the client is easily fatigued and their immunity seems to be particularly challenged. ENERGY work and similar supportive techniques can be helpful until the acute stage has passed.

 Clients routinely self-medicate in addition to prescription medications for this condition. Closely check all medications and their precautions.

 In the subacute stage of the common cold, LIGHT and ENERGY massage techniques may speed healing. Be sure to inform the client, however, that they must support the massage with good nutrition and rest, or the body will struggle and symptoms may worsen.

Sinusitis

Sinusitis is an irritation of the membranes lining the sinuses. The irritation can be from inhaled irritants, allergies, or infections like viruses (or rarely, bacteria). It is classified as acute sinusitis when the irritation has been present less than thirty days, subacute sinusitis lingers for less than three months, and chronic sinusitis is when the irritation lasts longer than three months.

Symptoms of sinusitis can include headache, facial tenderness or pain, and occasionally fever.

Sinusitis Precautions

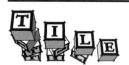 **Tolerance, Incremental, Light and Energy techniques are all encouraged.**

 If the client has recently developed any of the following warning symptoms, stop or avoid massage and have the client seek emergency attention: Extreme headache with vomiting or vision disturbances, sudden or severe dizziness, difficulty breathing, chest or abdominal pain, lethargy, confusion, or a fever with a rash.

 If you as the therapist have infectious sinusitis, be extremely cautious with whom you choose to massage. Postpone massage for immunocompromised individuals, including those on corticosteroids, pregnant women, and those who are battling cancer, HIV, allergies, etc.

 Warning: Adjust the face cradle if pressure on the face is uncomfortable, and consider alternative positions if the discomfort persists. Clients may be unable to stay in the prone position due to increasing pressure in the sinuses.

 Check the precautions listed for all current medications.

 Improving the body's ability to function will have a positive effect on the client's healing energy.

Acute Bronchitis

Bronchitis is an irritation and inflammation of the large air passages leading to the lungs (the trachea and bronchi). It most commonly follows an upper respiratory infection such as a cold or flu. The irritation may encourage a secondary infection. Symptoms include a deep cough, which produces thick sputum. Achy chest pain, shortness of breath and possibly fever may also accompany the coughing. Recurring bronchitis is covered under *chronic obstructive pulmonary disease* later in this chapter.

Acute Bronchitis Precautions

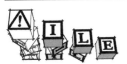 **Restrict massage to Incremental, Light and Energy techniques.**

 If the client has recently developed any of the following warning symptoms, stop or avoid massage and have the client seek emergency attention: Sudden or severe dizziness, difficulty breathing or catching their breath, chest or abdominal pain, lethargy, confusion, or a fever with a rash.

 If you as the therapist have acute bronchitis, be extremely cautious with whom you choose to massage. Postpone massage for immunocompromised individuals, including those on cortico-steroids, pregnant women, and those who are battling cancer, HIV, allergies, etc.

 Limit or avoid pressure techniques if the client is easily fatigued and their immunity seems to be particularly challenged. ENERGY work and similar supportive techniques can be helpful until the acute stage has passed.

 Clients routinely self-medicate in addition to prescription medications for this condition. Closely check all medications and their precautions.

 Improving the body's ability to function will have a positive effect on the client's energy to heal.

Chronic Obstructive Pulmonary Disease (COPD)

COPD is a degenerative condition in which a reduction of airflow to the lungs occurs because of blockage or excess mucus secretion. The two main types of COPD are *chronic bronchitis* and *emphysema*. Inhaled irritants are the number one cause, and smoking heads that list by far. The American Lung Association states that smoking is the cause of up to 90 percent of COPD cases annually. There is no cure for this condition, however, elimination of the irritant can slow the progression if the condition has not become too severe. Medications are designed to decrease symptoms and complications. Supplemental oxygen is administered as this disease progresses. This condition strains the cardiovascular system and causes secondary conditions such as cor pulmonale (see the cardiovascular system).

Chronic Bronchitis

Chronic bronchitis is repeated or persistent irritation and inflammation of the large air passages leading to the lungs (the *trachea* and *bronchi*). The body develops increased mucus production as a protective response to irritation, which further decreases airflow and makes the client more prone to infection. Scarring of the bronchial tubes develops as this disease progresses.

Emphysema

Emphysema destroys the tissue walls between the air sacs of the lungs (the *alveoli*). As the ability of the lungs to expand and contract is reduced, the air sacs enlarge and fill up the chest cavity. This diseased tissue presses on healthy lung tissue, which must then work harder to exchange oxygen and carbon dioxide.

Chronic Obstructive Pulmonary Disease Precautions

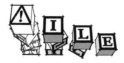 **Restrict massage to Incremental, Light and Energy techniques.**

Chronic Obstructive Pulmonary Disease Precautions, cont'd.

 If the client has recently developed any of the following warning symptoms, stop or avoid massage and have the client contact their physician: Swollen hands, ankles, or feet, muscle cramps or weakness, increased fatigue, increasingly difficult breathing, chest pain while coughing, or bloody, green or yellow phlegm.

 Postponing the session is recommended if the therapist is unwell. The client's immune system is compromised from COPD and they are at higher risk of contracting infections.

 Warning: Fatigue and endurance are factors in COPD. Consider how to limit the scope and duration of your massage to avoid overwhelming the client.

 Warning: Clients afflicted with COPD may have difficulty lying reclined. Ask them what positions are most comfortable and adapt your techniques to best suit their needs.

 Clients will have certain medications prescribed in case of crisis. Be sure to place these close by in case they are needed during a session. Closely check all medications and their precautions.

 A consistent massage schedule can improve your client's immune system and provide extra comfort for this chronic condition.

Asthma and Allergies

Asthma and allergies are caused by a sensitivity to certain allergens (or triggers) like pollen, mold spores, dust mites, dairy, etc., and may be irritated or aggravated by colds, flu or other respiratory infections. Emotional stress can also trigger attacks. As a result of the body's learned response to an allergen (asthma and allergies are not hereditary), it creates an overabundance of one or more immune chemicals called histamines and immunoglobulins. *Histamine* is the chemical responsible for producing inflammation. *Immunoglobulins* are specialized proteins (antibodies) that circulate in the blood and lymph and attack foreign substances. The five types of immunoglobulins are IgA, IgD, IgE, IgG, and IgM.

Asthma is a disease that is primarily allergic in nature, although the triggers may be abundant and complex. Asthma results in wheezing and shortness of breath due to a narrowing of the bronchial tubes. Attacks can range from a mild shortness of breath to a life-threatening *anaphylactic shock*. Anaphylactic shock is a severe restriction in airflow to the lungs with a sudden drop in blood pressure. Inhaled medications are prescribed and carried by clients afflicted with asthma to help counteract such attacks.

Allergies also affect the respiratory system in many people. Skin allergies are also common, and clients can be affected by an allergic reaction in one system and not the other. Inflammatory bowel disease (IBD) is also frequently explained as an allergic reaction to certain foods.

Asthma and Allergy Precautions

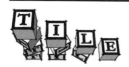 **Tolerance, Incremental, Light and Energy techniques are all encouraged.**

 If the client has recently developed faintness, nausea and/or vomiting, wheezing or difficulty breathing, stop or avoid massage and have the client utilize whatever medication they have been prescribed. Remain with the client until symptoms have subsided or it becomes clear they need additional medical assistance. Resume massage only when the symptoms have passed and both you and the client feel they are strong enough to proceed.

 Postponing the session is recommended if the therapist is unwell. The client's immune system is compromised from asthma and they have a higher risk of contracting infections.

 Warning: Discuss possible triggers that the client may be aware of (before they arrive for your session if possible), and scrutinize your materials and lubricants to ensure that fragrances are limited or eliminated. Offering hypoallergenic, scent-free lubricants can be emotionally reassuring to your client even if not specifically requested.

Asthma and Allergy Precautions, cont'd.

 Warning: Clients afflicted with asthma or allergies may have difficulty lying reclined. Ask them what positions are least likely to aggravate their asthma and adapt your techniques to best suit their needs.

 Clients will have certain medications prescribed in case of crisis. Be sure to place these close by in case they are needed during a session. Closely check all medications and their precautions.

 Your ability to relax the torso and neck muscles can have a significant effect on the client's quality of breathing and improve their total physical health potential.

Pneumonia

Pneumonia is a potentially life-threatening infection of the lungs. The inflammation and fluid buildup in the air sacs (the *alveoli*) and air passages dramatically reduces the ability to transfer oxygen to the blood. In severe cases the infection can spread to other parts of the body. A century ago it was the leading cause of death, but the advent of modern medicines has made survival far more likely. Pneumonia is currently ranked by the American Lung Association as the seventh leading cause of death when combined with influenza.

Symptoms include a painful cough with greenish, yellow or rust-colored mucus, fever with shaking chills, sharp chest pains, and shortness of breath.

Those at heightened risk for contracting pneumonia include the very young or old and those with other conditions such as HIV, congestive heart failure, COPD or diabetes.

Pneumonia Precautions

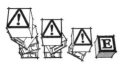 **Energy techniques only. Avoid all pressure and circulatory massage techniques.**

Pneumonia Precautions, cont'd.

 If the client has recently developed any of the following warning symptoms, stop or avoid massage and have the client seek emergency attention: Sudden or severe dizziness, difficulty breathing or catching their breath, chest or abdominal pain, lethargy, confusion, or a fever with a rash.

 Postponing the session is recommended if the therapist is unwell. The client's immune system is already compromised and they are at increased risk of secondary infections.

 When the client is past the acute stage for pneumonia, and after they have been cleared for massage by their physician, LIGHT and ENERGY techniques are appropriate. Be aware of the client's decreased endurance and modify the length of your session to avoid overwhelming them.

 Warning: Clients afflicted with pneumonia may have difficulty lying reclined. Ask them what positions are least likely to aggravate their condition and adapt your techniques to best suit their needs.

 Clients will have certain medications prescribed in case of crisis. Be sure to place these close by in case they are needed during a session. Closely check all medications and their precautions.

 Your ability to relax the torso and neck muscles can have a significant effect on the client's quality of breathing and improve their total physical health potential.

Tuberculosis (TB)

Tuberculosis is a disease caused by bacterium *Mycobacterium Tuberculosis*. The bacteria can attack any part of the body, but it is usually limited to the lungs. It produces fibrous capsules (*tubercules*) filled with dead, infected tissue. Early symptoms are not unlike a mild flu. In active TB disease, symptoms are far more severe and include a chronic severe cough with bloody sputum, recurring fever, night sweats, fatigue and weight loss.

It is not easy to become infected with tuberculosis. Usually a person has to be close to someone with TB disease for a long period of time, like those living or working with an infected person.

The American Lung Association reports that about 10 million Americans are infected with TB. 90 percent of those who become infected will not develop TB disease because their body's immune system protects them. Keeping the immune system strong is critically important in preventing the onset of TB disease.

Treatments including long courses of antibiotics are effective over 90 percent of the time when patients are consistent with their medication. Unfortunately, it is so common for patients to fail to follow through consistently with the regime that a program called DOTS is now the norm. DOTS stands for *Directly Observed Therapy, Short course*. Failure to follow through with therapy trains the bacteria to become resistant to the medication, creating *MultiDrug-Resistant Tuberculosis* (MDR TB). Less than half survive this aggressive form of TB.

Tuberculosis Precautions

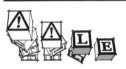 **Restrict massage to Light and Energy techniques.**

 Discuss your client's condition and current status with their physician before agreeing to perform massage. Be absolutely certain your client is not contagious before working with them.

 When the client is undergoing treatment for TB, and after they have been cleared for massage by their physician, LIGHT and ENERGY techniques are appropriate. Gentle stretching is also recommended. Be aware of the client's decreased endurance and modify the length of your session to avoid overwhelming them.

 Many medications are used in the treatment of TB, including antibiotics and antituberculars. In addition, a wide range of supportive medication is used to ease the client's discomfort. Check all medications for additional precautions.

Tuberculosis Precautions, cont'd.

 Utilizing massage for relaxation as well as stress relief will boost their immune system. Use your advanced knowledge to guide them towards an immune-building lifestyle.

Pulmonary Embolism (PE)

(also called pulmonary thromboembolism)

Pulmonary embolism describes a condition in which a blood clot lodges in one of the arteries in the lung. It is technically not a disease in and of itself, but rather, a common complication of deep vein thrombosis (DVT). When a blood clot (thrombus) breaks free of the vein wall in the leg, it travels through widening veins until reaching the heart. The blood is then pumped into the lungs to receive oxygen, carrying the embolism to a smaller artery where it becomes jammed.

PE is one of the most common causes of unexpected death, second only to heart attacks. Autopsy results show that as many as 60 percent of patients dying in the hospital have had a PE, but the diagnosis was been missed 70 percent of the time. If a PE goes undiagnosed and untreated, it has more than a 30 percent fatality rate. However, if correctly diagnosed and promptly treated, less than 10 percent are fatal.

There is a classic triad of signs and symptoms for PE which include coughing up blood (*hemoptysis*), breathing difficulties, and chest pain, but one should not wait for all three to be present before taking action. Other symptoms of PE can include back, shoulder, or upper abdominal pain, excessive sweating, a rapid heartbeat, and lightheadedness or fainting.

Acute Pulmonary Embolism Precautions

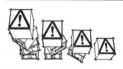 **Client is in critical condition.
Avoid all therapy until approved
by their physician.**

Pulmonary Embolism, Rehabilitative Precautions

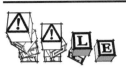 **Restrict massage to Light and Energy techniques.**

 Do not begin massage with any client having breathing difficulties, no matter how minor they may appear. If this occurs during a massage, stop and help the client sit. If the breathing does not return to normal within a few minutes, or if any additional symptoms appear, call emergency assistance immediately.

 Warning symptoms for PE: Coughing up blood, breathing difficulties, chest pain, back, shoulder, or upper abdominal pain, excessive sweating, a rapid heartbeat, and lightheadedness or fainting.

 Massage may be appropriate once client has been discharged from critical care. Avoid all pressure techniques for the entire body until the treating physician has stated that the threat of embolism has passed. Treatment may take months; ENERGY techniques can be freely utilized during this time.

 Follow the precautions listed under *deep vein thrombosis* as permanent restrictions for massage therapy for anyone with a history of PE.

 Anticoagulant and antithrombotic medications are commonly prescribed for an extended period of time. Be sure to ask about current medications and check their precautions.

 PE is life threatening, and prompt action is critical when suspicious. Risk being wrong; act on your instincts and you may very well save a life.

Respiratory System Medications

Antitubercular Medications

Antitubercular medications are oral chemotherapeutic agents used in the treatment of tuberculosis.

 If the client has recently developed any of the following, avoid massage and call the physician immediately: An unexplained skin rash, increased difficulty breathing, ringing in the ears, sudden severe headache, recent muscle weakness, unusual bleeding or bruising or swelling of the lips, tongue, or face. (This is a massage-specific list; refer to the documentation that was included with the medication for a complete list of side effects.)

 Warning: Begin massage cautiously, and use your own sense of appropriate pressure. Avoid relying upon the client to determine their limits. The client is likely to have a reduced perception of pressure and pain as a result of this medication.

 Side Effects: Headaches, dizziness, increased flatulence and intestinal cramping, dizziness and drowsiness all can occur with this class of medication. Take these into consideration as they may limit your ability to achieve your client's massage goals.

 Postural hypotension can occur as a side effect of this class of medication. Help the client to change positions and be on guard for dizziness or blacking out.

 Antitubercular medications include: <u>ethambutol</u> (Myambutol), <u>isoniazid</u> (INH, Laniazid, Nydrazid), and <u>pyrazinamide</u> (Tebrazid).

Sleep Disorder Medications

Sleep disorder medications are is used to improve wakefulness in people with *sleep apnea, narcolepsy, Obstructive Sleep Apnea/Hypopnea Syndrome* (OSAHS) and *Shift Work Sleep Disorder* (SWSD).

Sleep Disorder Medication Precautions

 If the client has recently developed any of the following, avoid massage and call the physician immediately: An unexplained skin rash, increased difficulty breathing, chest pain, ringing in the ears, sudden severe headache, unusual bleeding or bruising or swelling of the lips, tongue, or face. (This is a massage-specific list; refer to the documentation that was included with the medication for a complete list of side effects.)

 Side Effects: Headaches are a common side effect of this class of medication. Take this into consideration as it may limit your ability to achieve your client's massage goals.

 Sleep disorder medications include <u>modafinil</u> (Provigil).

Antihistamines, Decongestants, and Antitussives

Decongestants (such as pseudoephedrine) constrict blood vessels. Therefore, when a decongestant is used, the blood vessels in the nose (and other areas of the body) tighten, causing the linings of the nose to be less swollen and stuffy.

Antihistamines are the most effective medications for reducing the symptoms of sneezing, itchiness, and runny nose. They are not as effective in treating nasal congestion. Histamine stimulates the production of mucus and the dilation of blood vessels. Antihistamines prevent histamine from binding to histamine (H1) receptors, thereby blocking the histamine reaction.

 If the client has recently developed any of the following, avoid massage and call the physician immediately: Prolonged dizziness or drowsiness, severe back or neck weakness, unusual or uncontrolled movements, unexplained skin rash, severe headache, increased tremors, increased difficulty breathing, ringing in the ears, recent muscle weakness, unusual bleeding or bruising or swelling of the lips, tongue, or face. (This is a massage-specific list; refer to the documentation that was included with the medication for a complete list of side effects.)

Antihistamine, Decongestant, and Antitussive Medication Precautions, cont'd.

 All heat therapies should be avoided (including hot stone massage, heat pads, saunas, steam rooms, etc.) as the client's ability to control their body temperature is compromised.

 Warning: Decongestants and antihistamines are often combined with pain relievers. Check each individual medication for precautions in addition to those listed here.

 Side Effects: Headaches, drowsiness and fatigue, dizziness, urine retention, constipation, upset stomach, nervousness or a fast pulse can occur with these medications. Take these into consideration as they may limit your ability to achieve your client's massage goals.

 Postural hypotension can occur as a side effect of this class of medication. Help the client to change positions and be on guard for dizziness or blacking out.

 Antihistamine and decongestant medications include: <u>acrivastine</u>, <u>azatadine</u>, <u>azelastine</u>, <u>bromodiphenhydramine</u>, <u>brompheniramine</u>, <u>carbinoxamine</u>, <u>cetirizine</u>, <u>chlorpheniramine</u>, <u>clemastine</u>, <u>cromolyn</u>, <u>cyproheptadine</u>, <u>cyclizine</u>, <u>desloratadine</u>, <u>dexbrompheniramine</u>, <u>dex-chlorpheniramine</u>, <u>dimenhydrinate</u>, <u>diphenhydramine</u>, <u>diphenylpyra-line</u>, <u>doxylamine</u>, <u>fexofenadine</u>, <u>hydroxyzine</u>, <u>loratadine</u>, <u>meclizine hydrochloride</u>, <u>methapyrilene</u>, <u>methdilazine</u>, <u>oxymetazoline</u>, <u>phen-indamine</u>, <u>pheniramine</u>, <u>phenyltoloxamine</u>, <u>promethazine</u>, <u>pyrilam-ine</u>, <u>pseudoephedrine</u>, <u>terpin</u> <u>hydrate</u>, <u>trimeprazine</u>, <u>tripelennamine</u>, and <u>triprolidine.</u>

 Antitussive medications include: <u>benzonatate</u>, <u>codeine</u>, <u>carbeta-pentane</u>, <u>dextromethorphan</u>, <u>hydrocodone.</u>

 Combination brand name medications include: Actagen, Actamine, Actifed, Afrin, Alavert, Alka-Seltzer, Allegra, Aller-Chlor, Allercon, Allerfrim, Allerphed, Altryl, Aprodine, Astelin, Atridine, Banophen, Beldin, Belix, Benadryl, Benylin, BroveX, Calmydone, Calmylin, Cenafed, Cheracol, Chlo-Amine, Chlor-Pheniton, Chlor-Trimeton, Clarinex, Claritin, CoActifed, Comtrex, (continued next page)

Antihistamine, Decongestant, and Antitussive Medication Precautions, cont'd.

 (Combination brand name medications continued) Congestac, Contac, Coristex, Cotridin, Dayhist, DayQuil, Dimetane, Dimetapp, Diphedryl, Diphenhist, Dristan, Duratuss, Efidac, Entex, Genac, Genahist, Genatuss, Guaifenex, Histenol, Hycomine, Kolephrin, Lodrane, Mersyndol, Nasalcrom, Novahistex, Novahistine, Nucofed, Nucotuss, NyQuil, Nytcold, Nytime, PediaCare, Penntuss, Pharmasave, Phenergan, Pneumotussin, Primatuss, ProfenII, Prometh, Protuss, Quelidrine, Rentamine, Rescon, Respa, Respaire, Rhinosyn, Robafen, Robitussin, Rondec, Ru-Tuss, Ryna, Rynatuss, Scot-Tussin, Silafed, Sinufed, Sinutab, Sudafed, Tanta, Tavist, Teldrin, TheraFlu, Tolu-Sed, Touro, Triac, Triacin, Triafed, Triafed, Triaminic, Triofed, Triposed, Triptifed, Tussafed, Tussilyn, Tussionex, Tussi-Organidin, Tussirex, Tusso, Uni-Tussin, Vanex, Versacaps, Vicks, Zephrex, and Zyrtec.

Beta-2 Agonists

(also called respiratory sympathomimetics)

Beta-2 agonists work in a manner similar to adrenaline by relaxing smooth muscles and opening airways. They create a sympathetic reaction, which can cause irritation, nervousness, and other symptoms similar to taking too much caffeine.

 If the client has recently developed any of the following, avoid massage and call the physician immediately: An unexplained skin rash, severe headache or muscle cramping, increased difficulty breathing, ringing in the ears, recent muscle weakness, unusual bleeding or bruising or swelling of the lips, tongue, or face. (This is a massage-specific list; refer to the documentation that was included with the medication for a complete list of side effects.)

 If the client complains of a full bladder and an inability to urinate, seek emergency medical attention immediately.

Beta-2 Agonist Precautions, cont'd.

 Side Effects: Headaches, muscle cramping, tremors, dizziness or drowsiness all can occur with this class of medication. Take these into consideration as they may limit your ability to achieve your client's massage goals.

 Side Effects: Isoproterenol may cause saliva and sputum to turn pink. This is a normal and harmless response.

 Postural hypotension can occur as a side effect of this class of medication. Help the client to change positions and be on guard for dizziness or blacking out.

 Beta-2 agonist medications include: <u>albuterol</u> (Alti-Salbutamol, Apo-Salvent, Novo-Salmol, Proventil, Ventolin, Volmax), <u>bitolterol</u> (Tornalate), <u>ephedrine</u>, <u>formoterol</u> (Foradil), <u>isoproterenol</u> (Isuprel, Medihaler), <u>levalbuterol</u> (Xopenex), <u>mephentermine</u> (Wyamine Sulfate), <u>metaraminol</u> <u>bitartrate</u> (Aramine), <u>methoxamine</u>, <u>meta-proterenol</u> (Alupent), <u>phenylephrine</u> (Despec-SF, Neo-Synephrine, Rhinall), <u>pirbuterol</u> (Maxair), <u>salmeterol</u> (Serevent), and <u>terbutaline</u> (Brethaire, Bricanyl).

Respiratory Anticholinergics

Anticholinergics are moderately fast acting medications that open the airway by blocking nerves that control the smooth muscle around the airways. Slower-acting than the beta-agonists, they can take 15 to 20 minutes to show a significant effect.

 If the client has recently developed any of the following, avoid massage and call the physician immediately: An unexplained skin rash, severe headache, increased difficulty breathing, ringing in the ears, recent muscle weakness, unusual bleeding or bruising or swelling of the lips, tongue, or face. (This is a massage-specific list; refer to the documentation that was included with the medication for a complete list of side effects.)

 Side Effects: Headaches, dizziness, upset stomach, constipation a skin rash all can occur with this class of medication. Take these into consideration as they may limit your ability to achieve your client's massage goals.

Respiratory Anticholinergic Precautions, cont'd.

 Postural hypotension can occur as a side effect of this class of medication. Help the client to change positions and be on guard for dizziness or blacking out.

 Respiratory anticholinergic medications include: <u>ipratropium</u> <u>bromide</u> (Atrovent), and <u>ipratropium</u> <u>bromide</u> with <u>albuterol</u> (Combivent).

Inhaled Steroids

Steroids (corticosteroids) suppress the body's production of substances that trigger inflammation and reduce the production of substances that maintain inflammation. This lowers the body's immunity, making the client vulnerable to infection and disease.

 If the client has recently developed any of the following, avoid massage and call the physician immediately: An unexplained skin rash, severe headache, increased difficulty breathing, ringing in the ears, recent muscle weakness, unusual bleeding or bruising or swelling of the lips, tongue, or face. (This is a massage-specific list; refer to the documentation that was included with the medication for a complete list of side effects.)

 Warning: Begin massage cautiously, and use your own sense of appropriate pressure. Avoid relying upon the client to determine their limits. The client is likely to have a reduced perception of pressure and pain as a result of this medication.

 Side Effects: Peripheral edema and neuropathy, cold extremities, neck, back or joint pain, nausea, and/or vomiting all can occur with this class of medication. Take these into consideration as they may limit your ability to achieve your client's massage goals.

 Postural hypotension can occur as a side effect of this class of medication. Help the client to change positions and be on guard for dizziness or blacking out.

Inhaled Steroid Precautions, cont'd.

 Inhaled steroid medications include: <u>beclomethasone</u> (Beclovent, QVAR, Vanceril), <u>budesonide</u> (Pulmicort), <u>flunisolide</u> (Aerobid), <u>fluticasone</u> (Flovent), <u>fluticasone</u> with <u>salmeterol</u> (Advair), <u>methylprednisolone</u> (Depo-Medrol, Solu-Medrol, Adlone), <u>tiotropium</u> (Spiriva), and <u>triamcinolone</u> (Azmacort).

Leukotriene Modifiers

Leukotrienes cause airway obstruction through smooth muscle contraction, mucous production, and swelling of the airways. Leukotriene modifiers block the action or production of leukotrienes and subsequently inhibit the inflammatory process.

 If the client has recently developed any of the following, avoid massage and call the physician immediately: An unexplained skin rash, severe headache, increased difficulty breathing, ringing in the ears, recent muscle weakness, unusual bleeding or bruising or swelling of the lips, tongue, or face. (This is a massage-specific list; refer to the documentation that was included with the medication for a complete list of side effects.)

 Side Effects: Headaches, tremors, dizziness and drowsiness all can occur with this class of medication. Take these into consideration as they may limit your ability to achieve your client's massage goals.

 Postural hypotension can occur as a side effect of this class of medication. Help the client to change positions and be on guard for dizziness or blacking out.

 Leukotriene modifier medications include: <u>montelukast</u> (Singulair), <u>zafirlukast</u> (Accolate) and <u>zileuton</u> (Zyflo).

Mast Cell Stabilizers

Mast cell stabilizers interfere with the inflammatory process by stabilizing membranes and inhibiting the histamine response. They are not used to relieve acute asthma attacks. They are taken as preventive medicine and may take 4 to 6 weeks of continuous use before the maximum benefit is achieved.

 If the client has recently developed any of the following, avoid massage and call the physician immediately: An unexplained skin rash, severe headache, increased difficulty breathing, ringing in the ears, recent muscle weakness, unusual bleeding or bruising or swelling of the lips, tongue, or face. (This is a massage-specific list; refer to the documentation that was included with the medication for a complete list of side effects.)

 Side Effects: Headaches can occur as a result of this class of medication. Take this into consideration as it may limit your ability to achieve your client's massage goals.

 Mast cell stabilizer medications include: <u>cromolyn</u> <u>sodium</u> (Intal) and <u>nedocromil</u> (Tilade).

Mucolytics and Expectorants

Mucolytics and expectorants thin the mucus making it easier to expel.

 If the client has recently developed any of the following, avoid massage and call the physician immediately: An unexplained skin rash, severe headache, increased difficulty breathing, ringing in the ears, recent muscle weakness, unusual bleeding or bruising or swelling of the lips, tongue, or face. (This is a massage-specific list; refer to the documentation that was included with the medication for a complete list of side effects.)

 Side Effects: Headaches and drowsiness can occur as a result of this class of medication. Take these into consideration as they may limit your ability to achieve your client's massage goals.

 Postural hypotension can occur as a side effect of this class of medication. Help the client to change positions and be on guard for dizziness or blacking out.

Mucolytic and Expectorant Precautions, cont'd.

 Mucolytic and expectorant medications include: <u>acetylcysteine</u> (Airbron, Mucomyst, Mucosil, Parvolex), and <u>guaifenesin</u> (Anti-Tuss, Bidex, Consin, Tussin EX, Duratuss, Fenesin, Glycotuss, Glytuss, Guaifenex, Guiadrine, Guiatuss, Humibid, Hytuss, Liquibid, Pneumomist, Robitussin, Scot-Tussin, Siltussin, Tusibron).

Methylxanthines

(also called xanthines)

Methylxanthines produce bronchial smooth muscle relaxation, which helps to dilate constricted airways, stimulates the increased secretion of urine by the kidneys (*diuresis*) to help relieve congestion, and acts as a mild cardiac and central nervous system stimulant. They also occur naturally in cocoa, tea and coffee plants.

 If the client has recently developed any of the following, avoid massage and call the physician immediately: An unexplained skin rash, severe headache, increased difficulty breathing, ringing in the ears, recent muscle weakness, unusual bleeding or bruising or swelling of the lips, tongue, or face. (This is a massage-specific list; refer to the documentation that was included with the medication for a complete list of side effects.)

 Side Effects: Headaches, dizziness, restlessness and anxiety can occur with this class of medication. Take these into consideration as they may limit your ability to achieve your client's massage goals.

 Postural hypotension can occur as a side effect of this class of medication. Help the client to change positions and be on guard for dizziness or blacking out.

 Methylxanthine medications include: <u>aminophylline</u> (Phyllocontin), <u>caffeine</u>, <u>oxtriphylline</u> (Brondelate, Choledyl), <u>theophylline</u> (Accurbron, Aquaphyllin, Asmalix, Bronkodyl, Elixomin, Elixophyllin, Lanophyllin, Quibron, Dividose, Respbid, Slo-Phyllin, Theo-Dur, Theo-Sav, Theo-X, Theobid, Theochron, Theoclear, Theolair, Theospan, Theostat, Theovent, Uni-Dur, Uniphyl).

Chapter 9

Endocrine and Reproductive Systems

Diabetes

The primary form of energy in the body is produced by metabolizing glucose in the blood. This is known as *blood sugar*. When the blood sugar levels get too low, the liver secretes sugar to bring the level back to healthy levels. Likewise, when the blood sugar level is too high, insulin is secreted from the pancreas to transport sugar from the blood into all the cells of the body.

Diabetes is a chronic disorder in which the body cannot keep the blood sugar levels from rising. In *Type 1 diabetes*, the pancreas is subjected to an autoimmune attack and becomes unable to make insulin in sufficient quantities. This type was formerly known as *juvenile diabetes* or *Insulin-Dependent Diabetes Mellitus* (IDDM), and only accounts for 5 percent of all diagnosed cases of diabetes.

95 percent of people have *Type 2 diabetes*, where the body builds a resistance to insulin, requiring ever increasing amounts to entice the cells to accept sugar. When the pancreas reaches its limit and the insulin resistance becomes high enough, sugar is drained from the blood into the kidneys and out the urine. Type 2 was formerly known as *Non-Insulin Dependent Diabetes Mellitus* (NIDDM), or *Adult Onset Diabetes Mellitus* (AODM).

The trend for Type 2 diabetes is alarming. The U.S. Centers for Disease Control and Prevention report that in the last 20 years the number of diabetes cases have almost doubled. The National Institutes of Health reports that up to one half of all new clinical diagnoses for Type 2 diabetes are now children, a type that only recently was reserved for adults over 40.

Uncontrolled blood sugar levels damages the vascular system. Damage to the smaller vessels can cause blindness, loss of sensation in the extremities (*peripheral neuropathy*), and damage to the kidneys. Larger vessels become inflexible and clogged (*atherosclerosis*), leading to heart attacks and stroke.

Throughout this progression, the body struggles to heal and provide nutrition as the blood supply is hampered.

Diabetic KetoAcidosis (**DKA**) is an acute crisis in which the lack of insulin and extremely high blood sugar causes the release of *ketones* into the blood. Ketones turn the blood acidic, and symptoms of diabetic ketoacidosis include nausea, vomiting, and abdominal pain. Shock and even coma can result without a quick medical response.

An opposite crisis can result from a lack of food or too much insulin in the blood in a short amount of time. Low blood sugar can lead to nervous system symptoms such as dizziness, confusion, weakness, and tremors. Untreated, severely low blood sugar levels can also lead to *"insulin shock"*, seizures and coma.

Diabetes Precautions

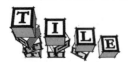 **Tolerance, Incremental, Light and Energy techniques are all encouraged within the client's limits.**

 If the client has any of the following symptoms the massage should be delayed until they have confirmed that their blood sugar levels are with normal range: Nausea, vomiting, abdominal pain, headache, shakiness, dizziness, rapid heartbeat, sweating or confusion, or blurred vision. The client should eat or inject some sugar without delay to resolve the issue. They should call their physician if symptoms do not improve within 20 minutes.

 Ask if the client carries glucagon in case of emergency. If so, ask them to explain the steps you should take if ever the client should become unconscious. *Glucagon* causes the release of glucose from the liver, and is usually administered by intramuscular injection.

 Limit or avoid TOLERANCE and INCREMENTAL massage techniques as the client's age or condition progresses. Cardiovascular and nerve losses are so prevalent that 15 percent of those with diabetes eventually require at least a partial lower extremity amputation. Sensation and circulation can be severely hampered. While the need for massage is obvious, caution and a gentle approach is also necessary.

Diabetes Precautions, cont'd.

 Warning: During the session if the client develops a headache, rapid heartbeat, significant perspiration, shakiness, and/or anxiety, stop the massage and have the client check their blood sugar levels. Resume the massage only when both you and the client determine that it is safe.

 Warning: Secondary conditions are the norm, including edema, ulcers, heart, kidney and vascular conditions. Be thorough in your notetaking and check all conditions for precautions.

 Ask the client where their last injection was placed and avoid the region around the site to prevent accelerating the absorption of insulin. In addition, recent injection sites may be inflamed; use discretion when massaging these areas. Oral medicines do not require this precaution.

 Take whatever time necessary to list the precautions for the client's medications. Ask each session which medications have changed, and keep your list updated.

 Clients with diabetes may be your most complex of cases, requiring the greatest forethought and care. They also may be the clients most in need of your skilled compassionate healthcare.

Hypoglycemia

Hypoglycemia is a condition in which the blood sugar levels are too low for normal healthy functioning. When levels rise the pancreas secretes insulin, which transports sugar from the blood into the cells. If the blood sugar is too low, the liver secretes glucose (sugar) into the blood.

As the amount and concentration of sugars increase in our diet, the pancreas becomes hyperactive and secretes more and more insulin. It increasingly overreacts to dietary sugars, effectively producing lower blood sugar levels than before the meal. If a person goes too long between meals, the liver is forced into secreting sugar, which also incites a response by the pancreas. A "rollercoaster" of sugar highs and lows can last days and be extremely difficult to stop. Attempting to ease the symptoms by eating sugar only compounds the problem.

It is estimated that over 100 million people in the U.S. suffer from the effects of hypoglycemia. Physical symptoms commonly include headaches, dizziness, and fatigue, and cold hands and feet, blurred vision, and heart palpitations can occur. Mood swings are almost universal and can be mild to extreme. Depression, anxiety, slow thinking and confusion are common. For those with diabetes, hypoglycemia can lead to severe *insulin shock* and even coma (see diabetes). Some say that many of the symptoms of low blood sugar are misdiagnosed and treated with medications that cover up the underlying condition.

Hypoglycemia Precautions

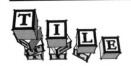 **Tolerance, Incremental, Light and Energy techniques are all encouraged.**

 During the session if the client develops a headache, shakiness, persistent dizziness, rapid heartbeat, sweating or confusion, stop the massage and have the client eat something. Seek medical attention if the symptoms persist or worsen, and only continue the session when symptoms go away.

 Warning: Wounds slow to heal, edema or peripheral neuropathy can all be indications of a more severe condition like diabetes. Bring your concerns to your client's attention as soon as you suspect a problem may exist.

 Diet is typically the recommended treatment unless the condition is secondary to another such as diabetes, although the client may be taking medication for symptomatic relief. Check all medications for specific precautions.

 Even without specific training in this condition, your guidance in basic nutrition and skills in stress relief will encourage the client to be more proactive and healthy.

Hyperthyroidism

(also called thyrotoxicosis)

Hyperthyroidism is a condition in which an overactive thyroid gland is producing an excessive amount of thyroid hormones. *Grave's disease* is the most common cause of hyperthyroidism. It is an autoimmune disorder producing antibodies that stimulate overgrowth of the gland and overproduction of thyroid hormones.

Since the thyroid essentially "runs" your metabolism, hyperthyroidism causes symptoms of excess metabolism. These can include tremors, fatigue, muscle weakness, weight loss despite an increased appetite, a racing heartbeat (*tachycardia*), increased sweating, restlessness and irritability, and often an enlarged thyroid gland (called a *goiter*). If the excess metabolism gets too far out of hand due to stress or other immune challenges, a *thyroid storm* can develop with a critical intensification of the symptoms listed above. In over half the cases a storm includes dramatic weight loss of over 40 pounds.

Radioactive iodine is used to destroy a portion of the thyroid gland to reduce output to normal levels. If this is unsuccessful, surgery to remove some of the gland may be required.

Hyperthyroidism Precautions

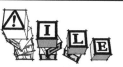 **Restrict massage to Incremental, Light and Energy techniques.**

 Abdominal pain, sudden confusion, severe agitation, high fever, or recent dramatic weight loss can be signs of a medical emergency. Stop or avoid massage and have the client call their physician or seek medical attention immediately.

 Avoid techniques that may stimulate the immune response (especially TOLERANCE techniques). Reducing tension and stress should be the focus of each session.

 Beta blockers and antithyroid medications are used to treat hyperthyroidism. Be sure to ask about current medications and check their precautions.

Hyperthyroidism Precautions, cont'd.

 Stress is a major reason for increasing symptoms with hyperthyroidism. Your support and skill in stress relief can make a significant difference in controlling this disease.

Hypothyroidism

Hypothyroidism is a group of medical conditions in resulting in an insufficient amount of thyroid hormones. When it results from part of the thyroid gland failing to work properly, it is referred to as *primary hypothyroidism* (or *cretinism*). The pituitary gland is the organ responsible for telling the thyroid gland to produce thyroid hormone. When a malfunctioning pituitary gland is the cause for low thyroid hormone levels, the condition is called *secondary hypothyroidism* (or *myxedema*).

Hypothyroidism results in mental retardation, decreased metabolism and weight gain. Physical development may be severely retarded in children. Other symptoms include muscle cramps, aches and weakness, fatigue, intolerance to cold, swelling in the legs (*edema*) and the abdomen (*ascites*), constipation, weight gain and dry skin. An enlarged thyroid gland (called a *goiter*) may also be present.

Hypothyroidism Precautions

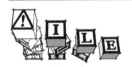 **Restrict massage to Incremental, Light and Energy techniques.**

 If the client cannot get warm and acts lethargic or drowsy, stop or avoid massage and have client call their physician or emergency medical care. They are in no condition to drive and need treatment without delay.

 Avoid deep pressure techniques. Limit the duration and intensity of your sessions until you and the client recognize their limitations.

Hypothyroidism Precautions, cont'd.

 Warning: Cardiovascular conditions are common due to the influences of insufficient thyroid hormone levels. Be thorough in your client history to best determine all necessary precautions.

 Thyroid replacement hormones are the drugs of choice in hypothyroidism often accompanied by long-term corticosteroid use. Medicines for individual symptoms or other conditions may complicate this condition; review all medicines and their precautions for massage.

 Consistent massage may play a vital role in the emotional and physical quality of life for the client suffering from hypothyroidism.

Erectile Dysfunction (ED)

While obviously beyond the scope of practice for the massage profession, ED has been included in this section because of the increasing prevalence of the U.S. population to treat it with medication. A complete list of these drugs is at the end of this chapter.

Erectile dysfunction (also called *impotence*) is the inability to achieve or maintain an erection for sexual intercourse. ED may be a result of a variety of factors, ranging from chronic diseases and medications to psychological factors. Common diseases such as diabetes, high blood pressure, atherosclerosis (hardening of the arteries), thyroid problems, and alcoholism may also cause erectile dysfunction. Up to 25 percent of cases of erectile dysfunction can result from medication side effects.

Erectile Dysfunction Precautions

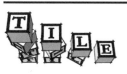 **Tolerance, Incremental, Light and Energy techniques are all encouraged within the scope of professional massage.**

Erectile Dysfunction Precautions, cont'd.

 Undiagnosed ED can be a warning sign of advanced diabetes, peripheral artery disease, or a dangerous medication side effect. Have the client consult with their physician in all cases.

 Within the scope of massage practice there are no precautions for any full body technique.

 Medication classes used in the treatment of erectile dysfunction include alkaloids, phosphodiesterase enzyme inhibitors, and certain androgens. Check the client's medications for specific precautions.

 Whether you became aware of your client's condition through your examination of their medications or through discussion with the client, it should be considered strictly taboo. Following this guideline is best for professional liability as well as ethical reasons, and you are likely to be regarded with appreciation by your client for your discretion.

Infertility

While obviously beyond the scope of practice for the massage profession, infertility has been included in this section primarily because of the medication involved. A complete list of these drugs is at the end of this chapter.

Infertility affects the male or female reproductive system almost equally. 25 percent of infertile couples have more than one factor that contributes to their infertility, including physical, emotional and lifestyle challenges.

Up to 90 percent of infertility cases are treated with medication or surgery. *Assisted reproductive technologies* (ART) are laboratory procedures to successfully induce conception. This includes *in-vitro fertilization* (IVF), which accounts for only 5 percent of all treatments for infertility.

Infertility Precautions

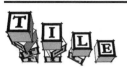

Tolerance, Incremental, Light and Energy techniques are all encouraged within the scope of professional massage.

 Consult with the physician about any procedure that you are unfamiliar with before your massage session in order to have a complete understanding of the necessary precautions.

 Avoid deep abdominal massage, as you have no way of knowing if conception has occurred.

 Warning: Be knowledgeable and very specific in your techniques concerning the hands, feet, and Achilles tendons to avoid the possibility of stimulating abortion triggers.

 Many drugs can be used to treat infertility, including biguanides, dopamine agonists, estrogen agonist-antagonists, gonadotropin-releasing hormone agents, gonadotropin-releasing hormone analogs, gonadotropins, and thiazolidinediones. Be sure to ask about current medications and check their precautions.

 Supporting both partners in reducing their stress and tension through massage for those dealing with fertility challenges will be appreciated.

Pregnancy

An amazing and awe-inspiring metamorphosis occurs at the moment of conception. The ingrained self-awareness, survival instincts, physical and emotional growth and mental values of a woman are now forced to compete with a powerful new reality. A pregnant female has arguably the most vital job on earth, and the conflicts between the old rules and the new can be dramatic and disconcerting. Nutrients used for maintenance and growth are now redirected for fetal development, even if the mother suffers from the loss. Hormone levels change dramatically throughout the development of the infant, wreaking havoc on mental and physical stability.

Many conditions temporarily disappear during pregnancy, such as those that are driven by monthly hormonal changes (e.g. endometriosis and dysmenorrhea). A wide array of new conditions develop, however, and the therapist must be on guard for these. Do not be lulled into a sense of complacency stemming from knowledge of a client's condition before they became pregnant. Be alert and responsive to the following pregnancy-specific conditions.

Pregnancy-induced diabetes (*gestational diabetes*) is possible, causing circulatory and nervous system challenges (see diabetes). *Pregnancy-induced hypertension* (PIH) is a common and potentially serious malady. Most often it is limited to hypertension, causing elevated stress on the heart and a reduced ability to deliver nutrients to the baby. *Pre-eclampsia* is more serious. It combines the challenges of hypertension with systemic edema and excess proteins in the urine. The most severe form of PIH is *eclampsia*, which involves seizures and multiple organ dysfunctions and threatens the life of both the mother and child.

Pregnancy Precautions

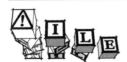 **Restrict massage to Incremental, Light and Energy techniques.**

 If the client has developed any of the following warning symptoms, stop or avoid massage and seek emergency medical attention immediately: Chest discomfort, pain or discomfort in one or both arms, the back, neck, jaw or stomach, labored breathing, breaking out in a cold sweat, nausea or lightheadedness, seizure or loss of consciousness. Stop the massage and assist them in seeking immediate medical attention.

 Avoid deep abdominal massage throughout the pregnancy term.

 Avoid TOLERANCE techniques and aggressive stretching as ligament instability and fatigue are both increased. Work within the restrictions imposed by the client and their physician. If edema is present, limit the duration and intensity of lower extremity pressure massage.

Pregnancy Precautions, cont'd.

 Warning: Carefully consider your options before laying the pregnant mother prone during any stage, even before she is actually showing. Increased pressure on the infant is always of high concern even if the client verbally gives consent, and alternative positions will allow for a more relaxing experience both mentally and physically.

 Warning: Reduce the duration and intensity of pressure techniques to guard against overworking the cardiovascular system. Be knowledgeable and very specific in your techniques concerning the hands, feet, and Achilles tendons to avoid the possibility of stimulating abortion triggers.

 Reactions to medications change with pregnancy and become potentially more dangerous. Thoroughly check each current medication for massage precautions.

 Gentle massage can offer wonderful stability to the pregnant woman at a time of great mental and physical instability. Give the gift of relaxation and it will be gratefully received -- by the mother as well as her infant.

Dysmenorrhea

Approximately 40 percent of adult females in the U.S. have menstrual pain, and 10 percent are incapacitated for up to 3 days each month. Dysmenorrhea means painful menstrual cramps. *Primary dysmenorrhea* is the direct result of peak levels of *prostaglandins* at menses. Prostaglandins are naturally occurring body chemicals that induce pain, inflammation and fever. This results in increased painful uterine contractions. *Secondary dysmenorrhea* may be from excessive prostaglandin production, as well as an underlying pathology such as endometriosis, pelvic inflammatory disease, infection or other underlying disease.

Dysmenorrhea Precautions

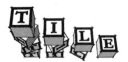 **Tolerance, Incremental, Light and Energy techniques are all encouraged.**

 Severe, debilitating pain, severe or abnormal bleeding, pain radiating down one or both legs, or pronounced vomiting are all signs of a possible medical emergency. Postpone massage until the client has been cleared for massage by a physician.

 Avoid abdominal massage during any pain cycle because there is no way the therapist can distinguish between primary and secondary dysmenorrhea. Abdominal massage may be helpful during other times of the cycle, as long as there is no discomfort with pressure.

 Prostaglandin inhibitors such as NSAIDS are commonly prescribed, as are contraceptive medications. Be sure to ask what medications the client has taken in the last 24 hours and check their precautions.

 Dysmenorrhea can be perplexing to treat. Remember that no other health care profession approaches the body as you do, and your techniques may very well be the hidden key to providing lasting relief.

Pelvic Inflammatory Disease (PID)

Pelvic inflammatory disease is caused by organisms ascending to the upper female genital tract from the vagina and cervix. It encompasses a group of infections including *endometritis*, *salpingitis*, *tuboovarian abscess*, and *peritonitis*. PID is the single most frequent serious infection encountered by women in the U.S., afflicting more than 1 million women each year.

Symptoms include lower abdominal pain, low back pain, vaginal discharge and bleeding, nausea, vomiting and fever. Often the beginning symptoms are mild and not recognized as dangerous until the infection has gained a dangerous foothold. Untreated, PID causes scarring and can lead to infertility, tubal pregnancy, chronic pelvic pain, and other serious consequences.

Immediate treatment upon diagnosis includes antibiotics, pain medication, and IV fluids if dehydrated.

Pelvic Inflammatory Disease Precautions

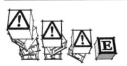 **Energy techniques only. Avoid all pressure and circulatory massage techniques.**

 Avoid all pressure massage until the infection has been eliminated and the physician has given approval.

 Warning: Pelvic and abdominal pain with pressure massage is a symptom in many conditions and must be investigated without delay.

 The client may remain on medication even after the physician feels that massage is safe. Check all current medications for precautions.

 The client recovering from **PID** will welcome the stress relieving and relaxing benefits that your techniques have to offer. Even during their ordeal, ENERGY techniques can provide a nurturing environment for accelerated healing.

Endometriosis

Endometriosis occurs when tissue like that which lines the uterus (the *endometrium*) grows outside the uterus. When menses occurs the endometrium sheds cells and builds new tissue. Because it is outside the uterus, but inside the abdominal cavity, the blood and tissue shed from endometrial growths has no way of leaving the body.

Before and during menses, endometriosis commonly causes increased pain, as well as painful urination and defecation. Other symptoms can include fatigue, diarrhea, constipation, nausea, and pain during intercourse. Infertility is often a result of endometrial growths outside the uterus.

The causes of endometriosis are yet unclear. Hormone replacement therapy can accelerate the growths. There is a genetic likelihood that children of those with endometriosis will develop the condition, as well as those exposed to environmental toxins such as *dioxin* (found in pesticides and paper manufacturing waste). It is a chronic condition that frequently results in surgery after an extended trial of medication. Surgery to remove endometrial tissue can range from a minimally invasive procedure through the bellybutton (called *laparoscopy*), to a far more invasive removal of reproductive organs (called a *hysterectomy*).

Endometriosis Precautions

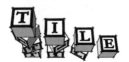 **Tolerance, Incremental, Light and Energy techniques are all encouraged.**

 Severe, debilitating pain, severe or abnormal bleeding, pain radiating down one or both legs, or pronounced vomiting are all signs of a possible medical emergency. Postpone massage until the client has been cleared for massage by a physician.

 Avoid abdominal massage after any surgery until the physician has given specific approval.

 Avoid abdominal massage before and during menses, as the increased circulation will likely aggravate their condition. Avoid deep abdominal massage at other times, for the same reason.

 Medications used to treat endometriosis include NSAIDS, contraceptives, androgens and gonadotropin-releasing hormone analogs. Check the client's medications for specific precautions.

 Techniques that calm and relax the body and minimize the inflammatory nature of the endometrial tissue can provide a safe harbor for the client with this chronic, challenging condition.

Polycystic Ovary Syndrome (PCOS)

(also called ovarian cysts, Stein-Leventhal syndrome)

When one of the eggs in the ovaries matures but does not drop into the fallopian tube, it produces a fluid filled sac known as an *ovarian cyst*. Up to 10 percent of U.S. women of childbearing age develop one or more cysts on their ovaries. This is known as polycystic ovary syndrome.

Symptoms of PCOS include infrequent or absent menstrual periods, infertility, chronic pelvic pain, weight gain, insulin resistance, high blood pressure, excessive hair growth on the face, chest, and torso with thinning scalp hair, patches of thick, darkened skin on the neck, groin, underarms, and skin tags. Women with PCOS are at a higher risk of developing cardiovascular disease type 2 diabetes, and symptoms of depression.

A laparoscopic surgery called *ovarian drilling* is available to treat PCOS. A physician makes several punctures in the ovary with an electrified probe to destroy a small portion of the ovary. The success rate is less than 50 percent, and there is a risk of developing adhesions or scar tissue on the ovary. More invasive surgery includes total removal of one or both ovaries.

Polycystic Ovary Syndrome Precautions

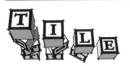 **Tolerance, Incremental, Light and Energy techniques are all encouraged.**

 Avoid abdominal massage after any surgery until the physician has given specific approval.

 Avoid deep abdominal massage, and avoid any massage in the area of the ovaries. An increase in pressure can result in an inflammatory reaction or rupture of a cyst.

 Warning: Secondary conditions are common, including cardiovascular diseases and diabetes. Be thorough in your notetaking and check all conditions for precautions.

Polycystic Ovary Syndrome Precautions, cont'd.

 Warning: Be extra cautious with pressure. If the client appears to have difficulty determining appropriate pressure, recommend they see their physician for a checkup.

 Biguanides are often used in the treatment of PCOS, as are blood sugar regulating medications and contraceptives. Be sure to ask about all current medications and check their precautions.

 Precautions are limited to the abdomen, unless there are complicating conditions as discussed above. Your full range of massage techniques are welcome, and will help minimize the mental and physical stresses associated with PCOS.

Fibroid Tumors

(also called uterine fibroids, leiomyomas, and myomas)

Fibroid tumors affect more than 30 percent of women in their childbearing years, yet since they rarely cause symptoms, most are unaware of their presence until revealed by examination. Fibroids tend to grow as a woman gets older and shrink after the onset of menopause.

Possible symptoms include bleeding between periods, heavy menstrual periods, or pain during intercourse. The fibroid may grow large enough to aggravate the functioning of the reproductive system and may be a cause of infertility.

Most fibroids do not cause symptoms, and do not require treatment. If the fibroid appears to be growing rapidly or is causing other health concerns, medications controlling the gonadotropin-releasing hormone are initially used. Surgery to remove the fibroid can range from minimally invasive laparoscopy to a complete removal of the uterus and full hysterectomy.

Fibroid Tumor Precautions

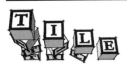 **Tolerance, Incremental, Light and Energy techniques are all encouraged.**

 Avoid abdominal massage after any surgery until the physician has given specific approval.

 Avoid deep abdominal massage for diagnosed cases of fibroid tumors to avoid the possibility of trauma.

 GnRH medications are the drugs of choice, along with other medications to treat the symptoms as needed. Be sure to ask about current medications and check their precautions.

 Fibroid tumors are largely unrelated to the practice of massage. With the above precautions in mind, you can best help the client attain a sense of normalcy by focusing on full-body therapies without restriction.

Perimenopause and Menopause

Perimenopause is not a disease. It is a label describing changes in the menstrual cycle with women ages 35 to 55, including changes in the discomfort intensity, flow or timing. It causes a wide range of symptoms including hot flashes, night sweats, vaginal dryness, sleep problems, mood changes, pain during intercourse, urinary incontinence, an increase in body fat, and problems with concentration or memory.

Menopause has been reached when there has been 12 consecutive months without menses. It is a natural stage in life, not a disease, unless something acts to hasten its arrival. Induced menopause occurs suddenly after a complete hysterectomy in which the ovaries (one major source of estrogen), uterus and fallopian tubes are removed. Premature menopause occurs in women under the age of 40 who have had cancer, medicines or other conditions that accelerate the loss of female hormones. The symptoms are the same as in perimenopause, with the addition of an increased likelihood of bone loss (see osteoporosis) and cardiovascular disease.

Perimenopause and Menopause Precautions

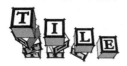 **Tolerance, Incremental, Light and Energy techniques are all encouraged.**

 If there has been a recent history of falling (in the last few weeks), avoid massage until the client has consulted a physician. Do not trust that all fractures are accompanied by pain, as there may be medications or other conditions (such as peripheral neuropathy) that mask the discomfort.

 Avoid TOLERANCE and INCREMENTAL techniques for those with a history of osteoporosis, and be especially careful with pressure on the torso. There are no visible signs to determine if a client has bone loss. Because osteoporosis is so hidden and so common, extra care should be taken with women over 50 years of age.

 Medications to improve bone density, hormone replacements, and antidepressives are all likely to be prescribed during this stage of life. Check all medications for additional precautions.

 The nurturing effect of massage can have dramatic effects, especially for a woman going through this change in their life.

Hernias

A hernia is an abnormal protrusion of one body part from one anatomic space to another. More than a half million hernia operations are performed in the United States each year. Hernias are the leading cause of intestinal obstruction in the world. Some are dangerous and require prompt medical attention. For example, *intestinal strangulation* (where blood supply is cut off) can lead to death of the tissue (called *gangrene*) in as little as 6 hours!

Common types of hernias include the following:

Inguinal Hernia

These make up 75 percent of all abdominal wall hernias and occur up to 25 times more often in men than women. They occur in the area where the skin crease at the top of the thigh joins the torso (the inguinal crease), and they may appear as a bulge in the inguinal crease. The *"indirect" inguinal hernia* follows the path leading to and may protrude into the scrotum. The *"direct" inguinal hernia* occurs slightly to the inside of the site of the indirect hernia, in a place where the abdominal wall is slightly thinner. It rarely protrudes into the scrotum.

Inguinal hernias show as a bulge in the groin or scrotum, which may or may not be tender to the touch. The bulge may appear gradually over a period of several weeks, or it may form suddenly after strenuous activity.

Surgery is often performed through an incision near the bulge or through the bellybutton. Gentle activity like walking may resume within days, but strenuous activities are discouraged for several weeks.

Femoral Hernia

The femoral canal is the way that the femoral artery, vein, and nerve leave the abdominal cavity to enter the thigh. A loop of intestine may be forced into this tight canal and is then in danger of being strangulated. Symptoms include groin discomfort or pain aggravated by bending or lifting, with a tender lump in the groin or upper thigh.

Surgery occurs through a small incision near the bulge or possibly through the bellybutton, and a mesh is often used to patch the weakened abdominal wall. Gentle activity like walking may resume within days, but strenuous activities are discouraged for several weeks.

Umbilical Hernia

This type of hernia is caused when an opening in the abdominal wall, which normally closes before birth, doesn't close completely, forming a protrusion at the bellybutton. It may be present at birth, or may be revealed much later in pregnancy or the elderly when extra pressure is exerted on the weakened area. If it appears after age 3 it will not go away on its own and strapping or taping it is not recommended. If the bulge becomes firm and unyielding, it often means a blockage has occurred and is a signal for immediate medical attention.

Surgery is minimally invasive and often includes a mesh to prevent reoccurrence, and full activity can be resumed in two to four weeks.

Hiatal Hernia

This common condition can be the underlying cause of gastroesophageal reflux disease (see GERD). It often occurs during or soon after eating, when the esophageal opening in the diaphragm is relaxed to allow food to enter the stomach. If the neck of the stomach is forced up into the diaphragm opening it can become trapped. This prevents the lower esophageal sphincter from working properly, which can allow acidic stomach contents to irritate the esophagus. It can also eliminate the protective bend in the esophagus as it attaches to the stomach (called the angle of His), making it even easier for acids to reflux.

Symptoms of a hiatal hernia are similar to those with GERD, including cramping or nausea after eating, heartburn or an acid taste in the back of your throat, and constipation or bowel changes.

Unlike the other hernias listed above, conservative treatments are strongly recommended before surgical intervention. Massage to relax the diaphragmatic spasm has been very effective when combined with postural restrictions. Staying in an upright posture without slouching throughout the meal and for an hour after is vital to the success of both conservative and medical treatments. Surgery to widen the diaphragm opening and attach the stomach is largely ineffective without post-surgical training.

Hernia Precautions

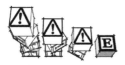 **Avoid all pressure and circulatory massage techniques in the affected area(s). Energy techniques only. Your full technique range is encouraged for the rest of the body.**

 Avoid massage on or around a suspected hernia, and avoid positions that place pressure on the area. Any suspicious area should be examined by a physician without delay, and any firm, tender bulge in the areas listed above should be considered a medical emergency.

Hernia Precautions, cont'd.

 Avoid local massage near recently repaired hernias for a minimum of 6 weeks (both the incision scar and the area where the hernia resulted). Be cautious with stretching these tissues for two to four months, and avoid deep tissue techniques to the area until the physician has given approval.

 The client may be on temporary post-surgical medications that have specific precautions for massage. Those with hiatal hernias have a myriad of medication choices that may change frequently. Keep up on your client's current medicines and their precautions.

 Once massage is approved for post-surgical hernia repair it can be extremely helpful to minimize the restrictive adhesions formed from inactivity. Your techniques may also be very much appreciated with clients suffering from hiatal hernia.

Benign Prostatic Hyperplasia (BPH)

It is common for the prostate gland to become enlarged as a man ages. This is a condition known as benign prostatic hyperplasia. More than half of men over age 60 will have symptoms from BPH, and this increases to a 90 percent likelihood after age 70. The cause is not known, but some researchers believe that factors related to aging and the testes may spur the development of BPH. It is unrelated to prostate cancer.

Symptoms of BPH involve the urinary system: Weak, difficult urinary stream, an inability to hold urine without leakage, and increasingly frequent urges to urinate. Most treatment begins with medicines to control the inflammation and possible infection. If drugs alone aren't effective, a surgical process called TURP is used. *Trans-Urethral Resection of the Prostate* is a procedure in which prostate tissue is removed to allow space for the urethra. It is performed by inserting the instruments through the urethra, thereby eliminating the need for external scarring.

Another surgical procedure is called *Trans-Urethral Incision of the Prostate* (TUIP). Instead of removing prostate tissue, this procedure widens the urethra by making a few small cuts in the bladder neck, where the urethra joins the bladder, and in the prostate gland itself.

Benign Prostatic Hyperplasia Precautions

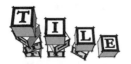 **Tolerance, Incremental, Light and Energy techniques are all encouraged.**

 Avoid abdominal massage for clients who have undergone BPH surgery until you have specific approval from their physician. In addition, during this time avoid all techniques that may require the client to hold their breath, especially TOLERANCE techniques. This increases internal pressure and can be dangerous.

 If the client complains of a full bladder and an inability to urinate, seek emergency medical attention immediately. Additionally, complaints of burning upon urination or pain in the back of the ribs (kidney pain) can be signs of an infection. Avoid massage and seek medical attention.

 The client may be unable to last through an entire session without a bathroom break. Anticipate this possibility and offer the break to eliminate the need for the client to ask. This will allow the client to relax more completely.

 Drug classes used to treat benign prostatic hyperplasia include alpha blockers, antihypertensives, benzodiazepines, 5-alpha reductase inhibitors and antiprostatitis medications. Infections are treated with antibiotics. Be sure to ask about current medications and check their precautions.

 Being proactive with the special needs of your elderly clients while offering them a relaxing, healing environment will surely earn their gratitude and loyalty.

Endocrine and Reproductive System Medications

5-Alpha Reductase Inhibitors

This class of medication inhibits the production of the hormone *dihydrotestosterone* (DHT), a hormone that may be responsible for prostate enlargement.

 If the client reports any of the following serious side effects, stop or avoid all massage and seek emergency medical attention: Mental confusion, a severe headache, difficulty breathing, closing of the throat, swelling of the lips, tongue, or face, or hives. (This is a massage-specific list; refer to the documentation that was included with the medication for a complete list of side effects.)

 Side Effects: Skin rash, impotence, and *gynecomastia* (increase in breast size) all can occur with this class of medication.

 5-alpha reductase inhibitor medications include: <u>dutasteride1</u> (Avodart) and <u>finasteride</u> (Proscar).

Anticonvulsants

The medications in this class act on the body in a slightly different fashion, and so a client may have used one or more in the past and switched when its effectiveness wanes. Primarily used for controlling seizures, they can also be prescribed for chronic pain or severe pain (like shingles) when other pain relievers have failed.

 If the client has developed any of the following, avoid massage and have them call their doctor immediately: An unexplained or sudden rash, easy bruising, swelling of the feet or lower legs, difficulty breathing; swelling of the lips, tongue, throat, or face, difficulty with concentration, speech, or language, excessive sleepiness or fatigue, loss of coordination, difficulty walking, or blurred vision. (This is a massage-specific list; refer to the documentation that was included with the medication for a complete list of side effects.)

Anticonvulsant Precautions, cont'd.

 Schedule the session at a time when the medication is at its peak effectiveness (e.g. carbamazepine peaks at least four hours after taking a dose, so a massage would best be scheduled at least four hours after ingestion).

 Side Effects: Headaches, peripheral edema, tremors, dizziness, stomach pain, and constipation all can occur with this class of medication. Take these into consideration as they may limit your ability to achieve your client's massage goals.

 Postural hypotension can occur as a side effect of this class of medication. Help the client to change positions and be on guard for dizziness or blacking out.

 Anticonvulsant medications include: <u>carbamazepine</u> (Atretol, Carba-trol, Depitol, Epitol, Tegretol), <u>divalproex</u> (Depakote, Epival), <u>ethotoin</u> (Peganone), <u>felbamate</u> (Felbatol), <u>fosphenytoin</u> (Cerebyx), <u>gabapentin</u> (Neurontin), <u>lamotrigine</u> (Lamictal), <u>levetiracetam</u> (Keppra), <u>oxcarbazepine</u> (Trileptal), <u>phenytoin</u> (Dilantin, Phenytek), <u>primidone</u> (Mysoline), <u>tiagabine</u> (Gabitril), <u>topiramate</u> (Topamax), <u>valproic acid</u> (Depakene), and <u>zonisamide</u> (Zonegran).

Alkaloid Medications

Alkaloid medications are used in the management of erectile dysfunction (ED).

 If the client reports any of the following serious side effects, stop or avoid all massage and seek emergency medical attention: Mental confusion, a severe headache, difficulty breathing, closing of the throat, swelling of the lips, tongue, or face, or hives. (This is a massage-specific list; refer to the documentation that was included with the medication for a complete list of side effects.)

Alkaloid Medication Precautions, cont'd.

 Side Effects: Headaches, increased heart rate, sweating, nervousness, tremor, irritability, dizziness and flushing all can occur with this class of medication. Take these into consideration as they may limit your ability to achieve your client's massage goals.

 Alkaloid medications include <u>yohimbine</u> (Aphrodyne, Dayto Himbin, Yocon, Yohimex).

Alopecia and Antiprostatitis Medications

There are two medical hair loss treatments available. Finasteride prevents the conversion of testosterone to dihydrotestosterone (DHT) in the body. DHT is involved in the development of benign prostatic hyperplasia (BPH) and hair loss. Minoxidil is a lotion and works by stimulating new hair growth.

 If the client reports any of the following serious side effects, stop or avoid all massage and seek emergency medical attention: Mental confusion, a severe headache, difficulty breathing, closing of the throat, swelling of the lips, tongue, or face, or hives. (This is a massage-specific list; refer to the documentation that was included with the medication for a complete list of side effects.)

 Side Effects: Skin rash, impotence, and *gynecomastia* (increase in breast size) all can occur with this class of medication.

 Alopecia and antiprostatitis medications include <u>finasteride</u> (Propecia, Proscar) and <u>minoxidil</u> (Rogaine, Ronoxidil).

Androgens

(also called anabolic androgenic steroids, (AAS), anabolic steroids)

Androgens are prescribed to replace deficiencies in the production of testosterone. They stimulate red blood cell production, stimulate cells that produce male sex characteristics and suppress the production of estrogen.

Individual medications in this class are used to treat endometriosis, fibrocystic breast disease, osteoporosis, anemia, and other conditions. Androgens are also used by athletes and bodybuilders to dramatically stimulate muscle growth. Non-prescribed usage of anabolic steroids poses a life-threatening health risk.

 This class of medication can create breathing difficulties, angina, and abnormal heart rate. Pay special attention to the client's breathing patterns and blood pressure throughout the visit. These are considered medical emergencies. Stop massage and call physician or emergency assistance if abnormalities occur.

 If the client has developed the following, avoid massage and have them call their doctor immediately: An unexplained skin rash, persistent or severe headache, persistent upset stomach or abdominal pain.

 Limit your massage to LIGHT and ENERGY techniques if the client is also taking anticoagulants, as the combination increases the chance of excessive bruising and internal bleeding.

 Side Effects: Headaches, muscle cramps, weight gain, and edema are side effects that may occur as a result of this class of medication. Take these into consideration as they may limit your ability to achieve your client's massage goals.

 Androgen medications include: <u>aldosterone</u>, <u>danazol</u> (Cyclomen, Danocrine), <u>ethylestrenol</u> (Orabolin), <u>fludrocortisone</u> (Florinef), <u>fluoxymesterone</u> (Halotestin), <u>methyltestosterone</u> (Android, Methitest, Testred, Virilon), <u>nandrolone</u>, <u>oxandrolone</u> (Oxandrin), <u>oxymetholone</u> (Anadrol), <u>stanozolol</u> (Winstrol), and <u>testosterone</u> (Andro, Androderm, AndroGel, Andronate, Andropository, Andryl, Delatest, Delatestryl, Depotest, Durabolin, Everone, Hybolin, Kabolin, Methitest, Oreton, Testamone, Testaqua, Testex, Testoderm, Testopel, Testrin).

Anterior Pituitary Medications

Hormones secreted by the anterior pituitary gland and regulated by the hypothalamus control the adrenals, testes and ovaries. An imbalance can cause fertility and menstrual difficulties as well as growth abnormalities.

 If the client reports any of the following serious side effects, stop or avoid all massage and seek emergency medical attention: Painful urination, testicular or prostate pain, or pain in the legs or groin; A severe headache; difficulty breathing; closing of the throat; swelling of the lips, tongue, or face; or hives. (This is a massage-specific list; refer to the documentation that was included with the medication for a complete list of side effects.)

 Long-term or ongoing medication use: Avoid deep pressure massage and stretching techniques. There is an increased likelihood of trauma with long-term use, as the soft tissues and bones become increasingly fragile. Consider limiting the session to LIGHT and ENERGY techniques if there is concern about tissue strength.

 Side Effects: Headaches, stomach pain, nausea or vomiting, mood changes, breast tenderness or breast swelling all can occur with this class of medication. Adjust your massage therapy accordingly to take these into account. Take these into consideration as they may limit your ability to achieve your client's massage goals.

 Anterior pituitary medications include: corticotropin (Acthar), cosyntropin (Cortrosyn), follitropin (Follistim, Gonal-F), Human Chorionic Gonadotropin (APL, Chorex, Choron, Gonic, Novarel, Pregnyl, Profasi), menotropins (Humegon, Pergonal, Repronex), somatrem (Protropin), thyrotropin (Thyrogen, Thyroid Stimulating Hormone), and urofollitropin (Bravelle, Fertinex, Metrodin).

Posterior Pituitary Medications

Hormones secreted by the posterior pituitary gland regulate fluid volumes. They are also used in some circumstances to stimulate smooth muscle contraction.

 If the client reports any of the following serious side effects, stop or avoid all massage and seek emergency medical attention: Severe headache; difficulty breathing; closing of the throat; swelling of the lips, tongue, or face; or hives. (This is a massage-specific list; refer to the documentation that was included with the medication for a complete list of side effects.)

 Long-term or ongoing medication use: Avoid deep pressure massage and stretching techniques. There is an increased likelihood of trauma with long-term use, as the soft tissues and bones become increasingly fragile. Consider limiting the session to LIGHT and ENERGY techniques if there is concern about tissue strength.

 Side Effects: Headaches, stomach pain, nausea or vomiting, mood changes and genital tenderness all can occur with this class of medication. Take these into consideration as they may limit your ability to achieve your client's massage goals.

 Postural hypotension can occur as a side effect of this class of medication. Help the client to change positions and be on guard for dizziness or blacking out.

 Posterior pituitary medications include: <u>antidiuretic hormone</u> (ADH), <u>desmopressin</u> (DDAVP, Octostim, Stimate), <u>oxytocin</u> (Pitocin, Syntocinon), and <u>vasopressin</u> (Pitressin, Pressyn).

---

*Your client places great value
in the extra effort you take in
researching their condition.*

Emergency Contraception Medications

(also called "the morning after pill," RU-486)

This medication causes termination of a pregnancy by blocking the effects of the progesterone hormone, which is necessary to maintain a pregnancy.

 If the client reports any of the following serious side effects, stop or avoid all massage and seek emergency medical attention: Mental confusion, a severe headache, difficulty breathing, closing of the throat, swelling of the lips, tongue, or face, or hives. (This is a massage-specific list; refer to the documentation that was included with the medication for a complete list of side effects.)

 Side Effects: Cramps, upset stomach, headaches, diarrhea and vomiting, pelvic pain, dizziness and fainting are possible side effects of this medication. Take these into consideration as they may limit your ability to achieve your client's massage goals.

 Emergency contraception medications include <u>mifepristone</u> (Mifeprex).

Menstrual Regulation and Contraceptive Medications

(also called birth control pills, BCP)

This grouping of medications are all used to prevent pregnancy or to regulate the menstrual cycle.

 If the client reports any of the following serious side effects, stop or avoid all massage and seek emergency medical attention: Pain in the calves, numbness or tingling in the arms or legs, A severe headache; difficulty breathing; closing of the throat; swelling of the lips, tongue, or face; or hives. (This is a massage-specific list; refer to the documentation that was included with the medication for a complete list of side effects.)

Menstrual Regulation and Contraceptive Medication Precautions, cont'd.

 Side Effects: Swelling of the hands or feet, skin rash, and brown or black skin patches all can occur with this class of medication. Take these into consideration as they may limit your ability to achieve your client's massage goals.

 Postural hypotension can occur as a side effect of this class of medication. Help the client to change positions and be on guard for dizziness or blacking out.

 Menstrual regulation and contraceptive medications include: ethinyl estradiol (Estinyl), norgestrel (Ovrette), beta-estradiol with norgestimate (Ortho-Prefest), ethinyl estradiol with desogestrel (Apri, Cyclessa, Desogen, Kariva, Mircette, Ortho-Cept, Velivet), ethinyl estradiol with drospirenone (Yasmin), ethinyl estradiol with ethynodiol diacetate (Demulen, Zovia), ethinyl estradiol with levonorgestrel (Aviane, Aviave, Enpresse, Lessina, Levlen, Levlite, Levora, Nordette, Portia, Seasonale, Tri-Levlen, Triphasil, Trivora), ethinyl estradiol with norgestimate (Mononessa, Ortho Tri-Cyclen, Ortho-Cyclen, Sprintec, Tri-Sprintec, TriNessa), ethinyl estradiol with norgestrel (Cryselle, Lo/Ovral, Low-Ogestrel, Ogestrel, Ovral), and ethinyl estradiol with norelgestromin (Ortho Evra).

Dopamine Agonists

Dopamine agonists are used to inhibit the production of prolactin by the pituitary gland. They are used in women whose infertility is caused by high levels of *prolactin*, a hormone produced by the pituitary gland that (along with estrogen and progesterone) stimulates breast development and milk production during pregnancy. If prolactin levels are too high, a lack of menses (*amenorrhea*) may occur. Prolactin is also present in males, and if levels get too high it can cause reduced sexual potency or impotence.

Dopamine Agonist Precautions

 If the client reports any of the following serious side effects, stop or avoid all massage and seek emergency medical attention: Mental confusion, a severe headache, difficulty breathing, closing of the throat, swelling of the lips, tongue, or face, or hives. (This is a massage-specific list; refer to the documentation that was included with the medication for a complete list of side effects.)

 Side Effects: Unusual weakness or fatigue, nausea or vomiting, constipation, headache, drowsiness, tingling or numbness in the extremities all can occur with this class of medication. Take these into consideration as they may limit your ability to achieve your client's massage goals.

 Postural hypotension can occur as a side effect of this class of medication. Help the client to change positions and be on guard for dizziness or blacking out.

 Dopamine agonist medications include <u>cabergoline</u> (Dostinex).

Estrogens and Progesterones

These medications mimic the effects of the naturally occurring hormones. In addition to balancing hormone levels, some (like medroxyprogesterone) are used as an injected temporary contraceptive.

 If the client has developed any of the following symptoms, avoid massage and have them call their doctor immediately: Sudden, severe headache, severe vomiting, sudden partial or complete loss of vision, speech problems, weakness or numbness of an arm or leg, sudden shortness of breath or chest pain, calf pain, severe abdominal pain, or any unexplained rash.

 Side Effects: Edema of hands, feet, or lower legs, stomach cramps, diarrhea, increased blood pressure, brown or black skin patches, bleeding or spotting between menstrual periods, and breast tenderness all can occur with this class of medication. Take these into consideration as they may limit your ability to achieve your client's massage goals.

Estrogen and Progesterone Precautions, cont'd.

 Postural hypotension can occur as a side effect of this class of medication. Help the client to change positions and be on guard for dizziness or blacking out.

 Estrogen and progesterone medications include: <u>calcitonin</u> (Calcimar, Miacalcin), <u>estrogens</u> (Alora, Cenestin, Climara, Estraderm Patch, FemPatch, Vivelle, DepoGen, DepGynogen, Estrace, Estradiol, Estratab, Gynodiol, Menest, Premarin), <u>estradiol</u> with <u>norethindrone</u> (Activella), <u>medroxyprogesterone</u> (Amen, Depo-Provera, Curretab, Cycrin, Premphase, Prempro, Provera), <u>progesterone</u> (Crinone, Gesterol, Prochieve, Progestasert) <u>raloxifene</u> (Evista), <u>teriparatide</u> (Forteo).

Estrogen Agonist-Antagonists

Estrogen agonist-antagonists work by stimulating the pituitary gland to release certain hormones that trigger ovulation.

 If the client reports any of the following serious side effects, stop or avoid all massage and seek emergency medical attention: Stomach pain and/or vomiting, a severe headache, difficulty breathing, closing of the throat, swelling of the lips, tongue, or face, or hives. (This is a massage-specific list; refer to the documentation that was included with the medication for a complete list of side effects.)

 Side Effects: Headaches, dizziness, nausea, tiredness, bleeding or spotting between menstrual periods and breast tenderness all can occur with this class of medication. Take these into consideration as they may limit your ability to achieve your client's massage goals.

 Postural hypotension can occur as a side effect of this class of medication. Help the client to change positions and be on guard for dizziness or blacking out.

 Estrogen agonist-antagonist medications include <u>clomiphene</u> (Clomid, Milophene, Serophene).

Gonadotropin-Releasing Hormone (GnRH)

GnRH is a hormone that is secreted by the hypothalamus. It works to regulate gonadotropins. GnRH replacement therapy can be used to induce ovulation in women whose hypothalamus isn't working properly.

 If the client reports any of the following serious side effects, stop or avoid all massage and seek emergency medical attention: Skin rash or hives, difficulty in breathing, persistent skin flushing, or a rapid heartbeat. (This is a massage-specific list; refer to the documentation that was included with the medication for a complete list of side effects.)

 Side Effects: Headaches, nausea, and abdominal discomfort all can occur with this class of medication. Take these into consideration as they may limit your ability to achieve your client's massage goals.

 Gonadotropin-releasing hormone medications include gonadorelin (Factrel, Lutrepulse, Relisorm).

Gonadotropin-Releasing Hormone Analogs (GnRHa)

These drugs work basically the same way as gonadotropin-releasing hormone (GnRH) but are more potent. They are also used to help treat endometriosis and certain types of cancer.

 If the client reports any of the following serious side effects, stop or avoid all massage and seek emergency medical attention: Painful urination, testicular or prostate pain, or pain in the legs or groin. Be alert for signs of an allergic reaction, such as a severe headache, difficulty breathing, closing of the throat, swelling of the lips, tongue, or face, or hives. (This is a massage-specific list; refer to the documentation that was included with the medication for a complete list of side effects.)

 Side Effects: Headaches, bone pain, hot flashes, weight gain, constipation, breast swelling and tenderness, numbness or tingling of the lower extremities, or unstable moods all can occur with this class of medication. Take these into consideration as they may limit your ability to achieve your client's massage goals.

Gonadotropin-Releasing Hormone Analog Precautions, cont'd.

 Postural hypotension can occur as a side effect of this class of medication. Help the client to change positions and be on guard for dizziness or blacking out.

 Gonadotropin-releasing hormone analog medications include: goserelin (Zoladex), leuprolide (Lupron), and nafarelin (Synarel).

Hormone Replacement Medications

Natural thyroid hormone replacement therapies are derived from pig, cow, or sheep thyroid glands, which are similar to thyroid hormones found in humans. Natural thyroid hormone replacement products work by simply replacing or supplementing low thyroid hormone levels. Synthetic thyroid hormones are created by a pharmaceutical company to mimic the naturally occurring human hormone.

 If the client has recently developed any of the following, avoid massage and call the physician immediately: An unexplained skin rash, severe headache, increased difficulty breathing, ringing in the ears, recent muscle weakness, unusual bleeding or bruising or swelling of the lips, tongue, or face. (This is a massage-specific list; refer to the documentation that was included with the medication for a complete list of side effects.)

 Side Effects: Headaches, edema, sensitivity to heat, tremors, vomiting, diarrhea, stomach cramps and excessive sweating all can occur with this class of medication. Take these into consideration as they may limit your ability to achieve your client's massage goals.

 All heat therapies should be avoided (including hot stone massage, heat pads, saunas, steam rooms, etc.) if the client is on any thyroid medication, as the client's ability to control their body temperature is compromised.

Hormone Replacement Medication Precautions, cont'd.

 Natural thyroid hormone medications include: <u>thyroglobulin</u> (Proloid), and <u>thyroid</u> (Armour Thyroid, Desiccated thyroid, S-P-T, Thyrar, Thyroid Strong, Westhroid).

 Synthetic thyroid hormone medications include: <u>levothyroxine</u> (Eltroxin, Levothroid, Levoxine, Levoxyl, Synthroid, Unithroid), <u>liothyronine</u> (Cytomel, L-Triiodothyronine), and <u>liotrix</u> (Thyrolar).

Insulins

Increasing the amount of insulin in the blood allows more glucose to be absorbed from the blood stream and into body tissue cells to provide energy.

 If the client has recently developed any of the following, avoid massage and call the physician immediately: An unexplained skin rash, severe headache, increased difficulty breathing, ringing in the ears, recent muscle weakness, unusual bleeding or bruising or swelling of the lips, tongue, or face. (This is a massage-specific list; refer to the documentation that was included with the medication for a complete list of side effects.)

 If the client has any of the following symptoms the massage should be delayed until they have confirmed that their blood sugar levels are with normal range: Nausea, vomiting, abdominal pain, headache, shakiness, dizziness, rapid heartbeat, sweating or confusion, or blurred vision. The client should eat or inject some sugar without delay to resolve the issue. They should call their physician if symptoms do not improve within 20 minutes.

 Warning: Massage is often a stress reducer, and this can change the body's need for this class of medication. Inform the client to be aware that massage may change their insulin needs, and have them contact their physician if necessary.

 Rapid acting insulin medications include <u>insulin</u> <u>glulisine</u> (Apidra), <u>insulin</u> <u>lispro</u> (Humalog), and <u>insulin</u> <u>aspart</u> (NovoLog).

Insulin Precautions, cont'd.

 Short acting insulin medications include <u>insulin regular</u>.

 Combination insulins include: <u>Actraphane HM, Humulin 50/50, Humulin 70/30,</u> and <u>Novolin 70/30.</u>

 Intermediate acting medications include: <u>insulin isophane</u> (Humulin N, Humulin N Pen, Iletin II NPH Pork, Insulin Purified NPH Pork, Novolin N, Novolin N Innolet, Novolin N PenFill, Velosulin), and <u>insulin zinc</u> (Humulin L, Iletin Lente, Insulin Lente Pork, Novolin L).

 Long acting insulin medications include <u>Insulin Zinc Extended</u> (Humulin U).

 Very long acting insulin medications include <u>Insulin Glargine</u> (Lantus).

Meglitinides

Meglitinides stimulate the pancreas to produce insulin.

 If the client has recently developed any of the following, avoid massage and call the physician immediately: An unexplained skin rash, severe headache, increased difficulty breathing, ringing in the ears, recent muscle weakness, unusual bleeding or bruising or swelling of the lips, tongue, or face. (This is a massage-specific list; refer to the documentation that was included with the medication for a complete list of side effects.)

 Side Effects: Back or joint pain and flu-like symptoms are side effects that may occur as a result of this class of medication. Take these into consideration as they may limit your ability to achieve your client's massage goals.

 Postural hypotension can occur as a side effect of this class of medication. Help the client to change positions and be on guard for dizziness or blacking out.

 Meglitinide medications include <u>nateglinide</u> (Starlix) and <u>repaglinide</u> (Prandin).

Alpha-Glucosidase Inhibitors

Alpha-glucosidase inhibitors temporarily block enzymes that digest carbohydrates. Since your body cannot turn the carbohydrates into sugar, your blood sugar levels remain closer to normal after eating.

 If the client has recently developed any of the following, avoid massage and call the physician immediately: An unexplained skin rash, severe headache, increased difficulty breathing, ringing in the ears, recent muscle weakness, unusual bleeding or bruising or swelling of the lips, tongue, or face. (This is a massage-specific list; refer to the documentation that was included with the medication for a complete list of side effects.)

 Side Effects: Diarrhea, stomach pain, and skin rash can occur as a result of this class of medication.

 Alpha-glucosidase inhibitor medications include <u>acarbose</u> (Precose) and <u>miglitol</u> (Glyset).

Biguanides

Biguanides reduce insulin resistance in muscle cells and decrease the release of glucose from the liver. They also reduce the absorption of glucose in the small intestine, stimulate the disposal of glucose, and enhance insulin sensitivity inside the cell.

 If the client has recently developed any of the following, avoid massage and call the physician immediately: An unexplained skin rash, severe headache, recent muscle weakness or unexplained pain, increased difficulty breathing, ringing in the ears, unusual bleeding or bruising or swelling of the lips, tongue, or face. (This is a massage-specific list; refer to the documentation that was included with the medication for a complete list of side effects.)

 Side Effects: Nausea and stomach aches can occur with this class of medication.

 Biguanide medications include <u>metformin</u> (Glucophage).

Phosphodiesterase Enzyme Inhibitors

Phosphodiesterase enzyme inhibitors are used to treat erectile dysfunction (ED). These medications do not directly cause an erection of the penis, but they alter the body's response to sexual stimulation by enhancing the effect of *nitric oxide*, a chemical that is normally released during stimulation. Nitric oxide causes relaxation of the muscles in the penis, which allows for better blood flow to the penile area.

 If the client has developed a sudden rash, fainting, chest pain, itching or burning during urination, avoid all massage and have them call their doctor immediately. These drug side effects are considered very serious and require medical attention. (This is a massage-specific list; refer to the documentation that was included with the medication for a complete list of side effects.)

 Side Effects: Headaches, dizziness and diarrhea all can occur with this class of medication. Take these into consideration as they may limit your ability to achieve your client's massage goals.

 Postural hypotension can occur as a side effect of this class of medication. Help the client to change positions and be on guard for dizziness or blacking out.

 Phosphodiesterase enzyme inhibitor medications include sildenafil (Viagra), tadalafil (Cialis), and vardenafil (Levitra).

Sulfonylureas

Sulfonylureas lower glucose levels in the blood by stimulating cells in the pancreas to release more insulin.

 If the client has recently developed any of the following, avoid massage and call the physician immediately: An unexplained skin rash, severe headache, increased difficulty breathing, ringing in the ears, recent muscle weakness, unusual bleeding or bruising or swelling of the lips, tongue, or face. (This is a massage-specific list; refer to the documentation that was included with the medication for a complete list of side effects.)

Sulfonylurea Precautions, cont'd.

 Side Effects: Headaches, skin rash, nausea, vomiting and diarrhea all can occur with this class of medication. Take these into consideration as they may limit your ability to achieve your client's massage goals.

 Sulfonylurea medications include: <u>acetohexamide</u> (Dymelor), <u>chlorpropamide</u> (Diabinese), <u>glimepiride</u> (Amaryl), <u>glipizide</u> (Glucotrol), <u>glyburide</u> (DiaBeta, Glynase, Micronase), <u>tolazamide</u> (Tolinase), and <u>tolbutamide</u> (Orinase).

Thiazolidinediones

(also called glitazones)

In most people suffering from type 2 diabetes, the cells have developed an insulin resistance, which means that they do not respond to insulin in the way they should. Thiazolidinediones alter the metabolism of fatty acids so that they do not compete with glucose for metabolism in the cell, making the cells more responsive to insulin.

 If the client has recently developed any of the following, avoid massage and call the physician immediately: Nausea, vomiting, stomach pain, unexplained skin rash, severe headache, increased difficulty breathing, ringing in the ears, recent muscle weakness, unusual bleeding or bruising or swelling of the lips, tongue, or face. (This is a massage-specific list; refer to the documentation that was included with the medication for a complete list of side effects.)

 Side Effects: Headaches, muscle pain and sinus congestion all can occur with this class of medication. Take these into consideration as they may limit your ability to achieve your client's massage goals.

 Thiazolidinedione medications include <u>pioglitazone</u> (Actos) and <u>rosiglitazone</u> (Avandia).

Biguanide Combination Medications

A new trend in diabetes therapy is to combine commonly used medications into one product. Many patients require more than one medication to control their diabetes. Taking multiple medications can be difficult to remember and to plan for proper timing of doses. While combining medications into one product may help with patient compliance, it also may make dosing adjustments trickier.

Biguanides reduce insulin resistance in muscle cells and decrease the release of glucose from the liver. They also reduce the absorption of glucose in the small intestine, stimulate the disposal of glucose, and enhance insulin sensitivity inside the cell. Thiazolidinediones alter the metabolism of fatty acids so that they do not compete with glucose for metabolism in the cell, making the cells more responsive to insulin. Sulfonylureas lower levels of glucose in the blood by stimulating cells in the pancreas to release more insulin.

 If the client has recently developed any of the following, avoid massage and call the physician immediately: An unexplained skin rash, severe headache, increased difficulty breathing, ringing in the ears, recent muscle weakness, unusual bleeding or bruising or swelling of the lips, tongue, or face. (This is a massage-specific list; refer to the documentation that was included with the medication for a complete list of side effects.)

 Side Effects: Headaches, fatigue, nausea, vomiting and diarrhea all can occur with this class of medication. Take these into consideration as they may limit your ability to achieve your client's massage goals.

 Postural hypotension can occur as a side effect of this class of medication. Help the client to change positions and be on guard for dizziness or blacking out.

 Sulfonylurea and biguanide combination medications include: glipizide with metformin (Metaglip) and glyburide with metformin (Glucovance).

 Thiazolidinedione and biguanide combination medications include rosiglitazone with metformin (Avandamet).

Thyroid Antagonists

This class of medication prevents the thyroid gland from producing too much thyroid hormone. These medications can also be prescribed for people with autoimmune disorders such as psoriasis.

 If the client has recently developed any of the following, avoid massage and call the physician immediately: An unexplained skin rash, severe backache or headache, increased difficulty breathing, ringing in the ears, recent muscle weakness, unusual bleeding or bruising or swelling of the lips, tongue, face, feet or legs. (This is a massage-specific list; refer to the documentation that was included with the medication for a complete list of side effects.)

 Avoid massage if the client has recently developed a fever, sore throat, coughing, or painful or difficult urination, black, bloody, or tarry stools, blood in urine, or unusual tiredness or weakness. These are serious signs of abnormal blood cell or platelet populations, and a physician should be consulted without delay.

 Postponing the session is recommended if the therapist is unwell. The client's immune system is compromised from this medication.

 Avoid all contact with the client for one week after radioactive iodine treatment to allow sufficient time for the radiation to dissipate and for the immune system to recover.

 Side Effects: Headaches, muscle pain, nausea, vomiting and stomach pain all can occur with this class of medication. Take these into consideration as they may limit your ability to achieve your client's massage goals.

 Healing after tissue damage will be extended. Adjust your treatment schedules and goals to account for the slower than normal time frame.

 Thyroid antagonist medications include: <u>methimazole</u> (Tapazole), <u>propylthiouracil</u> (Propyl-Thyracil), and <u>radioactive iodine</u> (Iodotope, Sodium Iodide).

The quality of food, combined with the quality of digestion, is one of the the most powerful long-term factors in the quality of one's life.

Consistent massage has much to offer in the improvement of digestion.

Chapter 10

Digestive System

Gastroesophageal Reflux Disease (GERD)

(also known as, heartburn, hiatal hernia)

GERD is a condition where acidic stomach contents repeatedly come in contact with the sensitive lining of the esophagus.

Causes range from stress, poor dietary intake, poor posture during and after eating (which increases pressure on the stomach), slow movement of food through the gastrointestinal system, over or under production of stomach acids, and improper functioning of the esophageal sphincter. A hiatal hernia occurs when the neck of the stomach is forced up into the diaphragm opening. This pressure prevents the sphincter from working properly and allows stomach contents to reflux (see hernias).

Medications are used to improve the speed that the stomach empties, to neutralize the acids, and to reduce or eliminate the production of stomach acids. Unfortunately, this allows partially undigested and unabsorbable food to move through the intestines. Long-term results of medical treatment are thought to result in irritable bowel disease and complications due to malnutrition. Other recent innovations in the treatment of GERD include a permanently implanted sponge-like device (called *Enteryx*) to prevent the reflux of stomach acids. Tubes (called *stents*) can be inserted to act as a barrier between the acid and esophagus.

Symptoms commonly begin as a burning sensation in the throat, chest or stomach (called heartburn, even though it is not associated with the heart), a sour or bitter taste in the mouth, and chest pain or pain with swallowing.

Gastroesophageal Reflux Disease Precautions

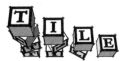 **Tolerance, Incremental, Light and Energy techniques are all encouraged.**

Gastroesophageal Reflux Disease Precautions, cont'd.

 After any surgical test or procedure, have the client seek approval from their physician before performing abdominal massage.

 Warning: Be cautious with pressure in the upper half of the abdominal cavity, and stop if the client reports discomfort. Your full range of techniques are acceptable elsewhere unless another condition requires caution.

 It may be best to schedule the session more than two hours after a meal, and they may be uncomfortable in certain positions. Be flexible and talk with your client about the alternatives available for their comfort. A massage chair may be an optimal solution if available.

 Antacids, histamine blockers, proton pump inhibitors, and promotility agents are all used both prescription and non-prescription. Since medications vary and are frequently combined, be sure to update your precautions before each session.

 You can undoubtedly help your client's general health through massage; consider how they also may benefit from learning what you know about stomach physiology and health.

Peptic Ulcer Disease (PUD)

An ulcer is a crater-like sore in the lining of the stomach or upper part of the small intestine. Stress, ethanol, bile, and nonsteroidal anti-inflammatory drugs (NSAIDs) disrupt the mucous lining, making the stomach and small intestine vulnerable to normal stomach acid secretions. Infection with *Helicobacter pylori* bacteria is the leading cause of PUD and is associated with virtually all ulcers not induced by NSAIDs. Peptic ulcer disease is the single most common disorder diagnosed in the United States today, and over 25 million Americans will suffer from an ulcer at some point during their lifetime.

Symptoms include recurring pain localized in the central to left upper abdomen, with a burning sensation occurring one to five hours after eating, and possible pain radiating to the back. NSAID-induced ulcers usually occur without any symptoms until they become severe.

Peptic Ulcer Disease Precautions

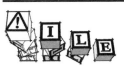 **Restrict massage to Incremental, Light and Energy techniques in the upper abdomen. Your full technique range is encouraged for the rest of the body.**

 Stop or avoid massage if the client reports any blood visible when vomiting, and have them consult their physician without delay. Symptoms similar to those listed above should also be investigated by medical personnel.

 Avoid deep pressure in the upper half of the abdominal cavity. Your full range of techniques are acceptable elsewhere unless another condition requires caution.

 Histamine blockers, antacids, proton pump inhibitors and antiulcer medications are just some of the classes utilized in the treatment of PUD. Since medications vary and are frequently combined, be sure to update your precautions before each session.

 Work your magic to help your client relieve stress, and know that you play a significant role in improving their quality of life!

Increasing their water intake will help the client's massage last longer. This is a free way to add value to your sessions!

Inflammatory Bowel Disease (IBD)

(also called regional ileitis, irritable bowel syndrome, IBS)

Crohn's disease is a chronic inflammatory disease of both the small and large intestines. *Ulcerative colitis* causes inflammation only in the large intestine and rectum. Differentiating between Crohn's disease and ulcerative colitis is sometimes difficult due to similar symptoms, including abdominal pain, diarrhea, and weight loss. Less common symptoms include poor appetite, fever, night sweats, rectal pain and bleeding. *Celiac disease* (CD) is a genetic autoimmune disorder in which the body reacts to foods containing gluten. Damage to the mucous lining in the small intestine prevents the proper absorption of nutrients. Those afflicted with CD are more likely to have additional diseases caused by malnutrition.

The cause of Crohn's disease and ulcerative colitis cannot be currently pinpointed. The most popular theory is that the body's immune system reacts to a virus or a bacterium causing ongoing inflammation in the intestinal wall. Complications of IBD can include skin conditions, joint pains (and arthritis), and liver inflammation (hepatitis).

Inflammatory Bowel Disease Precautions

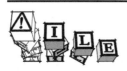 **Restrict massage to Incremental, Light and Energy techniques for the abdomen. Your full technique range is encouraged for the rest of the body.**

 Avoid massage and have them consult their physician without delay if the client reports any blood visible with fecal material. Symptoms related to those listed above should also be investigated by medical personnel.

 Postponing the session is recommended if the therapist is unwell. This is especially important if the client is having an acute attack or is reporting a fever.

 Warning: Be especially careful with pressure techniques if the client has had a history of long-term steroid use, as this predisposes the client to advanced osteoporosis.

Inflammatory Bowel Disease Precautions

 Warning: Gentle abdominal massage can be very helpful, however, the client will have low endurance and a reduced tolerance for pressure. Be brief and light in your technique to prevent an inflammatory reaction.

 Warning: Permanent peripheral neuropathy is a complication with long-term use of metronidazole (an antibiotic used to treat IBD). Be extra cautious with pressure, as the client may not be able to accurately determine their limits.

 A complex and ever shifting array of medications are utilized in the treatment of IBD. Medications include antibiotics, antimetabolites, biologic response modifiers, corticosteroids, DMARDs, etc. Be sure to ask about current medications and check their precautions.

 The client suffering from IBD is likely to be emotionally as well as physically exhausted from struggling daily with this many-faceted disease. Give sustenance to their emotional flame while strengthening their physical vitality, and watch them thrive in your nurturing care.

Diverticular Disease

(also called diverticulosis)

Diverticular disease is a common disorder in which one or more pouches form in the large intestine. It can be any part of the colon, however, 95 percent of the time it involves the *sigmoid colon*. One third of the general U.S. population develops diverticulosis by age 45 and two thirds by age 85. When a pouch becomes inflamed it is called *diverticulitis*. The exact causes of diverticular disease are unknown, but it is well understood that a low fiber diet increases the chance of creating diverticulosis.

Most people with diverticulosis do not have any discomfort or symptoms. Symptoms that do appear may include include mild abdominal cramping, bloating, and constipation. Diverticulitis results in moderate to severe abdominal pain and cramping, typically centering on the left lower portion of the abdomen. Fever, nausea and vomiting may also occur if there is an infection. Occasionally, diverticulitis will produce bleeding, perforation, or intestinal blockages. Surgery to repair the intestine is usually successful for that area, but does not stop the formation of new pouches.

Diverticular Disease Precautions

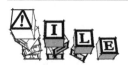 **Restrict massage to Incremental, Light and Energy techniques in the lower abdomen. Your full technique range is encouraged for the rest of the body.**

 Avoid massage and have the client contact their physician if they report nausea or vomiting, abdominal pains, blood in their stool or any other alarming symptoms.

 Avoid all pressure massage during acute diverticulitis. ENERGY techniques are encouraged.

 Avoid TOLERANCE techniques, and limit the duration of each session to guard against overwhelming the client. INCREMENTAL, LIGHT and ENERGY techniques during phases of remission are encouraged.

 Avoid deep pressure in the lower half of the abdominal cavity. Your full range of techniques are acceptable elsewhere unless another condition requires caution.

 Be sure to ask about current medications and check their precautions.

 You are especially knowledgeable about the benefits of water and proper diet; guide your client to better health with your words as well as your skills.

Appendicitis

The appendix is a small, dead-end tube that attaches to the first few inches of the large intestine. The inner lining of the appendix produces a small amount of mucus that flows into the intestines, and the wall of the appendix contains lymphatic tissue that is part of the immune system for making antibodies.

Appendicitis begins when the opening from the appendix into the cecum becomes blocked from fecal material. Bacteria from the blockage irritates the appendix and can cause it to rupture. Symptoms usually begin as a diffuse abdominal pain that intensifies and becomes localized between the bellybutton and right hip bone. Pressure on the area may or may not increase pain, but acute appendicitis is clearly suspected when the pain is sharply worse after quickly removing the pressure.

Surgery is performed within hours of diagnosis, but since many diseases can mimic appendicitis (like pelvic inflammatory disease or a kidney abscess) physicians may opt for a period of hospitalized observation before a decision has been reached. If the appendix ruptures it can cause *peritonitis* (inflammation of the membrane that lines the wall of the abdomen) or even a life-threatening bacterial infection of the blood (called *sepsis*).

Appendicitis Precautions

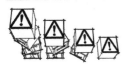 **Client is in critical condition. Avoid all therapy until approved by their physician.**

 Always avoid massage if a client complains of moderate to severe abdominal pain, especially if you are uncertain of the cause. Appendicitis is a medical emergency and prompt action is critical.

 Avoid deep tissue techniques directly over scars. Reduce and closely monitor pressure intensity and duration to avoid damaging the scar tissue. Your full range of techniques are acceptable elsewhere unless another condition requires caution.

 No medicines are used to directly treat appendicitis other than those for pain after surgical removal. As always, check each medicine the client is taking for precautions to massage.

 The trauma of appendicitis followed by surgical intervention can sap the strength of the hardiest of clients. Once massage has been approved, techniques that help rebuild their energy and vitality will be especially well received.

Hepatitis

Hepatitis simply translated means inflammation of the liver. This damages the liver and can lead to cirrhosis. The vast majority of cases of hepatitis involve infection with some form of virus, however, other causes do exist. Autoimmune hepatitis is a serious condition in which the body attacks and destroys liver cells. Approximately 10 percent of the people who contract infectious mononucleosis develop hepatitis as a complication.

There are seven types of hepatitis virus, labeled Hepatitis A, B, C, D, E, F, and G. The first three are by far the most common in the U.S. and will be the types discussed here.

Hepatitis A virus (HAV) is primarily spread through food or water contaminated by feces containing the virus, although may be spread by blood. It is self-limiting, resolving within weeks of infection and immunizes the person from becoming infected with HAV again.

Hepatitis B virus (HBV) is spread through contact with infected blood either by injection or through intercourse. HBV is 100 times more infectious than HIV, and unlike the virus that causes AIDS, HBV can stay active in a dry speck of blood for up to a week. Symptoms are chronic in about 5 percent of those affected, but are far less frequent or as severe as HCV.

Hepatitis C virus (HCV) is also spread through contact with infected blood either by injection or through intercourse. It is also a chronic disease and by far the most damaging of the three, with more than 75 percent having long-term effects. 25 percent of this group eventually have liver failure.

There is a variable incubation period from a few weeks to 6 months before symptoms begin. Symptoms for all forms of hepatitis include yellowing of the skin and eyes (called *jaundice*), headache, fever, fatigue, abdominal pain, nausea, vomiting, and diarrhea.

Hepatitis Precautions

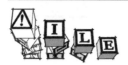 **Restrict massage to Incremental, Light and Energy techniques.**

Hepatitis Precautions, cont'd.

 Avoid massage until the physician has given the approval that the acute stage has passed. ENERGY techniques are acceptable. Avoid massage in any individual you are concerned about that exhibits significant symptoms as listed above, and have them seek medical attention.

 Postponing the session is recommended if the therapist is unwell for clients with chronic hepatitis, as their immune system is less capable of withstanding the exposure to infection.

 Avoid TOLERANCE techniques, and limit the duration of each session to guard against overwhelming the client. INCREMENTAL, LIGHT and ENERGY techniques during phases of remission are acceptable.

 Avoid all areas of broken skin along with a generous margin for safety even if you do not see blood. Keep that area of the body covered with bandages or the client's clothing to limit contamination.

 Warning: Touching the skin under linens or clothing is acceptable as long as you have visually inspected the skin that day. Never touch an area of skin that you have not seen.

 Follow the Standard Precautions (see the integumentary system) for all equipment and linen that may have been in contact with blood or fecal material.

 Interferons, antivirals, and steroids are all common medications used in the treatment of hepatitis. Be sure to ask about current medications and check their precautions.

 With the precautions listed above in place, turn your focus to nurturing the healing energy within your client. Treat your client, not the condition. Massage has a lot to offer in their quest for maintaining a good quality of life.

Gallstones

(also called cholelithiasis)

Bile is a substance produced by the liver and stored in the gallbladder. It removes waste from the liver and breaks down fats as food is digested. *Gallstones* occur when the bile in the gallbladder becomes over concentrated and forms crystal stones in the gallbladder or bile ducts. 80 percent of the time these stones are made up of cholesterol. The remaining 20 percent are comprised of *calcium bilirubinate*, a pigment resulting from certain infections and liver cirrhosis.

More than 60 percent of people diagnosed with gallstones have no symptoms. The classic symptom is right upper abdomen pain lasting one to five hours, with pain radiating to the right shoulder or upper back. They may also have chronic indigestion, belching, bloating, and/or intolerance with fatty foods. If symptoms persist or other complications are present, surgical removal (called *cholecystectomy*) is often performed.

Gallstone Precautions

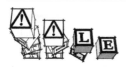 **Restrict massage to Light and Energy techniques in the right upper abdomen. Your full technique range is encouraged for the rest of the body.**

 If the client reports acute pain in the abdomen, possibly radiating to the right shoulder, back or upper ribs, avoid pressure massage techniques and have them seek medical attention if it persists. Resume normal massage once they have been cleared by their physician.

 Avoid moderate or deep pressure to the right upper abdomen with any client diagnosed with gallstones to prevent inflammation or irritation.

 Clients may self-medicate based upon symptoms associated with this condition. Check precautions for any current medication the client may be taking.

 Other than a local precaution in the area surrounding the liver, this client can benefit from the full range of techniques at your disposal.

Cirrhosis

In cirrhosis of the liver, scar tissue replaces normal, healthy tissue, blocking the flow of blood through the organ and preventing proper functioning. This produces a variety of symptoms, including fatigue, weakness, nausea, loss of appetite, weight loss, abdominal pains, spider veins, increased bruising and bleeding, jaundice, intense itching, swelling of the lower extremities (*edema*) and abdomen (*ascites*).

However, these symptoms pale in comparison to the complications of cirrhosis. Blood flow through the scarred liver becomes sluggish, backing up into other vessels in the abdomen. These enlarged blood vessels (called *varices*) have thin walls and higher pressure and are more likely to rupture. The reduced liver function increases the likelihood of hypertension, diabetes, medication hypersensitivities, gallstones and eventually, kidney failure, brain degeneration and liver cancer. The immune system relies heavily on normal liver function, and the person with cirrhosis has greater difficulty battling infections and maintaining muscle tone and strength.

Today, cirrhosis is caused by the hepatitis C virus as often as it is from chronic alcoholism. Rarely, an autoimmune response by the body can attack the liver and cause cirrhosis. Treatment focusing on the liver is limited to stopping or slowing the degeneration. Most treatments are to battle the various complications caused by the disease. Liver transplants are typically reserved for those with aggressive cirrhosis who have few complications.

Cirrhosis Precautions

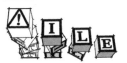 **Restrict massage to Incremental, Light and Energy techniques within the client's limits.**

 Avoid massage and have the client contact their physician if they report recent dramatic weight loss, nausea or vomiting, abdominal pains or any other alarming symptoms.

 Postponing the session is recommended if the therapist is unwell for clients with advanced cirrhosis as their immune system is challenged.

Cirrhosis Precautions, cont'd.

 Take time before beginning your session for a full visual inspection of the areas you intend to massage. Note general skin health and look up any conditions (like edema) for a complete understanding of the client's limitations.

 Avoid deep pressure and deep abdominal massage and reduce the duration of massage to any area, as the client will likely bruise more easily.

 Warning: Reduce the duration of all pressure techniques, as toxin elimination relies heavily on the already overtaxed liver.

 A variety of medications are utilized to treat this condition as well as the complications that arise, including beta blockers, insulins, digestive aids, and antivirals. Check the client's current medications each session to maintain a complete list of precautions.

 The client suffering from cirrhosis will likely benefit as much from your nutritional knowledge as from your physical techniques.

Consistent, compassionate massage within the client's limits will stimulate their physical well being, boost their healing response and bolster their emotional strength.

Digestive System Medications

Antacids

Antacids reduce or neutralize the acidic secretions present in the stomach. They do not have a significant effect on future acid production.

 If the client reports any of the following serious side effects, stop or avoid all massage and seek emergency medical attention: A severe headache; difficulty breathing; closing of the throat; swelling of the lower extremities; swelling of the lips, tongue, or face; or hives. (This is a massage-specific list; refer to the documentation that was included with the medication for a complete list of side effects.)

 Side Effects: Significant side effects are common with many of these medications: Headaches, muscle stiffness, bone or joint pain, trembling, fatigue, increased bruising, vomiting and diarrhea. Take these into consideration as they may limit your ability to achieve your client's massage goals. If any of these symptoms are severe or persistent, have the client contact their physician.

 Antacid medications include: aluminum hydroxide (AlternaGEL, Alu-Cap, Alu-Tab, Amphojel, Dialume), aluminum with magnesium hydroxide (Alamag, Aludrox, Di-Gel, Maalox, Magnalox, Mylanta, Rulox), bismuth subsalicylate (Pepto-Bismol), calcium carbonate (Alka-Mints, Amitone, Calel-D, Caltrate, Chooz, Dicarbosil, Equilet, Mallamint, Os-Cal, Rolaids, Titralac, Tums), magaldrate (Losopan, Lowsium, Ri-Mag, Riopan), magnesium gluconate (Almora, Mago-nate, Magtrate), magnesium hydroxide (Milk of Magnesia, Phillips Chewable), sodium bicarbonate (Alka-Seltzer, Baking Soda, Bell-Ans, Citrocarbona).

Appetite Suppressant Medications

These drugs are used to decrease appetite in overweight patients. Combined with a reduced calorie diet, they can help you reduce weight. They are typically meant to be used only for a short period of time (8 to 12 weeks). They should not be used along with other diet medications. These medicines should not be shared with anyone else.

Appetite Suppressant Medication Precautions

 If the client reports any of the following serious side effects, stop or avoid all massage and seek emergency medical attention: a severe headache, difficulty breathing, closing of the throat, swelling of the lips, tongue, or face, or hives. (This is a massage-specific list; refer to the documentation that was included with the medication for a complete list of side effects.)

 Side Effects: Headaches, tremors, dizziness or drowsiness, increased flatulence and intestinal cramping all can occur with this class of medication. Take these into consideration as they may limit your ability to achieve your client's massage goals.

 Appetite suppressant medications include: benzphetamine (Didrex), diethylpropion (Tenuate), mazindol (Mazanor, Sanorex), orlistat (Xenical), phendimetrazine (Bontril, Melfiat, Prelu-2), phentermine (Adipex, Anoxine, Fastin, Ionamin, Obephen, Obermine, Obestin, Phentrol), and sibutramine (Meridia).

Histamine-2 Receptor Blockers

Histamine-2 receptor blockers prevent histamine from being produced, which reduces the amount of acid released into the stomach.

 If the client reports any of the following serious side effects, stop or avoid all massage and seek emergency medical attention: Mental confusion, a severe headache; difficulty breathing; closing of the throat; swelling of the lips, tongue, or face; or hives. (This is a massage-specific list; refer to the documentation that was included with the medication for a complete list of side effects.)

 Side Effects: Headaches, muscle pain, constipation, diarrhea, drowsiness and breast soreness all can occur with this class of medication. Take these into consideration as they may limit your ability to achieve your client's massage goals.

 Postural hypotension can occur as a side effect of this class of medication. Help the client to change positions and be on guard for dizziness or blacking out.

Histamine-2 Receptor Blocker Medication Precautions, cont'd.

 Histamine-2 receptor blocker medications include: <u>cimetidine</u> (Tagamet), <u>famotidine</u> (Pepcid AC), <u>nizatidine</u> (Axid) and <u>ranitidine</u> (Zantac).

Promotility Agents

Promotility agents are used to improve symptoms for patients with slow gastric emptying. Some of these medications are used for irritable bowel syndrome in reducing constipation.

 If the client reports any of the following serious side effects, stop or avoid all massage and seek emergency medical attention: A severe headache, difficulty breathing, closing of the throat, swelling of the lips, tongue, or face, or hives. (This is a massage-specific list; refer to the documentation that was included with the medication for a complete list of side effects.)

 Side Effects: Headaches, stomach discomfort and diarrhea all can occur with this class of medication. Take these into consideration as they may limit your ability to achieve your client's massage goals.

 Promotility agent medications include: <u>alosetron</u> (Lotronex), <u>cisapride</u> (Propulsid), <u>metoclopramide</u> (Apo-Metoclop, Clopra, Maxeran, Maxolon, Octamide, Reclomide, Reglan), and <u>tegaserod</u> (Zelnorm).

Clients treasure the compassion in your attitude as much as they benefit from your techniques.

Proton Pump Inhibitors

Hydrochloric acid is released by the *proton pump* (*ATPase pump*) located within the parietal cells of the stomach. Proton pump inhibitors bind to the *ATPase enzyme*, suppressing gastric acid output.

 If the client reports any of the following serious side effects, stop or avoid all massage and seek emergency medical attention: A severe headache, difficulty breathing, closing of the throat, swelling of the lips, tongue, or face, or hives. (This is a massage-specific list; refer to the documentation that was included with the medication for a complete list of side effects.)

 Side Effects: Headaches, constipation, increased flatulence and intestinal cramping all can occur with this class of medication. Take these into consideration as they may limit your ability to achieve your client's massage goals.

 Proton pump inhibitor medications include: esomeprazole (Nexium), lansoprazole (Prevacid), omeprazole (Prilosec), pantoprazole (Protonix), and rabeprazole (Aciphex).

Antiulcer Medications

Misoprostol protects the stomach lining and decreases stomach acid secretion. Sucralfate binds to and coats the ulcerative tissue, preventing further injury by acids.

 If the client reports any of the following serious side effects, stop or avoid all massage and seek emergency medical attention: A severe headache; difficulty breathing; closing of the throat; swelling of the lips, tongue, or face; or hives. (This is a massage-specific list; refer to the documentation that was included with the medication for a complete list of side effects.)

 Warning: Misoprostol may cause miscarriages, premature labor, or birth defects. Only the person to whom this medicine is prescribed should take this medicine.

Antiulcer Medication Precautions, cont'd.

 Side Effects: Headaches, constipation, increased flatulence and intestinal cramping all can occur with this class of medication. Take these into consideration as they may limit your ability to achieve your client's massage goals.

 Antiulcer medications include: <u>misoprostol</u> (Cytotec) and <u>sucralfate</u> (Carafate, Sulcrate).

Antiulcer Multi-Drug Regimens

Ulcers infected with the H. Pylori bacteria often require a multi-faceted approach for treatment. Physicians may customize a drug regimen, or may utilize one of two pre-packaged combination regimens listed below.

 If the client reports any of the following serious side effects, stop or avoid all massage and seek emergency medical attention: Clumsiness, dizziness, or unsteadiness, fever, numbness, tingling, pain or weakness in the hands or feet, a severe headache, difficulty breathing, closing of the throat, swelling of the lips, tongue, or face, or hives. (This is a massage-specific list; refer to the documentation that was included with the medication for a complete list of side effects.)

 Warning: Permanent peripheral neuropathy is a complication with long-term use of this class of antibiotics. Be extra cautious with pressure, as the client may not be able to accurately determine their limits.

 Side Effects: Dark brown or reddish urine, headaches, nausea, mild stomach pain or cramps and diarrhea often occur as a result of this class of medication. Take these into consideration as they may limit your ability to achieve your client's massage goals. If any of these symptoms are persistent or of concern, have the client contact their physician.

 Medications include: <u>bismuth</u> <u>subsalicylate</u> with <u>metronidazole</u> and <u>tetracycline</u> (Helidac), <u>lansoprazole</u> with <u>clarithromycin</u> and <u>amox-icillin</u> (Prevpac).

Antidiarrhea and Laxative Medications

These medications help control diarrhea and constipation by slowing down the movements of the intestines. The reduced smooth muscle contractions moderate the intestinal responses.

 If the client reports any of the following serious side effects, stop or avoid all massage and seek emergency medical attention: A severe headache; difficulty breathing; closing of the throat; swelling of the lips, tongue, or face; or hives. (This is a massage-specific list; refer to the documentation that was included with the medication for a complete list of side effects.)

 If the client has not had a bowel movement in several days, avoid massage and call the physician immediately. Bowel obstruction is a severe side effect of this class of medication.

 Side Effects: Constipation, drowsiness and fatigue can occur as a result of this class of medication. Take these into consideration as they may limit your ability to achieve your client's massage goals. If any of these symptoms are persistent or of concern, have the client contact their physician.

 Antidiarrhea and laxative medications include: <u>bismuth</u> <u>subsalicylate</u> (Bismatrol, Bismatrol Extra Strength, Children's Kaopectate, Extra Strength Kaopectate, Kaopectate, Pepto-Bismol, Pink Bismuth), <u>Difenoxin</u> with <u>Atropine</u> (Motofen), <u>diphenoxylate</u> with <u>atropine</u> (Diphenatol, Lomocot, Lomotil, Lonox), and <u>loperamide</u> (Diamode, Imodium, Imogen, Imotil, Imperim).

*Skillfully matching your
techniques with the client's
limitations and needs is
the true art of massage.*

Chapter 11

Urinary System

Kidney Stones

(also called nephrolithiasis)

A *kidney stone* is a hard crystal mass, usually made from calcium and *oxalate* or *phosphate*. These are chemicals normally found in the body, but when an abundance of them end up in the kidney they can crystallize into stones.

The formation of the stone is painless. The extreme pain often begins suddenly when a stone moves in the urinary tract, causing irritation or blockage. Typically, a person feels a sharp, cramping pain in the back and side in the area of the kidney or in the lower abdomen. Sometimes nausea and vomiting occur. As the stone travels down the urinary tract, the pain may spread to the groin area. There may also be visible blood in the urine.

Diuretics (like chlorothiazide) may be prescribed to prevent kidney stones in those with high levels of calcium in their blood. People affected by repeated kidney stones are encouraged to increase their daily water intake and limit their intake of foods that contain high oxalates and phosphates. These include beets, carbonated beverages, chocolate, coffee, nuts, rhubarb, spinach, strawberries, tea, and wheat bran. Studies published in the British Journal of Urology scientifically prove that (pure unsweetened) cranberry juice (not cranberry concentrate capsules or tablets) is an effective cure for kidney stones. The juice lowers the concentration of oxalate and phosphate, it increases the citrate concentration (which balances the urine pH levels), and it dilutes the concentration of calcium oxalate in the urine.

Kidney Stone Precautions

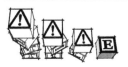 **Energy techniques only. Avoid all pressure and circulatory massage techniques until the stone has passed and the symptoms are gone.**

Kidney Stone Precautions, cont'd.

 Avoid massage and have the client seek emergency medical attention if they are experiencing severe pain in the midback or deep abdominal pain.

 Avoid all pressure techniques for the entire body until the stone has been passed or eliminated to avoid taxing the urinary system. ENERGY techniques are encouraged.

 Kidney stones are excruciatingly painful, but are temporary and not life threatening. Once the pain and stone are gone, your full range of techniques are encouraged unless another condition requires caution.

 The client may be taking ongoing diuretic medication to dilute the urine and flush the system. As always, check all your client's medications for massage precautions.

 Massage doesn't have a practical application in preventing the formation of kidney stones or for eliminating them. However, for those clients looking to avoid the excruciatingly painful stones in the future, your nutritional advice may be priceless.

Urinary Tract Infection (UTI)

Urinary tract infections are caused by bacteria in the urinary system. The name of the infection depends upon the area infected. *Pyelonephritis* is an infection of the entire kidney. An infection in the bladder is called *cystitis*.

Symptoms and signs include back, side, and groin pain, urgent, frequent and painful urination, fever, nausea and possibly vomiting. Treatment consists of controlling the symptoms with medication while eliminating the infection with antibiotics.

Urinary Tract Infection Precautions

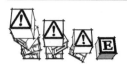 **Energy techniques only. Avoid all pressure and circulatory massage techniques.**

Urinary Tract Infection Precautions, cont'd.

 Pain that travels to the back or groin accompanied by fever, nausea or vomiting may be an indication of an infection complicating a UTI. Avoid massage and have client seek medical attention.

 Avoid all pressure techniques for the entire body until the active infection has been controlled to prevent taxing the urinary system further. ENERGY techniques are encouraged.

 Avoid deep techniques in the lower half of the abdominal cavity until the client is completely healed and there is no discomfort with pressure.

 Antibiotics, antispasmodics, and painkillers are all used to treat UTIs. Check current medications for additional precautions.

 Supportive techniques, carefully wielded by one skilled as you are, can bring relaxation and comfort to the client recovering from a urinary tract infection.

Interstitial Cystitis (IC)

The natural lining of the bladder is protected from toxins in the urine by a layer of protein called *glycoaminoglycan* (GAG). In IC this protective layer has broken down, allowing toxins to irritate the bladder wall. The bladder then becomes inflamed and tender, causing frequent, urgent, and painful urination and pelvic discomfort. According to the National Institutes of Health, interstitial cystitis affects about 700,000 people in the U.S.

Although it is known that IC is not an infectious disease like cystitis, there is no known common cause. Lupus, irritable bowel syndrome, endometriosis, fibromyalgia and food allergies have all been implicated as possible factors in the onset of IC. There is no treatment; the focus is on reducing the chronic symptoms.

Interstitial Cystitis Precautions

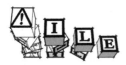 **Restrict massage to Incremental, Light and Energy techniques in the lower abdomen. Your full technique range is encouraged for the rest of the body.**

 Pain that travels to the back or groin accompanied by fever, nausea or vomiting may be an indication of an infection complicating IC. Avoid massage and have client seek medical attention.

 Avoid deep pressure in the lower half of the abdominal cavity. Your full range of techniques are acceptable elsewhere unless another condition requires caution.

 Antispasmodics, urinary analgesics and other pain medications may all be used in ever-changing variations as the body's needs change. Check current medications for additional precautions before each session.

 This client can benefit from the full range of techniques at your disposal. You'll earn their gratitude by being flexible with their need for frequent urination, as you will by reducing their body stress.

Glomerulonephritis

Glomerulonephritis is a type of kidney disease caused by inflammation of tiny internal kidney structures (called *glomeruli*) where the blood is cleaned. Damage to the glomeruli causes impaired filtering which leaks blood and protein into the urine and causes fluid and toxins to be retained in the body tissues. If it continues to degenerate it results in kidney failure. Systemic bacterial infections, diabetes, lupus, and AIDS are some of the conditions that produce glomerulonephritis.

Signs and symptoms include protein in the urine (*proteinuria*), blood in the urine (*hematuria*), and generalized edema. As this disease progresses, the fluid retention causes hypertension, and the buildup of toxins cause various secondary conditions, including chronic itchy skin, general tension, fatigue and a lowering of the body's immune system.

Treatment includes medication to control the symptoms, most importantly hypertension. *Dialysis* is a procedure in which an internal structure or external machine is used to filter waste from the blood and remove excess fluid from the body.

Glomerulonephritis Precautions

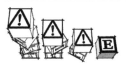 **Energy techniques only. Avoid all pressure and circulatory massage techniques.**

 Avoid all pressure massage during any stage of glomerulonephritis. ENERGY techniques that do not stimulate the circulatory system are encouraged. Only consider LIGHT techniques after the acute or infectious form of this disease has been eradicated and the client's physician has given approval.

 Avoid the region surrounding the area used in dialysis if LIGHT techniques are allowed.

 Carefully consider how much support your client can benefit from and how much may be overwhelming. Even ENERGY techniques can be physically and emotionally taxing.

 Be sure to ask about current medications and check their precautions.

 Keep in mind the power your range of techniques have in eliminating toxins and excess fluids, as well as the client's particular challenge in this area. They will appreciate your restraint as well as your supportive intent.

You are unique and special.
Keep focused on what you do
best to support your client.

Kidney Failure

Kidney failure is the phrase used when the kidneys are not able to regulate water and chemicals in the body or remove waste products from your blood. *Acute renal failure* (ARF) is the sudden onset of kidney failure. This can be caused by an accident that injures the kidneys, loss of a lot of blood, and poisons. ARF may lead to permanent loss of kidney function, but if the kidneys are not seriously damaged they may recover.

Chronic kidney disease (CKD) is the gradual reduction of kidney function that may lead to permanent kidney failure. Chronic kidney disease is the ninth leading cause of death in the U.S. and affects about 19 million American adults. Diabetes and high blood pressure are major causes of chronic kidney failure, accounting for 60 percent of new cases, says the U.S. Centers for Disease Control and Prevention. Drugs such as COX-2 inhibitors and NSAIDs are also major causes of CKD. The final degenerative stage of kidney failure is called *end-stage renal disease* (ESRD).

You may go several years without knowing you have CKD. Symptoms appear gradually and often are associated with other conditions or easily explained away. Symptoms include muscle twitches and cramps, headaches, persistent itching, high blood pressure, weight loss, anemia, chronic fatigue, nausea or vomiting, decreased urine output, and reduced mental functions.

Chronic kidney failure has no cure, but treatment can help control symptoms, reduce complications and slow the progress of the disease. For those with no other complications like heart disease or diabetes, a kidney transplant may offer a higher quality of life than dialysis.

Dialysis is a procedure in which an internal structure or external machine is used to filter waste from the blood and remove excess fluid from the body. Hemodialysis and peritoneal dialysis are two types of dialysis used to treat kidney failure.

Hemodialysis uses a special machine with a special filter (called a *dialyzer*) to clean your blood. During the 2 to 4 hour treatment, the blood travels through tubes (called catheters) into the dialyzer filtering out wastes and extra fluids. Then the newly cleaned blood flows through another set of tubes and back into your body. This procedure is performed three times per week.

Peritoneal dialysis is another dialysis procedure that uses the lining of the abdomen (the *peritoneum*) to filter your blood instead of a dialyzer. Special fluids are inserted by a permanent tube (*catheter*) into your abdomen, and waste products are later eliminated through the same tube. It may or may not require a machine, and is typically an ongoing 4 to 6 hour cycle.

Kidney Failure Precautions

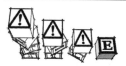 **Energy techniques only. Avoid all pressure and circulatory massage techniques.**

 Avoid all pressure massage during any stage of kidney failure. ENERGY techniques that do not stimulate the circulatory system are encouraged. Only consider LIGHT techniques after the acute or infectious form of this disease has been eradicated and the client's physician has given approval.

 Avoid the region surrounding the area used in dialysis if LIGHT techniques are allowed.

 Carefully consider how much support your client can benefit from and how much may be overwhelming. Even ENERGY techniques can be physically and emotionally taxing.

 Those suffering from kidney failure will likely have an extensive list of current medications. If you are given permission by the physician for LIGHT techniques, check each medication for any complicating precaution.

 Those suffering from CKD and ESRD must limit their water intake for obvious reasons. For a profession that relies heavily upon the urinary system to eliminate toxins, a condition such as this can effectively tie the therapist's hands. Carefully match your support with their limited endurance, recognizing that compassion may be your greatest tool.

Urinary System Medications

Antigout Medications

Uricosuric (*antigout*) agents help prevent recurring attacks of gout by helping the kidneys get rid of the excess uric acid produced in the body. Most are not used to treat an attack of gout once it has started, as they may make the condition worse. Allopurinol reduces the production of uric acid in the body, and colchicine is used to treat an acute attack of gout.

 If the client reports any of the following serious side effects, stop or avoid all massage and seek emergency medical attention: Lower back or side pain, skin rash and itching, mental confusion, pain or difficulty passing urine, a severe headache, difficulty breathing, closing of the throat, or swelling of the lips, tongue, or face. (This is a massage-specific list; refer to the documentation that was included with the medication for a complete list of side effects.)

 Side Effects: Common side effects from the medication include painful, swollen joints, heartburn, nausea and/or vomiting. Colchicine often causes numbness or tingling in the hands and feet. Take these into consideration as they may limit your ability to achieve your client's massage goals.

 Postural hypotension can occur as a side effect of this class of medication. Help the client to change positions and be on guard for dizziness or blacking out.

 Antigout medications include: allopurinol (Alloprim, Zyloprim), colchicine (Colgout), probenecid (Benemid, Probalan) and sulfinpyrazone (Anturane).

Antispasmodic Medications

Antispasmodics help decrease the muscle spasms that cause the urgency to urinate.

 If the client reports any of the following serious side effects, stop or avoid all massage and seek emergency medical attention: Mental confusion, a severe headache; difficulty breathing; closing of the throat; swelling of the lips, tongue, or face; or hives. (This is a massage-specific list; refer to the documentation that was included with the medication for a complete list of side effects.)

 Side Effects: Common side effects from the medication include headaches, decreased sweating, constipation, drowsiness and dry eyes. Take these into consideration as they may limit your ability to achieve your client's massage goals.

 Antispasmodic medications include flavoxate (Urispas), oxybutynin (Ditropan) and tolterodine (Detrol).

Urinary Analgesic Medications

These medications pass through the lining of the urinary tract and have a local anesthetic effect. This relieves the discomfort associated with bladder inflammation and infection.

 If the client reports any of the following serious side effects, stop or avoid all massage and seek emergency medical attention: Mental confusion, a severe headache; difficulty breathing; closing of the throat; swelling of the lips, tongue, or face; or hives. (This is a massage-specific list; refer to the documentation that was included with the medication for a complete list of side effects.)

 Side Effects: Common side effects from this medication include nausea and dark, orange to red urine. Take these into consideration as they may limit your ability to achieve your client's massage goals. If any of these symptoms are persistent or of concern, have the client contact their physician.

 Urinary analgesic medications include phenazopyridine hydrochloride (Azo-Standard, Baridium, Eridium, Geridium, Phenazodine, Pyridiate, Pyridium, Urodine, Urogesic, Viridium).

Your knowledge and wisdom,
combined with your innate desire
to make a positive impact
in someone's life, makes you
a rare and precious person.
You are a wellspring of hope
for your clients.

Medical Abbreviations

a	artery; before (Latin: ante)		**AB**	abdominal
A	anterior		**abd.**	abdomen; abduction; abductor
A & E	accident and emergency		**ABE**	activity before exercise; acute bacterial endocarditis
A & P	auscultation and percussion		**ABN**	abnormal
A & W	alive and well		**abs**	absent
a.c.	before meals (Latin: ante cenam)		**Ac**	acute
a.k.	above knee		**acc**	accident
a.p.	before dinner		**Acc.Inc.**	accidentally incurred
A.S.A. 1	normal healthy patient		**Acc.Inj.**	accidental injury
A.S.A. 2	patient with mild systemic disease		**accom.**	accommodation
A.S.A. 3	patient with severe systemic disease		**ACE**	angiotensin converting enzyme
A.S.A. 4	patient with incapacitating systemic disease that is a constant threat to life		**ACL**	anterior cruciate ligament
			ACM	acetaminophen
A/B	acid/base ratio		**Acous**	acoustic
A/O	alert and oriented		**ACS**	acute cervical sprain
AA	affected area		**ACT**	active motion
aa	equal part of each		**act**	activity
AAA	abdominal aortic aneurysm		**ACTH**	adrenocorticotrophic hormone
AAL	anterior axillary line		**AD**	right ear (Latin: auris dexter)
AAROM	active assisted range of motion		**ad lib**	as desired; at liberty (Latin: ad libitum)
AB	Ace Bandage; active bilaterally		**ADD**	attention deficit disorder
			ADH	antidiruetic hormone
ab	antibody		**ADHD**	attention deficit-hyperactivity disorder

ADL	activities of daily living	**amp.**	ampule; amputation
adm.	admission	**anes.**	anesthesia
ADR	adverse drug reaction	**ANF**	antinuclear factor
AE	above elbow	**ANS**	autonomic nervous system
AEA	above elbow amputation	**ant.**	anterior
AF	afebrile (no fever)	**ANX**	anxiety
AF	atrial fibrillation	**AO**	aorta
aI	active ingredient	**AOB**	alcohol on breath
AI	adequate intake	**A-P**	anteroposterior
AIDS	acquired immunodeficiency syndrome	**AP & L**	anteroposterior and lateral
		APAP	acetaminophen
AIDSKS	acquired immunodeficiency syndrome with Kaposi's sarcoma	**aph**	aphasia
		aq.	water (Latin: aqua)
		AR	active-resistance
AKA	also known as	**ARE**	active-resistance exercise
alb.	albumin	**AROM**	active range of motion
alc.	alcohol	**ART**	artery
ALL	anterior longitudinal ligament	**art**	arterial; articulation
		AS	left ear (Latin: auris sinistra)
ALL	acute lymphoblastic leukemia		
		ASA	aspirin (acetylsalicylic acid)
ALS	amyotrophic lateral sclerosis	**ASAP**	as soon as possible
		ASD	atrial septal defect
ALT	alternating with	**AT**	achilles tendon
AM	before noon (Latin: ante meridiem)	**ATN**	acute tubular necrosis
		ATP	adenosine triphosphate
AMA	against medical advice	**AU**	both ears (Latin: auris unitas); according to custom (Latin: ad usum)
amb.	ambulatory		
AMI	acute myocardial infarction		
		aud.	auditory
AML	acute myeloid anemia		

AV	aortic valve; atrioventricular
AW	able to work; above waist
Ax.	axial; axillary
B	born
B & C	biopsy and curettage
B & J	bone and joint
B.	bath
b.i.d.	twice daily (Latin: bis in die)
b.i.n.	twice a night (Latin: bis in nox)
B.U.O.	bleeding/bruising of undetermined origin
B/D	twice daily (Latin: bis in die)
B/N	twice a night (Latin: bis in nox)
BA	brachial artery
Barb	barbiturate
BAT	basic aid training
BBB	bundle branch block
BC	birth control
BCP	birth control pills
bd	twice daily
BD	birth date
BE	below elbow
Bic.	biceps
BID	brought in dead
bilat.	bilateral/bilaterally
BiW	twice weekly
BJM	bones joints muscles

BK	below knee
bk.	back
BL	blood loss
BL	baseline
Blad.	bladder
bld.	blood
BLE	both lower extremities
BLQ	both lower quadrants
BLS	basic life support
BLS-D	basic life support and defibrillation
BM	bowel movement; basal metabolism
BMI	body mass index
BMR	basal metabolic rate
BMT	bone marrow transplant
BND	barely noticeable difference
BOA	born on arrival
BoTox	botulinum toxin
BOW	bag of water
BP	blood pressure; body part
BPM	beats per minute
BPP	blood pressure and pulse
BR	bedrest
brach.	brachial
BRP	bathroom privileges
BS	blood sugar
BSA	body surface area
BsL	baseline

BT	blood type; body temperature	**CAPD**	chronic ambulatory peritoneal dialysis
BT	bedtime	**Caps**	capsules
BTE	behind the ear	**card.**	cardiac
BTU	British thermal unit	**CAT**	computerized axial tomography
BTW	by the way	**cath**	catheter
Buc	buccal	**CBC**	complete blood count
BUE	both upper extremities	**CBR**	complete bed rest
BUQ	both upper quadrants	**CC**	chief complaint
BV	blood vessel	**cc.**	cubic centimeter
BW	below waist; birth weight; body weight	**CCF**	congestive cardiac failure
Bx.	biopsy	**CCU**	coronary care unit.
C	cervical	**CD**	contagious disease
c	(with a bar on top) with (Latin: cum)	**CD**	cause of death (Latin: causa mortis)
C & S	culture and sensitivity	**CDC**	Center for Disease Control
C.	celsius	**CEA**	carcinoembryonic antigen
c.m.	cause of death (Latin: causa mortis)	**Cerv.**	cervical; cervix
c.v.	tomorrow night	**CF**	cardiac failure
C/O	care of	**cg.**	centigram
c/o	complains of	**Chem.**	chemotherapy
C1 - C7	cervical vertebra level	**CHO**	carbohydrate
Ca	calcium	**Chol**	cholesterol
CA	cancer	**Chr**	chronic
CABG	coronary artery bypass graft	**CI**	cardiac index
CAD	coronary artery disease	**CI-CXII**	1st to 12th cranial nerve
Caf.	caffeine	**CIS**	carcinoma in situ
Cal	calorie	**cl**	centiliter
Cap	capsule (Latin: capula)	**Cl**	chloride; clavicle

Clav.	clavicle
cldy	cloudy
CLL	chronic lymphoblastic leukemia
cm.	centimeter
CMass	center of mass
CML	chronic myeloid leukemia
CMV	cytomegalovirus
CNS	central nervous system
cnst.	constipation
CO	carbon monoxide
CO2	carbon dioxide
COD	cause of death (Latin: causa mortis)
COLD	chronic obstructive lung disease
comb.	combination
comm.	communicable
comp.	compound; compress
conc.	concentrated
cons.	consultation
cont.	continued
Cor	heart
CP	chest pain
CPAP	continuous positive airway pressure
CPR	cardiopulmonary resuscitation
cran.	cranial
CRF	chronic renal failure
CSF	cerebrospinal fluid
C-spine	cervical spine

CT	computed axial tomography; computed tomography
CU	cause unknown
CVA	cerebrovascular accident (stroke)
CVP	central venous pressure
Cx	cervix
CXR	chest X-ray
d	right (Latin: dexter)
D & C	dilation and curettage
D & E	dilation and evacuation
D & V	diarrhea and vomiting
D.O.B.	date of birth
d/c	discontinue
D/L	deciliter
D/S	discharge summary
D/W	discussed with
db.	decibel
DBE	deep breathing exercise
DC	discontinue
DD	discharge diagnosis
DDx	differential diagnosis
decr.	decreased
decub.	lying down
dehyd.	dehydrated
DH	drug history
DIAG.	diagnosis
diam.	diameter
DIC	disseminated intravascular coagulation

dil.	dilute		**EKG**	electrocardiogram
dim.	diminished		**elev.**	elevated
dis.	disease		**ELISA**	enzyme linked immunosorbent assay
disch.	discharge			
disp.	disposition		**elix.**	elixir
dist.	distal		**EMG**	electromyogram; electromyography
div.	divide			
DJD	degenerative joint disease		**EMS**	emergency medical service
DM	diabetes mellitus		**En.**	enema
DNA	deoxyribonucleic acid		**ENT**	ears, nose, throat
DNR	do not recussitate		**eq. pts.**	equal parts (Latin: equalis partis)
DNRCC	do not recussitate comfort care			
			ER	emergency room
DOA	dead on arrival		**ESR**	erythrocyte sedimentation rate
DOB	date of birth			
Dors	dorsal		**et**	and
dr.	dram		**Etio**	etiology
drsg.	dressing		**EVAL**	evaluation
DTR	deep tendon reflexes		**ex.**	example; exercise
DT's	delirium tremens		**expir**	expiration
DU	duodenal ulcer		**ext.**	extremity
DUI	driving under influence		**Ext.**	extract
DVT	deep venous thrombosis		**F**	fahrenheit; female
Dx	diagnosis		**F.A.**	first aid
e	without		**F.B.**	foreign body
e.g.	for example (Latin: exempli gratia)		**fem.**	femoral
			fet.	fetal
EBV	Epstein-Barr virus		**FFP**	fresh frozen plasma
ECG	electrocardiogram		**FH**	family history
ECHO	echocardiogram		**fl.**	fluids
EENT	eyes, ears, nose, throat		**fl. dr.**	fluid dram

fl. oz.	fluid ounce
flac.	flaccid
fld.	fluid
flex.	flexion
FR	fracture
FROM	full range of motion
FTT	failure to thrive
FU	follow-up
FUO	fever of unknown undetermined origin
FVC	forced vital capacity
Fx	fracture
g	gram
G	gravida (Latin: pregnant)
G.A.	general anesthesia
g/ml	grams per milliliter
GABA	gamma aminobutyric acid
Gal	gallon
GB	gallbladder
GC	general condition
GFR	glomerular filtration rate
gluc	glucose
gm	gram
gr.	grains (dosage)
GRAV	gravida (Latin: pregnant)
Grav.	pregnancy
gt.	drop (liquid)
gtt.	drops (liquid) (Latin: gutta)
H	history
h	hour (Latin: hora)

H & C	hot and cold
H & P	history and physical
h.d.	at bedtime
HRST	heat, reddening, swelling, tenderness
h.s.	at bedtime (Latin: hora somni)
H/A	headache
h/o	history of
H2O	water
H2O2	hydrogen peroxide
HA	headache
HBP	high blood pressure
HBV	hepatitis B virus
Hd	head
HEENT	head, eyes, ears, nose, throat
hern.	hernia
hgb	hemoglobin
hist.	history
HIV	human immunodeficiency virus
horiz.	horizontal
HRT	hormone replacement therapy
HS	bedtime
HS	at bedtime (Latin: hora somni)
HSV	herpes simplex virus
Ht	height
HT	hypertension
Hx	history

hypo	hypodermically		**int.**	internal
Hz	hertz (cycles per second)		**IQ**	intelligence quotient
I & D	incision and drainage		**irreg.**	irregular
I & O	intake and output		**ITP**	idiopathic thrombocytic purpura
i.c.	between meals (Latin: inter cenam)		**IV**	intravenous
i.d.	during the day		**IVC**	inferior vena cava
I.U.	international unit		**IVU**	intravenous urography
I/E	inspiratory/expiratory		**J**	joint
IBD	inflammatory bowel disease		**jt.**	joint
ICP	intracranial pressure		**JVP**	jugular venous pressure
ICU	intensive care unit		**K**	kidney; potassium
IDL	intermediate density lipoprotein		**Kg.**	kilogram
IgA	immunoglobulin A		**KUB**	kidney, ureter, bladder Xray
IgD	immunoglobulin D		**L**	left; lumbar
IgE	immunoglobulin E		**L.E.**	lower extremities
IgG	immunoglobulin G or Gamma Globulin		**L.N.**	lymph node
IgM	immunoglobulin M		**L.O.C.**	loss of consciousness
IHD	ischemic heart disease		**L.S.**	lumbosacral
IM	intramuscular		**l/min**	liter per minute
imp.	impression		**L1 – L5**	lumbar vertebra level
In.	inches		**LA**	left atrium
incr.	increased/increasing		**lab.**	laboratory
inf	inferior		**lac.**	laceration
inhal.	inhalation		**lat.**	lateral
inj	injection		**lax**	laxative
INR	international normalized ratio		**lb.**	pound
inspir	inspiration		**LBBB**	left bundle branch block
			LBP	lower back pain
			LFT	liver function test

lg	large		**MAL**	malignant
LH	lutenizing hormone		**max.**	maximum
lig.	ligament		**MCL**	midclavicular line
liq.	liquid		**MCV**	mean cell volume
LKS	liver, kidneys, spleen		**Mdnt.**	midnight
LLE	lower left extremity		**ME**	middle ear
LLQ	lower left quadrant (abdomen)		**Med.**	medicine
			Mets.	metastasis
LMP	last menstrual period		**mg.**	milligram
LOA	left occiput anterior		**mg/dl**	milligrams per deciliter
LOP	left occipital posterior		**MI**	myocardial infarction
LOS	length of stay		**micro**	microscopic
LOT	left occiput anterior		**min**	minute
LP	lumbar puncture		**ml.**	milliliter
LPN	licensed practical nurse		**mm**	muscles; millimeter
LRQ	lower right quadrant		**Mn.**	midnight
Ls.	loose		**mss**	massage
LSA	lateral sacrum anterior		**MSU**	midstream urine
LSB	left sternal border		**MVA**	motor vehicle accident
LSP	left sacrum posterior		**N & V**	nausea and vomiting
LST	left sacrum transverse		**N & W**	normal and well
Lt.	left; light		**n.**	nerve
LUE	left upper extremity		**n.p.o.**	nothing by mouth (Latin: nil per oris)
LUQ	left upper quadrant			
LVF	left ventricular failure		**N.S.**	nervous system
m	male; married; meter		**N/A**	not applicable
m.a.s.	patient is disagreeable and uncooperative		**N/T**	numbness & tingling
			NA	not available
m.b.	mix well		**NAD**	no abnormality detected; no apparent distress
M.T.	massage therapist; muscles and tendons			
			NBM	nothing by mouth

NED	no evidence of disease		**OCC.**	occasional; occipital
neg.	negative		**OCP**	oral contraceptive pill
NIP	no infection present		**od**	once daily
NKA	no known allergies		**OGTT**	oral glucose tolerance test
NM	neuromuscular		**oint.**	ointment
NMR	nuclear magnetic resonance		**OOB**	out of bed
no	number (Latin: numero)		**opt.**	best (Latin: optimus)
noct.	nocturnal		**OR**	operating room
NOS	not otherwise specified		**os**	bone (Latin: ossa); mouth (Latin: oris)
NS	nonspecific		**ot.**	ear
Ns.	nerves		**OTC**	over-the-counter (medication)
NSA	no significant abnormality		**OU**	both eyes; each eye (Latin: oculus uterqie)
NSAID	non-steroidal anti-inflammatory drug		**oz.**	ounce
NTP	normal temperature and pressure		**p**	after
NVD	nausea, vomiting, diarrhea		**P**	posterior
o	none		**p.c.**	after meals (Latin: post cenam)
O	oral		**P.M.**	afternoon (Latin: post meridiem); post-mortem
O.	pint (Latin: octarius)		**p.o.**	by mouth (Latin: per oris)
O.D.	right eye (Latin: oculus dexter)		**p.r.**	per rectum
O.L.	left eye		**p.r.m.**	according to circumstances
O.M.	otitis media		**p.r.n.**	as often as necessary (Latin: pro re nata)
O.S.	left eye (Latin: oculus sinister)		**p/c**	presenting complaint
O.T.	occupational therapy		**PA**	pulmonary artery
O/D	overdose		**PABA**	para- amino benzoic acid
O/E	on examination		**palp.**	palpable/palpated
O2	oxygen			
OC	oral contraceptive			

Pap	papanicolaou test (pap smear)
PAS	para-amino salicylic acid
Path.	pathology
PCL	posterior cruciate ligament
PCP	primary care physician
PCV	packed cell volume
PDA	patent ductus arteriosus
PDR	physician's desk reference
pdr.	powder
PEEP	positive-end expiratory pressure
PEFR	peak expiratory flow rate
per	Through; by
per/os	by mouth (Latin: per oris)
PERLA	pupils equal & responding to light & accomodation
PET	positron emission tomography
pH	potential of hydrogen (measure of acidity)
PH	past history
pharm	pharmacy
PHYS.	physical
PI	present illness
PID	pelvic inflammatory disease
PLL	posterior longitudinal lig.
PMH	past medical history
PNS	peripheral nervous system
POI	post operative instructions
pos.	positive
post.	posterior
POSTOP	postoperative
PP	per protocol
pp	post partum; post prandial
ppm	parts per million
ppt	part per trillion
pre-op	preoperative
prep.	prepare for; prepare as
PRICE	protection, rest, ice, compression, elevation
prod.	productive
Prog.	prognosis
PROM	passive range of motion
pron.	pronation
pros.	prostate
prosth.	prosthesis
PSH	past surgical history
psi	pounds per square inch
PT	physical therapy
pt.	patient
PTH	parathyroid hormone
PTT	partial thromboplastin time
Px	physical examination
q	each/every (Latin: quaque)
q.d.	once a day
q.h.	every hour
q.i.d.	four times a day (Latin: quarter in die)
q.i.w.	four times a week
q.l.	as much as desired

q.n.s.	quantity not sufficient
q.o.d.	every other day
q.o.n.	every other night
q.p.	as much as you please
q.q.	each; every (Latin: quaque)
q.q.h.	every four hours (Latin: quaque quarta hora)
q.s.	a sufficient quantity (Latin: quantum sufficiat)
q.v.	as much as you wish
q.w.	every week
q2H	every two hours
q4H	every four hours (Latin: quaque quarta hora)
q6H	every six hours
qhs	once in the evening
qn	every night (Latin: quaque nox)
QNS	quantity not sufficient
qt.	quart
qts.	drops
quant.	quantity
r.	rectal
R.	rub
R/O	rule out
RA	rheumatoid arthritis
rad.	radial; radiating
RAG	R antigen
RAtx	radiation therapy
RBC	red blood cell
rect.	rectal

reg.	regular
rehab.	rehabilitation
resp.	respirations
RFA	right frontoanterior
RFP	right frontoposterior
RFT	right frontotransverse
RLE	right lower extremity
RLQ	right lower quadrant
RMA	right mentoanterior
RML	right mediolateral
RMP	right mentoposterior
RMT	right mentotransverse
RNA	ribonucleic acid
RO	rule out
ROM	range of motion (joint)
ROP	right occipital posterior
ROS	review of systems
ROT	right occipital transverse
RRR	regular rate and rhythm
RSA	right sacrum anterior (fetal position)
RSP	right sacrum posterior (fetal position)
RST	right sacrum transverse (fetal position)
Rt.	right
RUE	right upper extremity
RUL	right upper lobe (lung)
RUQ	right upper quadrant
RVF	right ventricular failure

Rx	prescription; therapy; treatment
S	sensation
s	(with a bar on top) without (Latin: sans)
s.i.d.	once a day (Latin: semel in die)
s.l.	in a broad sense (Latin: sensu lato)
S.O.A.P.	subjective, objective, assessment, plan
S.O.S.	repeat once if urgent
S/S	signs and symptoms
SBE	subacute bacterial endocarditis
sec	second
SI	sacroiliac joint
sib.	sibling
SIDS	sudden infant death syndrome
Sig., S.	write on the label (Latin: signa)
SIJ	sacroiliac joint
skel.	skeletal
SL	under the tongue (Latin: sub lingua)
sl	in a broad sense (Latin: sensu lato)
Sl.	slightly
SLA	left sacroanterior (fetal position) (Latin: sacrolaeva anterior)
SLE	systemic lupus erythematosus

SLP	left sacroposterior (fetal position) (Latin: sacrolaeva posterior)
SLR	straight leg raise test
SLT	left sacrotransverse (fetal position) (Latin: sacrolaeva transversa)
sm	small
SO	superior oblique
SOA	swelling of ankles
SOB	shortness of breath
SOB (OE)	shortness of breath (on exercise)
sod.	sodium
SOL	space occupying lesion
Sol.	solution
sp.	spinal
sp.cd.	spinal cord
sp.fl.	spinal fluid
sp.gr	specific gravity
spec.	specimen
spin.	spinal
spont.	spontaneous
st.	stomach
stat.	immediately (Latin: statim)
STD	sexually transmitted disease
subcut.	subcutaneous
subling.	sublingual
sup.	superior
supin.	supination

supp	suppository
surg.	surgery
SVC	superior vena cava
SVT	supraventricular tachycardia
Sx	symptoms
sys.	system
syst.	systolic
T	temperature; thoracic
t.i.d.	three times a day (Latin: ter in die)
t.i.w.	three times per week
T.M.	ear drum (Latin: tympanum membrani)
T1–T12	thoracic vertebra level
tab.	tablet (Latin: tabella)
tbsp.	tablespoon
tds	three times daily
temp	temperature
TENS	transcutaneous electric nerve stimulation
THERAP	therapeutic
thor.	thoracic
TIA	transient ischemic attack
TLC	tender loving care
TMJ	temporomandibular joint
TNF	tumor necrosis factor
TNM	tumor, nodes, and metastases
TPN	total parenteral nutrition
tr	trace
TRH	thyroid releasing hormone

TSH	thyroid stimulating hormone
tsp.	teaspoon
TURP	transurethral resection of prostate
Tx	treatment
U & E	urea and electrolyte
U.	unit
u/o	under observation for
UC	ulcerative colitis
UCD	usual childhood diseases
UE	upper extremity (Latin: extremitas)
uln	ulnar
ULQ	upper left quadrant
umb.	umbilicus
ung.	ointment
unilat.	unilateral
Ur.	urine
URQ	upper right quadrant
URTI	upper respiratory tract infection
US	ultrasound
ut.	uterus
UTI	urinary tract infection
V	vein
V.S.	vital signs
vert.	vertical
VF	ventricular fibrillation
Via	by way of
vit.	vitamin

vol	volume
VS	vital signs
VSD	ventricular septal defect
VT	ventricular tachycardia
W	widowed
W/A	while awake
w/c	wheelchair; will call
w/n	within
WDWN	well developed, well nourished
wh.ch.	wheelchair
wk	week
WN	well nourished
WNL	within normal limits
wt.	weight
x	times
x/12	number of months
x/52	number of weeks
x/7	number of days
y.o.	years old
yrs.	years

A reporter, in an interview, asked Albert Einstein if he knew his own phone number. Mr. Einstein laughed and said that he did not.

The reporter then asked what the smartest man in the world would do if he needed to call home. Mr. Einstein's response was to lift a phone book, and state that it's not important to Know everything, rather, it's more important to Know Where to Find what you want.

Glossary

Abdominal cavity The part of the body between the bottom of the ribs and the top of the thighs.

Abduction Movement of the limb away from the medial plane.

ABO blood groups The system by which human blood is classified, based on proteins occurring on red blood cells. The four classification groups are A, AB, B, and O.

Abscess An accumulation of pus in a body tissue, usually caused by a bacterial infection.

Acetylcholine A chemical that works in the brain to transmit nerve signals.

Achilles tendon The tendon at the back of the lower leg that connects the calf muscle to the heel bone.

Acid base balance The mechanisms that the body uses to keep its fluids close to neutral (neither basic nor acidic) so that the body can function properly.

Acid reflux A disorder in which acid in the stomach backs up into the esophagus, because the valve separating the stomach and esophagus does not function properly. (See GERD.)

Acidosis A condition marked by abnormally high acid levels in the blood, associated with some forms of diabetes, lung disease, and severe kidney disease.

Acne A skin condition characterized by inflamed, pus-filled areas that occur on the skin's surface, most commonly occurring during adolescence.

Acquired A word describing any condition that is not present at birth, but developing at some point during life.

Acquired Immuno-Deficiency Syndrome Infection by the human immunodeficiency virus (HIV), which causes a weakening of the immune system. Also called AIDS.

Acute Describes a condition or illness that begins suddenly and includes inflammation.

Adduction Movement of the limb toward the medial plane.

Adenitis	Infection and inflammation of a gland, e.g. a lymph node.
Adipose	Another term for fatty tissue.
Adjuvant therapy	The use of drugs or radiation therapy in the treatment of cancer along with surgery.
Adrenal glands	Two small glands located on top of the kidneys that secrete several important hormones into the blood.
Adrenaline	A hormone produced by the adrenal glands in response to stress, exercise, or fear. Adrenaline increases the heart rate and opens airways to improve breathing. Also called epinephrine.
Adverse reaction	An unintended and unwanted side effect of some sort of treatment.
Afebrile	Without fever.
Affective disorder	A mental disorder involving abnormal moods and emotions, e.g. manic-depressive disorder, seasonal affective disorder (SAD).
Afferent nerve	Nerves that carry information about the body's senses toward the brain. Also called sensory nerve.
AIDS	See Acquired ImmunoDeficiency Syndrome.
AIDS-related complex	Symptoms including weight loss, fever, and enlarged lymph nodes experienced by people who are infected with HIV but do not yet have AIDS. Also called ARC.
Air embolism	The blockage of an artery by an air bubble which may have entered during surgery or after an injury.
Airway obstruction	Blockage of the passage of air through the windpipe to the lungs.
Albinism	A condition in which people are born with insufficient amounts of the pigment melanin, which is responsible for hair, skin, and eye color. Also called hypopigmentation.
Alimentary canal	Another term for the digestive tract.
Alkalosis	Dangerously decreased acidity of the blood, which can be caused by high altitudes, hyperventilation, and excessive vomiting.
Allergen	A substance that causes an allergic reaction.

Allergy	An excessive immune reaction to a substance.
Alopecia	Partial or complete lack of hair resulting from normal aging, physical disorders, drug reaction, anticancer medications, or skin disease.
Altitude sickness	Headaches, dizziness, and nausea usually experienced at heights above 8,000 feet because of reduced oxygen concentration in the air.
Alveoli	Tiny sac-like air spaces in the lung where carbon dioxide and oxygen are exchanged.
Amenorrhea	Absence of menstrual periods.
Anal fissure	A linear open sore on the skin of the anus.
Anal fistula	An abnormal tubelike passage connecting the anus to the surface of the surrounding skin.
Anal sphincter	A ring of muscle fibers at the opening of the rectum, controlling the opening and closing of the anus.
Anaphylactic shock	A life-threatening allergic reaction resulting in difficulty breathing and low blood pressure.
Anemia	A physical state in which there is a loss of red blood cells and/or hemoglobin.
Anesthesia	A loss of sensations, including the ability to sense heat, cold, pain or pressure. General anesthesia includes loss of consciousness.
Anesthetic	See anesthesia.
Aneurysm	An abnormal swelling of the wall of an artery, caused by a weakening in the vessel wall.
Angiogenesis	The process of creating new blood vessels.
Angioplasty	Surgically widening or reconstructing a blood vessel.
Annulus fibrosus	The thick ligamentous outer portion of a vertebral disc that contains the nucleus pulposus.
Anterior	At or toward the front of the body. Opposed to posterior.
Antibiotics	Bacteria killing substances that are used to fight infection.
Antibody	A protein made by white blood cells that reacts with a specific foreign protein as part of the immune response.

Anticoagulants	Drugs that reduce blood clotting to help prevent a heart attack or stroke.
Antiemetics	A substance used to treat nausea and vomiting.
Antihistamine	A substance that relieves an allergic reaction by reducing the production of histamine.
Antihypertensives	Drugs used to relieve the symptoms and prevent the damage that can occur from high blood pressure.
Antioxidants	Substances that protect against cell damage by guarding the cell from oxygen free radicals.
Antiseptics	Chemicals applied to the skin that prevent infection by killing bacteria and other harmful organisms.
Anus	The opening through which feces are passed from the body.
Aorta	The main artery in the body, carrying oxygenated blood from the heart to other arteries in the body.
Aortic stenosis	Narrowing of the opening of the aortic valve in the heart, which increases resistance to blood flow from the left ventricle to the aorta.
Aplasia	The complete failure of any organ or tissue to grow.
Apnea	A condition in which a person stops breathing for a period of time and then spontaneously resumes breathing.
Apoptosis	The self destruction of a cell at the end of its DNA programmed lifespan.
Appendectomy	Surgical removal of the appendix to treat appendicitis.
ARC	AIDS related complex: Symptoms including weight loss, fever, and enlarged lymph nodes experienced by people who are infected with HIV but do not yet have AIDS.
Arrhythmia	An irregular heartbeat.
Arteriosclerosis	A disorder causing thickening and/or hardening of artery walls.
Arteritis	Inflammation of the walls of an artery that causes the passageway to become narrower.

Artery	A large blood vessel that carries blood from the heart to tissues and organs in the body.
Arthroscopy	A procedure used to examine the inside of a joint using an endoscope.
Artificial respiration	The forcing of air into the lungs of a person who has stopped breathing (either by mouth-to-mouth or mouth-to-nose).
Ascites	Excess fluid in the abdominal cavity.
Asphyxia	The medical term for suffocation. It can be caused by choking on an object, by lack of oxygen in the air, or by chemicals such as carbon monoxide, which reduce the amount of oxygen in the blood.
Asthma	A disorder characterized by inflamed airways and difficulty breathing.
Astigmatism	A disorder in which the front surface of the eye (the cornea) is not correctly spherical, resulting in blurry vision.
Asymptomatic	Without obvious signs or symptoms of disease.
Atherectomy	A procedure performed to remove plaque that is blocking an artery.
Atheroma	Fatty deposits on the inner walls of blood vessels, which can cause narrowing and decrease blood flow.
Atresia	A birth defect in which a normal body opening or canal is absent; usually requires surgical repair soon after birth.
Atria	The two upper chambers of the heart; the singular form is atrium.
Atrial fibrillation	An irregular heartbeat in which the upper chambers of the heart (the atria) beat inconsistently and rapidly.
Atrial flutter	An irregular heartbeat in which the upper chambers of the heart (the atria) beat rapidly but consistently.
Atrophy	A wasting away or decrease in size of a cell, tissue, organ, or part of the body caused by lack of nourishment, inactivity or loss of nerve supply.

Audiogram	A graph showing a person's hearing ability, determined from a set of tests examining hearing acuity of different sound frequencies.
Aura	A "warning" signal that comes before a migraine headache or an epileptic seizure, which might include emotions or sensations of movement or discomfort.
Auscultation	The act of listening to sounds within the body, such as the heartbeat, with a stethoscope.
Autoantibody	A protein made by white blood cells that attacks the body's own tissues.
Autoimmune disease	A disorder in which the body's immune system attacks itself.
Autonomic nervous system	The part of the nervous system that controls automatic body functions, such as heart rate, sweating, pupil dilation, and digestion.
Autopsy	The examination of a body following death, possibly to determine the cause of death or for research.
Autosomal dominant	A term describing a gene on any chromosome other than the sex chromosomes that produces its effect whenever it is present; can also describe the effect of the gene itself.
Autosomal recessive	A term used to describe a gene on any chromosome other than the sex chromosomes that produces its effect only when two copies of it are present; can also describe the effect of the gene itself.
Avascular	Without blood vessels. e.g. cartilage is avascular.
Axilla	Medical term for the armpit.
B cell	A white blood cell that makes antibodies to fight infections caused by foreign proteins.
B lymphocyte	A type of white blood cell that makes antibodies and is an important part of the immune response.
Bacteremia	A condition in which bacteria are present in the bloodstream; may occur after minor surgery or infection and may be dangerous for people with a weakened immune system or abnormal heart valves.
Bacteriostatic	Term used to describe a substance that stops the growth of bacteria (such as an antibiotic).

Bacterium	A tiny, single-celled microorganism, commonly known as a germ; some bacteria, called pathogens, cause disease.
Bacteriuria	Bacteria in the urine; large amounts can indicate bladder, urethra, or kidney infection.
Balloon angioplasty	A technique that uses a balloon catheter to open arteries clogged with fatty deposits.
Balloon catheter	A hollow tube with a small, inflatable balloon at the tip; used to open a narrowed artery or organ that has become blocked.
Barium enema	A technique in which barium is placed into the large intestine and rectum and then X-rays are taken to check for possible disorders of these organs.
Basal metabolic rate	The lowest rate at which a person can possibly use energy and remain alive; at this rate, only absolutely necessary functions such as breathing are maintained.
Basement membrane	The thin boundary layer made of basal cells between the epidermis and the dermis that protects the internal tissues from surface infection.
BCG vaccine	A vaccine used to protect against tuberculosis.
Bed sore	An erosion or ulcer on the skin caused by prolonged pressure inhibiting blood supply. Also called decubitus ulcer.
Bends	See Decompression sickness.
Benign	Refers to a slow growing tumor that is not able to spread to distant tissues (metastasize) or invade nearby tissues.
Bicuspid valve	A two leaflet valve between the upper and lower chambers on the left side of the heart (the right atrium and right ventricle). Also called the mitral valve.
Bifocal	A lens that corrects both near and distant vision by having two parts with different focusing strengths.
Bilateral	Both sides of the body.

Bile
A yellow-green liquid produced in the liver and stored in the gall bladder whose function is to remove waste from the liver and break down fats as food is digested.

Bileduct
A tube that carries bile from the liver to the gallbladder and then to the small intestine.

Biliary atresia
A birth defect in which the bile ducts are not completely developed.

Biliary colic
A severe pain in the upper right section of the abdomen, usually caused by a gallstone passing out of the gallbladder or through the bile ducts.

Biliary tract
The system of organs and ducts through which bile is made and transported from the liver to the small intestine.

Bilirubin
The orange-yellow pigment in bile, causing jaundice if it builds up in the blood and skin; the levels of bilirubin in the blood are used to diagnose liver disease.

Bioavailable
The portion of a nutrient or other chemical that can be absorbed, transported, and utilized physiologically.

Biochemistry
The science that studies the chemistry of living organisms, including humans.

Bioequivalent
A drug that has the same effect on the body as another drug.

Biofeedback
A technique used to gain control over a function that is normally automatic (such as blood pressure or pulse rate); the function is monitored and relaxation techniques are used to change it to a desired level.

Biopsy
The use of a large hollow needle to remove a sample of tissue for examination.

Birth defect
An abnormality that is present when a baby is born.

Birthmark
Any area of discolored skin that is present at birth.

Bladder
An organ located in the pelvis whose function is to collect and store urine until it is expelled.

Blepharitis
Inflammation of the eyelids.

Blind spot	A spot in the field of vision that is not sensitive to light; it is a product of the entrance of the optic nerve into the eyeball, where no light receptors are present on the retina.
Blister	A lesion filled with clear, serous fluid that is larger than 5 millimeters in diameter. Also called a Bulla.
Blood clot	A mass of blood that forms to help seal and minimize bleeding.
Blood poisoning	See Septicemia.
Blood pressure	The tension in the main arteries that is created by the beating of the heart and the resistance to flow and elasticity of the blood vessels.
Blood transfusion	The transfer of blood or any of its parts to a person who has lost blood due to an injury, disease or surgery.
Blood type	A category used to describe a person's blood according to the kinds of proteins present on the surface of the red blood cells.
Blood-brain barrier	A layer of tightly bound cells that prevents certain substances carried in the bloodstream from entering the brain.
Bone marrow	The fatty yellow or red tissue inside bones that is responsible for producing blood cells.
Bone spur	Calcium deposits resulting from traumatic or repetitive stress to a tendon or ligament where it attaches to the bone.
Booster	An additional dose of a vaccine given after the first dose to maintain or renew the first one.
Botulism	Poisoning from poorly preserved food contaminated with a dangerous bacterial toxin that results in paralysis. Used in Botox treatment by injecting locally for intentional paralysis.
Bowel	See Intestine.
Bradycardia	A heart rate below 60 beats per minute in adults.
Bradykinesia	Abnormally slow movements, often associated with Parkinson's disease.

Brain damage	Death of brain cells resulting in decreased mental ability.
Brain death	The condition in which the brain stops functioning while the heart continues to beat.
Bronchiolitis	An infection caused by a virus in the bronchioles (the smallest airways in the lungs), mainly affecting young children.
Bronchitis	Inflammation of the bronchial tubes, which connect the trachea to the lungs.
Bronchoconstrictor	A substance that causes the lung airways to tighten up and become more narrow.
Bronchodilator	A drug that relaxes and widens the airways.
Bronchospasm	The temporary narrowing of the airways in the lungs, either as a result of muscle contraction or inflammation.
Bruise	See Contusion.
Bruxism	An unconscious clenching or grinding of the teeth, usually during sleep.
Bulimia	A disorder in which a person eats large amounts of food then forces vomiting or uses laxatives to prevent weight gain; see binging and purging.
Bulla	A lesion filled with clear, serous fluid that is larger than 5 millimeters in diameter. Commonly called a blister.
Bunion	Enlargement of the bone at one of the joints of the big toe, usually from improperly fitting footwear or excessive physical activity.
Bursa	A fluid-filled sac that cushions and reduces friction in certain parts of the body.
Bursitis	Inflammation of a bursa due to injury or repetitive trauma.
Bypass	A surgical technique in which the flow of blood or another body fluid is redirected around a blockage.
Cachexia	The malnutrition and wasting of bodily tissue that is produced by chronic diseases, such as the drain on host nutrients produced by the proliferation of cancer cells

Calcification	The depositing of calcium salts in the body, which occurs normally in teeth and bones but abnormally in soft tissues and arteries.
Calcitonin	A hormone made in the thyroid gland that controls calcium levels in the blood by slowing the loss of calcium from bones; used to treat hypercalcemia (excess calcium in the blood).
Callous formation	Calcium deposits connecting two fractured bones to stabilize while repairing the break.
Callus	A thickened area of skin due to consistent pressure or friction, or the area around a bone break where new bone is formed.
Calorie	A unit that is used to measure the energy content in food.
Canal	A tunnel-like passage.
Cancer	"Cancer" comes from the Latin word for "crab," and refers both to the tendency of a malignant neoplasm to grasp tissues firmly and not let go (like a crab) or their microscopic crab-shaped appearance (with growing extensions in several directions).
Candida	See candidiasis.
Candidiasis	A systemic yeast infection caused by the fungus Candida albicans.
Canker sore	Small, painful sore that usually occurs on the inside of the lip or cheek, or sometimes under the tongue; caused by bacteria, irritation, stress, allergies or a pH imbalance.
Capillary	A tiny blood vessel that connects the smallest arteries to the smallest veins and allows exchange of oxygen and other materials between blood cells and body tissue cells.
Carbohydrate	A substance comprised of sugar and starch that is a main source of energy for the body; found in food sources such as fruits, cereals, breads, pastas, grains, and vegetables.
Carbon dioxide	A colorless, odorless gas present in small amounts in the atmosphere and formed during respiration.
Carcinogen	Anything that can cause cancer.

Cardiac arrest	The sudden cessation of the heart's pumping action, possibly due to a heart attack, respiratory arrest, electrical shock, extreme cold, blood loss, drug overdose, or a severe allergic reaction.
Cardiogenic shock	A dangerous condition involving decreased blood output from the heart, usually as a result of a heart attack.
Cardiomegaly	A condition marked by enlargement of the heart, either because of a thickened heart muscle or an enlarged heart chamber; usually a result of the heart having to work harder than normal, as occurs with high blood pressure.
Cardiomyopathy	A heart disease where thickened muscle results in decreased output and reduced blood flow.
Cardiopulmonary resuscitation	The administration of heart compression and artificial respiration to restore circulation and breathing. Commonly called CPR.
Carditis	Inflammation of the heart.
Carotene	A pigment found in orange vegetables and fruits, which the body converts to vitamin A.
Carotid arteries	Arteries that carry blood to the head and neck.
Cast	A hard plaster or fiberglass shell that molds to a body part such as an arm and holds it in place for proper healing.
CAT scan	See Computerized Axial Tomography Scan.
Cataract	A disorder in which the lens of the eye becomes less transparent and in some cases a milky white, making vision less clear.
Catheter	A hollow, flexible tube inserted into the body to put in or take out fluid, or to open narrowed blood vessels.
Catheterization	A technique in which a hollow, flexible tube is used to drain body fluids (such as urine), to introduce fluids into the body, or to examine or widen a narrowed vein or artery.

Cat-scratch fever	An illness transmitted to humans through a cat's bite or scratch, which is thought to be caused by bacteria; characterized by swollen lymph nodes, a blister near the injury, fever, rash and headache.
Caudal	Inferior. Anatomically beneath, lower, or toward the bottom.
Cauliflower ear	A deformed ear caused by repeated injury.
Cauterization	The use of heat, laser, an electric current, or a chemical to destroy tissue or stop bleeding.
Cecum	The first portion of the large intestine.
Cell	The tiny structures that make up all the tissues of the body and carry out all of its functions.
Cellulitis	A skin infection caused by bacteria which can lead to tissue damage and blood poisoning if untreated.
Central nervous system	The brain and spinal cord.
Cerebellum	A region of the brain located at the back which is responsible for coordination of movement and maintaining balance.
Cerebrospinal fluid	A clear, watery fluid circulating in and around the brain and spinal column, which contains glucose, proteins, and salts for nutrition.
Cesarean section	An operation performed to remove a fetus by cutting into the uterus through the abdominal wall.
Chancre	A painless sore that has a thick, rubbery base and a defined edge.
Chemotherapy	The treatment of infections or cancer with drugs that act on disease-producing organisms or cancerous tissue.
Chlamydia	Microorganisms that cause several human infections and can be transmitted sexually.
Cholecystectomy	The surgical removal of the gallbladder.
Cholesterol	A fat-like substance that is made by the body and is found naturally in animal foods such as meat, fish, poultry, eggs, and dairy products.
Cholinesterase	A substance that breaks down acetylcholine.
Chondritis	Inflammation of cartilage.

Chondroma	A benign cartilage tumor.
Chorionic villus sampling	A method of diagnosing fetal defects in which a small amount of tissue is taken from the placenta and analyzed for abnormalities.
Choroiditis	Inflammation of the blood vessels that line the back of the eye.
Chronic	Term used to describe persistence for a long time. In some disorders, chronic is specified as persisting for 6 months or longer.
Cilia	Tiny, hairlike structures on the outside of some cells, providing mobility.
Cirrhosis	Gradual loss of liver function due to cell damage and internal scarring.
Claudication	Cramping, pain or fatigue in arms and legs due to poor supply of oxygen to the muscles.
Claustrophobia	Fear of being confined in an enclosed or crowded space.
Cleft lip	A birth defect in which the upper lip is split vertically, extending into one or both nostrils.
Cleft palate	A birth defect in which the roof of the mouth is split, extending from behind the teeth to the nasal cavity; often occurs with other birth defects such as cleft lip and partial deafness.
Clone	An exact DNA copy of a gene, cell, or organism.
Clotting factors	A group of substances in the blood that are needed for blood to harden and stop a wound from bleeding.
Clubfoot	A genetic disorder in which the foot is twisted and misshapen.
CNS	See Central Nervous System.
Coagulation	The conversion of blood from a liquid form to a solid form called a clot.
Cocarcinogen	A substance that does not cause cancer by itself, but increases the effect of a substance that does cause cancer.

Cochlea A coiled organ in the inner ear that plays a large role in hearing by picking up sound vibrations and transmitting them as electrical signals.

Colectomy The complete or partial surgical removal of the large intestine.

Colic A condition characterized by excessive crying in an otherwise healthy baby.

Colitis Inflammation of the large intestine (the colon), which usually leads to abdominal pain, fever, and diarrhea with blood and mucus.

Collagenase An enzyme secreted by a malignancy (cancer) that destroys healthy tissue. Also used as a cream in certain skin conditions.

Colon The main part of the large intestine, between the cecum and the rectum.

Colonoscopy Investigation of the inside of the colon using a long, flexible fiberoptic tube.

Color blindness Any vision disorder in which the person sees colors abnormally, has trouble distinguishing between them, or cannot see them at all.

Colostomy A surgical procedure in which some part of the colon is cut and redirected to the surface of the abdomen so that feces can be passed into a bag worn outside of the body.

Coma A condition in which the area of the brain involved in maintaining consciousness is somehow affected, resulting in a state of unconsciousness in which the patient does not respond to stimulation.

Communicable disease A disease that can be passed from one individual to another.

Computerized Axial Tomography Scan A technique for producing cross-sectional images of the body in which X-rays are passed through the body at different angles and analyzed by a computer; also called CT scanning or CAT scanning.

Concussion A short-term loss of consciousness due to physical head trauma or pressure.

Congenital Present or existing at the time of birth.

Conjunctiva	The clear membrane covering the white of the eye and the inside of the eyelid that produces a fluid that lubricates the cornea and eyelid.
Conjunctivitis	Inflammation of the conjunctiva; commonly called pinkeye.
Connective tissue	Connective tissue supports, binds, or separates more specialized tissues and organs of the body. Types of connective tissue include bone, cartilage, tendon, ligament, and adipose.
Constipation	Difficult or infrequent bowel movements of hard, dry feces.
Contagious	Able to be spread from person to person, or living object to nonliving object to living host.
Contraindication	An aspect of a patient's condition that makes the use of a certain drug or therapy an unwise or dangerous decision.
Contusion	Damage to the skin and underlying tissue as a result of a blunt injury. Commonly called a bruise.
Corn	A thickened callus on the foot that is caused by improper stress on a localized portion of skin.
Cornea	The clear, dome-shaped front portion of the eye's outer covering.
Coronal	A plane which divides the body into two parts by a plane passing at right angles to the sagittal plane.
Coronary	Describes structures that encircle another structure (such as the coronary arteries, which circle the heart); commonly used to refer to a coronary thrombosis or a heart attack.
Coronary arteries	The arteries that branch off from the aorta and supply blood to the heart muscle.
Coronary artery bypass surgery	An operation in which a piece of vein or artery is used to bypass a blockage in a coronary artery; performed to prevent myocardial infarction and relieve angina pectoris.
Coronary heart disease	Disorders that restrict the blood supply to the heart, including atherosclerosis.
Coronary thrombosis	The blockage of a coronary artery by a blood clot.

Corpuscle	A tiny, rounded structure in the body, such as a red or white blood cell.
Corticosteroids	Synthetic drugs that are used to replace natural hormones or to suppress the immune system and help prevent inflammation.
CPR	See Cardiopulmonary resuscitation.
Cranial	A position superior to another or closer to the head.
Creatinine	A waste product that is filtered from the blood by the kidneys and expelled in urine.
Croup	A usually mild and temporary condition common in children under the age of four in which the walls of the airways become inflamed and narrow, resulting in wheezing and coughing.
Cruciate ligaments	Two ligaments in the knee (anterior and posterior) that cross each other and stabilize the knee joint.
Crust	An area on the surface of the skin containing dried exudate. Also called a scab.
CT scanning	See Computerized Axial Tomography scan.
Culture	The artificial growth of cells, tissue, or microorganisms such as bacteria in a laboratory.
Curettage	Cleansing of a surface by scraping.
Cutaneous	When referring to skin, usually means the dermis.
CVS	See chorionic villus sampling.
Cyanosis	A bluish discoloration of the skin, caused by low levels of oxygen in the blood.
Cyst	A fluid filled sac.
Cystectomy	Surgical removal of the bladder; the bladder is often replaced with a short length of small intestine.
Cystic fibrosis	An inherited disorder in which the lungs are prone to infection, and fats and other nutrients cannot be absorbed into the body.
Cystitis	Inflammation of the lining and/or muscle of the bladder.
Cystoscopy	Examination of the urethra and bladder using a long, thin, fiberoptic tube.

Cystostomy	The surgical placement of a drainage opening in the bladder.
D and C	See Dilatation and Curettage.
Debridement	Surgical removal of dead, damaged, or infected tissue, or some foreign material from a wound or burn.
Decompression sickness	The formation of nitrogen gas bubbles in the body's tissues as a result of a scuba diver ascending too quickly from depth; also called the bends.
Decubitus ulcer	A craterlike ulceration of skin and subcutaneous tissue caused by prolonged pressure on the area. This occurs primarily over bony prominences of the lower back and hips in individual who are unable to care for themselves well and unable to roll or move periodically; also known as pressure sore or bedsore.
Deep	The structure is toward or near the center of the body or organ.
Deep tissue therapy	Slow strokes and intense, prolonged pressure on the deeper layers of muscles, tendons and fascia.
Defecation	The passing of feces out of the body through the anus; also called a bowel movement.
Defibrillation	A short electric shock to the chest to normalize an irregular heartbeat.
Dehydration	Excessive, dangerous loss of water from the body.
Dementia	A decline in mental ability.
Depilatory	A chemical hair remover.
Depot injection	Injection of a drug into a muscle, allowing the drug to absorb slowly into the bloodstream.
Dermabrasion	Removal of the surface layer of skin with a sanding wheel to treat scarring or to remove tattoos.
Dermatitis	See eczema.
Dermatomes	Sensory segments of the skin supplied by a specific nerve root.
Dermis	The layer of skin just underneath the epidermis that contains sensitive nerve endings, blood vessels, and hair follicles

Desensitization	The process of making a person less allergic to a substance by injecting gradually increasing amounts of the substance; sometimes done to prevent anaphylactic shock.
Detoxification	Treatment given either to fight a person's dependence on alcohol or other drugs or to rid the body of a poisonous substance and its effects.
Dextrocardia	A rare genetic condition in which the heart is located on the right side of the body, instead of the left.
Dextrose	Another name for the sugar glucose.
Diagnosis	the process of identifying a disease by its characteristic signs, symptoms, and lab findings.
Dialysis	A procedure in which an internal structure or external machine is used to filter waste from the blood and remove excess fluid from the body.
Diaphragm	The large, dome-shaped muscle separating the abdomen and chest that contracts and relaxes to make breathing possible; also, a thin, rubber dome that is used as a method of female contraception.
Diastolic pressure	The blood pressure measured when the heart is at rest between beats. It measures the pressure exerted by the artery walls.
Diathermy	The use of high-frequency currents, microwaves, or ultrasound to produce heat in the body in order to increase blood flow, relieve pain, or destroy diseased tissue.
Differentiation	The modification of a cell in terms of structure and/or function occurring during the course of development.
Dilatation and Curettage	A procedure in which the vagina and cervix are widened and the lining of the uterus is scraped away to diagnose and treat disorders of the uterus or as a method of abortion.
Diphtheria	A bacterial infection that causes a fever, headache, sore throat, and possibly death; diphtheria is rare in developed countries.
Disc	A flexible ligamentous pad with a gel center situated in the joint between vertebrae.

Disease	Any deviation from the normal structure or function of the human body that is manifested by a characteristic set of one or more signs or symptoms.
Dislocation	Complete separation of two bones in a joint.
Distal	At the end of, or in the area farthest from the center of the body.
Distention	Swelling, enlargement, or stretching.
Diuresis	The increased secretion of urine by the kidneys.
Diuretic	A substance that increases the amount of water in the urine, removing excess water from the body; also a drug used in treating high blood pressure and fluid retention.
Diverticulitis	Inflammation of diverticula (small sacs in the intestine's inner lining) which can cause fever and/or pain.
DNA	The particular sequence of four chemical building blocks (nucleotides) adenine, cytosine, guanine and thymine that make up a DNA chain and determines the unique genetic code of an individual.
Dominant gene	A gene that always produces its effect when it is present.
Dopamine	A chemical that transmits messages in the brain and plays a role in movement.
Dorsal	Toward posterior portion of the body.
Down syndrome	A genetic disorder in which a person's cells have one too many chromosomes, causing moderate to severe mental handicap and an altered appearance.
Duodenal ulcer	Erosion in the inner lining of the wall of the first part of the small intestine; see ulcer.
Duodenum	The first part of the small intestine, immediately following the stomach.
Dysentery	A severe intestinal infection causing abdominal pain and diarrhea with blood or mucus.
Dysphagia	Difficulty swallowing.
Dysplasia	An abnormal loss of cell differentiation. Dysplasia is a precancerous condition that may or may not turn into cancer at a later time.

Dyspnea	Difficulty breathing.
Dystrophy	Any disorder in which cells become damaged or do not grow properly.
Dysuria	Difficulty urinating.
ECG	Electrocardiogram: a record of the electrical impulses that trigger the heartbeat, used to diagnose heart disorders.
Echocardiogram	An image of the heart that is created by high-frequency (ultrasound) sound waves.
Ectopic	"Out of place;" referring to a pregnancy occurring elsewhere than in the cavity of the uterus, or a part of the heart rhythm that is out of place.
Eczema	Inflammation of the skin, usually causing itchiness and sometimes blisters and scaling; called dermatitis.
Edema	Abnormal buildup of fluid in the body's tissues.
EEG	Electroencephalography: A procedure for recording the electrical impulses of brain activity.
Efferent	A nerve that carries messages to a muscle that cause the muscle to contract. Also called a motor nerve.
Effleurage	A stroke generally used in a Swedish massage treatment. This smooth, gliding stroke is used to relax soft tissue and is applied using both hands.
Effusion	A collection of fluid in a body cavity, usually between two adjoining tissues.
EKG	Obsolete term for electrocardiogram.
Elective	Describes a treatment or procedure that is not urgent and can be arranged at the patient's convenience.
Electrocardiogram	A record of the electrical impulses that trigger the heartbeat, used to diagnose heart disorders. Also called an ECG.
Electroencephalography	A procedure for recording the electrical impulses of brain activity. Also called an EEG.
Electromyography	A test that measures muscle response to nervous stimulation (electrical activity within muscle fibers); also called an EMG or a myogram.

Embolism	The blockage of a blood vessel by an embolus.
Embolus	An abnormal particle (such as a blood clot or air bubble) circulating in the bloodstream.
Emetic	A substance that causes vomiting.
Emphysema	A chronic disease in which the small air sacs in the lungs (the alveoli) become damaged; characterized by difficult breathing.
Encapsulate	To enclose in a capsule.
Endarterectomy	Surgery performed to remove the lining of an artery that has been narrowed by fatty tissue buildup.
Endemic	Describes a disease that is always present in a certain population of people.
Endocarditis	Inflammation of the inner lining of the heart, usually the heart valves; typically caused by an infection.
Endocardium	The inner lining of the heart.
Endocrine gland	A gland that secretes hormones into the bloodstream.
Endogenous	Arising from inside of the body.
Endometriosis	A condition in which tissue similar to that normally lining the uterus develops in the ovaries, fallopian tubes, or other pelvic structures.
Endometrium	The membrane that lines the uterus.
Endorphin	A group of chemicals produced in the brain that are involved in coping with acute stress and modulating the perception of pain.
Endoscope	A lighted instrument used to view the inside of a body cavity.
Endothelium	The layer of flat cells that lines the blood and lymph vessels, the heart, and other structures in the body.
Endotracheal tube	A plastic tube that is fed down into the trachea through the mouth or nose to supply oxygen to a person who is not breathing properly.
Enteritis	Inflammation of the small intestine, usually causing diarrhea.
Enuresis	The medical term for wetting the bed.

Enzyme	Proteins that function as a catalyst to assist reactions in the body.
Epidemic	Term used to describe a disease affecting a disproportionately large number of individuals within a population, community or region at the same time.
Epidermis	The outermost layer of skin.
Epidural anesthesia	A method of pain relief in which a painkilling drug is injected into the space surrounding the spinal cord to block sensations in the abdomen and lower body.
Epinephrine	A hormone produced by the adrenal glands in response to stress, exercise, or fear; increases heart rate and opens airways to improve breathing; also called adrenaline.
Epithelium	Skin cells that cover the outside of the body and lining much of the respiratory and digestive tracts.
Erosion	An area in which part of the epidermis has been destroyed. The lesion has not disrupted the basement membrane.
Erythema	Redness of the skin.
Erythrocyte	A red blood cell.
Erythroplakia	Red patches in the mucous membranes of the mouth, throat, larynx that can become cancerous.
Esophageal spasm	Irregular contractions of the muscles in the esophagus, which lead to difficulty swallowing.
Esophageal varices	Swollen veins in the lower esophagus and possibly the upper part of the stomach; can cause vomiting of blood and passing of blackened stool.
Esophagus	A tube-shaped canal in the digestive tract, connecting the throat to the stomach.
Etiology	The study of what causes a disease; also the cause or causes of a certain disease.
Eustachian tube	The tube that connects the middle ear and the back of the nose, draining the middle ear and regulating air pressure.

Euthanasia	The act or practice of ending the life of an individual suffering from a terminal illness or an incurable condition.
Exacerbate	To increase the severity of; to aggravate or flare up; to make a chronic condition acute.
Excision	The surgical removal of diseased tissue.
Excoriation	A hollow, crusted area caused by scratching or picking at a primary lesion.
Excretion	The process by which the body rids itself of waste.
Exogenous	Arising from outside of the body.
Expectorant	A medication used to promote the coughing up of phlegm from the respiratory tract.
Extension	Increasing the angle of the joint.
Extracorporeal shock wave lithotripsy	See lithotripsy.
Extradural anesthesia	Injection of an anesthetic into the space outside the dura mater, the fibrous membrane that envelops the spinal cord.
Exudate	Drainage which comes from a wound.
Fainting	A sudden brief loss of consciousness, with loss of postural tone.
Familial	A term describing a disorder or characteristic (such as male pattern baldness) that occurs within a family more often than would be expected.
Fasciitis	Inflammation of the layer of connective tissue that covers, separates, and supports muscles.
Fatty acid	A class of compounds that contain a long chain composed of hydrogen and carbon atoms. In general, fatty acids refer to any compound derived from the breakdown of fats.
Febrile	Having a fever or increased body temperature.
Femoral artery	The main artery that supplies blood to the leg.
Fiberoptics	Thin, flexible instruments that transmit light and images, allowing structures inside of the body to be viewed.
Fibrillation	Rapid, inefficient contraction of muscle fibers.

Fibroblast	A cell which produces the collagen fibers that make up connective tissue.
Fibroid	A noncancerous tumor of the uterus made up of smooth muscle and connective tissue.
Fibroma	A benign tumor of connective tissue.
Fibrosis	Abnormal formation of connective or scar tissue.
Fissure	A linear ulcer.
Fistula	An abnormal passageway from one organ to another or from an organ to the body surface.
Flaccid	Weakness or loss of muscle tone. See hypotonic.
Flatulence	Excessive air or gas in the intestines, expelled through the anus.
Flexion	Decreasing the angle of a joint.
Floaters	Small spots that float across the field of vision, caused by debris floating in the gel-like substance that fills the eye.
Fluke	A parasitic flatworm that can infest humans.
Fluoroscopy	A method used to view organ structure and function by passing X-rays through the body and monitoring the resulting image on a fluorescent screen.
Folic acid	A vitamin essential to the production of red blood cells; plays an important role in the growth and development of the embryo.
Follicle	A tiny pouchlike cavity in a structure of the body, such as a hair follicle.
Follicle stimulating hormone	A hormone produced by the pituitary gland in the brain that stimulates the testicles to produce sperm in males, and in females stimulates the ovaries and causes eggs to mature. Also called FSH.
Folliculitis	The inflammation of hair follicles due to a bacterial infection.
Fontanelles	The two soft spots on a baby's scalp that are the result of gaps in the skull plates that have not yet joined.
Food poisoning	Stomach pain, diarrhea, and/or vomiting caused by eating contaminated food.

Forceps	Instruments resembling tweezers that are used to handle objects or tissue during surgery; an instrument that cups the baby's head (called an obstetric forceps), to help deliver a baby.
Foreign body	An object in an organ or body cavity that is not normally present.
Fraternal twins	Twins that develop from two different eggs fertilized by two different sperm. The twins are not identical as they have two different sets of DNA.
Free radical	See Oxygen free radical.
Friction	Deep, circular movements causing the underlying layers of tissue to rub against each other.
Frostbite	Tissue death as a result of freezing.
FSH	See follicle stimulating hormone.
Fulminant	Describes a disorder that begins suddenly and worsens quickly.
Fungus	An organism that is dependent on another organism for nourishment.
Gait cycle	The movement pattern of the lower limb in walking or running.
Galactocele	A milk-filled tumor in a blocked breast milk duct.
Galactorrhea	Breast milk production by a woman who is not pregnant and has not just given birth.
Galactose	A sugar that is formed from the breakdown of lactose.
Galactosemia	A genetic disorder in which galactose cannot be converted into glucose.
Gallbladder	A small, pear-shaped sac positioned under the liver, which concentrates and stores bile.
Gallstone	A round, hard mass of cholesterol, bile, or calcium salts that is found in the gallbladder or a bile duct.
Gamma globulin	A substance prepared from blood that carries antibodies to most common infections; also used in immunizations.
Ganglion	A fluid-filled cyst attached to a tendon sheath or joint.

Gangrene	Death of a tissue due to a lack of blood supply.
Gastrectomy	Surgical removal of all or part of the stomach.
Gastric acid	The digestive acid in the stomach.
Gastric juice	Digestive fluids (enzymes and acids) produced by the lining of the stomach that break down food and destroy harmful organisms.
Gastric lavage	Washing out of the stomach with water, often to treat poisoning; commonly called "stomach pumping".
Gastric ulcer	A peptic ulcer.
Gastrin	A hormone that stimulates the release of gastric acid in the stomach.
Gastrinoma	A tumor that produces gastrin, making the stomach and duodenum more acidic.
Gastritis	Inflammation of the mucous membrane lining of the stomach.
Gastroenteritis	Inflammation of the stomach and intestines.
Gastrointestinal tract	The part of the digestive system that includes the mouth, esophagus, stomach, and intestines.
Gastroscopy	Examination of the esophagus, stomach, and the first part of the small intestine (duodenum) using an endoscope inserted through the mouth.
Gastrostomy	The surgical creation of an opening in the abdominal wall into the stomach for drainage or a feeding tube.
Gate control theory	Nerve pain impulses, evoked by injury, are influenced in the spinal cord by other nerve cells (like pressure nerves) that act like gates, either preventing the impulses from getting through, or facilitating their passage.
Gaucher's disease	A genetic disorder in which lipids cannot be properly broken down and build up in certain cells; causes enlargement of the spleen and liver, bone damage, and anemia.
Gavage	An artificial feeding technique in which liquids are passed into the stomach by way of a tube inserted through the mouth or nose.

Gene	The basic unit of DNA, which is responsible for passing genetic information; each gene contains the instructions for the production of a certain protein.
Gene therapy	An experimental procedure in which disease-causing genes are replaced by normal, healthy genes.
General anesthesia	A method of preventing pain in which the patient is rendered unconscious.
Generic drug	A drug marketed under its chemical name instead of a brand name.
Genetic analysis	Examination of DNA in a laboratory to diagnose genetic disorders.
Genetic disease	A disorder caused partly or completely by a defect in genes, which carry hereditary information.
Genome	The complete set of an organism's genes.
Giardiasis	Infection with a single-celled parasite, causing abdominal cramps, diarrhea, and nausea.
Gingivectomy	Surgical removal of a diseased part of the gums.
Glaucoma	A disease in which eye damage is caused by an increase in the pressure of the fluid within the eye.
Glomerulosclerosis	Scarring of the filtering structures in the kidneys due to damage.
Glucagon	A hormone produced by the pancreas that converts stored carbohydrates (glycogen) into glucose.
Glucose	A sugar that is the main source of energy for the body.
Glucose tolerance test	A four to eight hour test that evaluates the body's response to glucose after a period of fasting; used to check for diabetes and hypoglycemia.
Glycogen	The main form that glucose takes when it is stored.
Glycosuria	Glucose in the urine.
Goiter	Enlargement of the thyroid gland, which produces a swelling on the neck.
Gonadotropic hormones	Hormones that stimulate activity in the ovaries and testicles.
Grading	Classifying tumor cells on the basis of their abnormality, invasiveness, and metastasis.

Graft

Healthy tissue that is used to replace diseased or defective tissue.

Grand mal

An older term for a tonic-clonic seizure, characterized by loss of consciousness, falling, stiffening, and jerking. See epilepsy.

Granuloma

A mass of tissue that forms at a site of inflammation, injury, or infection as a part of the healing process.

Growth Factor

Substances made by the body that function to regulate cell division and cell survival.

H1 blocker

A drug that blocks the action of histamine; used to treat inflammation.

H2 blocker

A drug used in the treatment of peptic ulcers that blocks histamine from causing acid production in the stomach.

Hammer toe

An abnormality in the tendons of the toe that causes the toe to be flexed at all times.

Hay fever

The common name for allergic rhinitis.

HDL

See High-density lipoprotein.

Heart rate

The rate at which the heart pumps blood, measured in the number of heartbeats per minute.

Heart valve

The structure at each exit of the four chambers of the heart that allows blood to exit but not to flow back in.

Heart-lung machine

A machine that takes over the functions of the heart and lungs during certain types of surgery.

Heat exhaustion

Fatigue, dizziness, and nausea experienced because of overexposure to heat; if not treated it can result in heat stroke.

Heat stroke

A life-threatening condition resulting from extreme overexposure to heat, which disrupts the body's system of regulating temperature.

Heel spur

An abnormal calcification of the portion of tendon or ligament that attaches to the bone. See bone spur.

Heimlich maneuver

A first-aid technique for choking; dislodges an object that is blocking a person's airway by force of air.

Helper T cells

White blood cells responsible for regulating other cells in the body's immune system.

Hemangioma	A purple-red mark on the skin, caused by an excess of blood vessels.
Hemarthrosis	Bleeding into and swelling of a joint.
Hematemesis	Vomiting of blood.
Hematocrit	The percentage of total blood volume that consists of red blood cells, which is determined by laboratory testing.
Hematoma	An accumulation of blood from a broken blood vessel.
Hematuria	Blood in the urine, which can be caused by urinary tract disorders (such as cysts, tumor, or stones) or by an infection.
Hemiparalysis	See Hemiplegia.
Hemiplegia	A condition in which there is paralysis on one side of the body. This paralysis may affect part of the body, such as one arm or leg, or the whole side of the body.
Hemochromatosis	A genetic disorder in which too much iron is absorbed from food.
Hemodialysis	See dialysis.
Hemoglobin	The iron in red blood cells that is responsible for carrying oxygen; hemoglobin bound to oxygen gives blood its red color.
Hemoglobinuria	Hemoglobin in the urine.
Hemolysis	The breakdown of red blood cells in the spleen.
Hemolytic	Destruction of blood cells.
Hemoptysis	Coughing up blood.
Hemorrhage	The medical term for bleeding.
Hemorrhoid	A bulging vein either at the opening of the anus or just inside the anus.
Hemospermia	Blood in the semen.
Hemostasis	The stopping of bleeding by the body's mechanisms.
Hemothorax	An accumulation of blood between the chest wall and the lungs.
Hepatectomy	Surgical removal of all or part of the liver.

Hepatic	A term used to describe something that is related to the liver.
Hepatomegaly	Enlargement of the liver.
Hereditary	Describes a genetic trait that is passed from parents to children.
Hermaphroditism	A rare condition in which an individual is born with both male and female reproductive organs.
Hernia	An abnormal protrusion of one body part from one anatomic space to another.
Herniated disc	A condition in which the jellylike nucleus of a vertebral disc is forced away from the center into the space where the nerve exits the spine. Also called prolapsed disc, bulging disc.
High-density lipoprotein	A type of protein found in the blood that removes cholesterol from tissues. Also called HDL.
Hirschsprung's disease	A condition that is present at birth in which nerve cells do not develop in parts of the intestine.
Hirsutism	Excessive hair growth.
Histamine	A chemical present in mast cells that is released during an allergic reaction and one of the substances responsible for the symptoms of inflammation.
Histoplasmosis	A respiratory disease acquired by inhaling the spores of a fungus found in soil.
HIV	Human immunodeficiency virus: a retrovirus that attacks helper T cells of the immune system and causes acquired immunodeficiency syndrome (AIDS); transmitted through sexual intercourse or contact with infected blood.
Hives	An itchy, inflamed rash of short duration. A single lesion is called a wheal. Also called urticaria.
Homeostasis	The body's coordinated maintenance of the stable, internal environment by regulating blood pressure, blood sugar, body temperature, etc.
Homocystinuria	A genetic disorder in which an enzyme deficiency causes a substance called homocystine to build up in the blood, leading to mental handicap and skeletal abnormalities.

Hormonal implant	Surgical insertion of a small object just under the skin that slowly releases a synthetic hormone for purposes such as birth control.
Hormone	A chemical produced by a gland or tissue that is released into the bloodstream; controls body functions such as growth and sexual development.
Hormone replacement therapy	The use of natural or artificial hormones to treat hormone deficiencies.
Hot flash	A sudden, temporary feeling of heat and sometimes sweating; usually occurs as a result of low estrogen levels in women because of menopause or after a hysterectomy.
Human immunodeficiency virus	HIV is a retrovirus that attacks helper T cells of the immune system and causes acquired immunodeficiency syndrome (AIDS); transmitted through sexual intercourse or contact with infected blood.
Hydrotherapy	The use of hot and/or cold temperatures to maintain and restore health.
Hyperactivity	A type of behavior characterized by excessive physical activity, sometimes associated with neurological or psychological causes.
Hyperalimentation	A method of providing nutrients by the use of a tube or intravenously to a person who cannot eat food or needs nutrients because of an illness.
Hyperbilirubinemia	A condition in which there is too much bilirubin, a substance produced when red blood cells are broken down; can lead to jaundice.
Hypercalcemia	A condition marked by abnormally high levels of calcium in the blood; can lead to disturbance of cell function in the nerves and muscles and, if not treated, can be fatal.
Hypercholesterolemia	An abnormally high level of cholesterol in the blood.
Hyperesthesia	Excessive sensory ability.
Hyperglycemia	A condition characterized by abnormally high levels of glucose in the blood.
Hyperkinesia	Excessive movements.

Hyperkyphosis	An excessive curvature of the thoracic spine.
Hyperlipidemia	A general term for a group of disorders in which lipid levels in the blood are abnormally high, including hypercholesterolemia.
Hyperlordosis	An exaggerated curve in the low back when viewed from the side. Also called sway back.
Hyperparathyroidism	Overactivity of the parathyroid glands, which increases calcium levels in the blood (called hypercalcemia) and decreases calcium in bones (causing osteoporosis).
Hyperplasia	The enlargement of an organ or tissue from an increase in the number of cells.
Hypersensitivity	An excessive response of the body's immune system to a foreign protein.
Hypertension	Abnormally high blood pressure, even when at rest.
Hyperthermia	An abnormally high body temperature.
Hypertonia	Abnormally high muscle tone.
Hypertrophy	Increase in the size of an organ or tissue due to an increase in cell size.
Hyperventilation	Abnormally rapid breathing.
Hypochondriac	One who has a chronic and abnormal anxiety about imaginary symptoms and ailments.
Hypochondriasis	A chronic and abnormal anxiety about imaginary symptoms and ailments.
Hypodermic needle	A thin, hollow needle attached to a syringe; used to inject a medication under the skin, into a vein, or into a muscle.
Hypoplasia	A reduced number of cells in a tissue or organ limiting full development.
Hypotension	The medical term for abnormally low blood pressure, which results in reduced blood flow to the brain, causing dizziness and fainting.
Hypothermia	An abnormally low body temperature.
Hypotonia	Abnormally low muscle tone.
Hypoventilation	A slower than normal breathing rate.

Hypovolemia	An abnormally low volume of blood circulating through the body.
Hypoxemia	A reduced level of oxygen in the blood.
Hypoxia	A reduced level of oxygen in tissues.
Hysterectomy	Surgical removal of the uterus.
Hysteria	A term used to describe symptoms that are caused by mental stress and occur in someone who does not have a mental disorder.
Hysterosalpingography	An X-ray examination performed to examine the inside of the uterus and fallopian tubes, in order to investigate infertility.
Hysteroscopy	A method used to examine the inside of the uterus and the cervix using a viewing instrument.
Iatrogenic	A term used to describe a disease, disorder, or medical condition that is a direct result of medical treatment.
Ichthyosis	A variety of diseases in which the skin is dry and scaly.
Identical twins	Twins that developed from one egg fertilized by one sperm which separated into two cells after mitosis. The DNA is the same in both persons.
Idiopathic	A disease of unknown origin or without apparent cause.
Ileostomy	A surgical procedure in which the lower part of the small intestine (the ileum) is cut and brought to an opening in the abdominal wall, where feces can be passed out of the body.
Ileum	The lowest section of the small intestine, which attaches to the large intestine.
Imaging	The technique of creating pictures of structures inside of the body using X-rays, ultrasound waves, or magnetic fields.
Immune deficiency	Impairment of the immune system, which reduces protection against infection and illness.
Immune system	The cells, substances, and structures in the body that protect against infection and illness.

Immunity	Resistance to a specific disease because of the responses of the immune system.
Immunization	The process of causing immunity by injecting antibodies or provoking the body to make its own antibodies against a certain microorganism.
Immunocompromised	Weakening of the body's immune system.
Immunodeficiency	Failure of the body's immune system to fight disease.
Immunoglobulin	A general term for antibodies, which bind to invading organisms, leading to their destruction. There are five classes of immunoglobulins: IgA, IgD, IgE, IgG, and IgM.
Immunology	The study of the immune system, including how it functions and disorders that affect it.
Immunostimulant	A drug that increases the ability of the body's immune system to fight disease.
Immunosuppressant	A drug that inhibits the activity of the immune system.
Impetigo	A highly contagious skin infection caused by bacteria.
Implant	An organ, tissue, or device surgically inserted and left in the body.
Impotence	The inability to acquire or maintain an erection of the penis (also called erectile dysfunction).
In situ	"in place"; the original or normal position of something. Often describes a cancer that has not grown beyond original tissue.
In vitro	"in glass"; A biological test or process that is carried out in a laboratory.
In vivo	"in the living body"; A biological process that occurs inside of the body.
Incontinence	Inability to hold urine or feces inside of the body.
Incubation period	The time period between when an infectious organism enters the body and when symptoms occur.
Indication	A therapy or act considered desirable or beneficial for a disease or condition.

Indigestion	Uncomfortable symptoms brought on by overeating or eating spicy, rich, or fatty foods; characterized by heartburn, pain in the abdomen, nausea, and gas.
Indurated	Hard, tough skin, usually referring to the edge of a specific lesion.
Infarction	Tissue death due to lack of blood supply.
Infection	Disease causing microorganisms that enter the body, multiply, and damage cells or release toxins.
Inferior	Anatomically beneath, lower, or toward the bottom. Also called caudal.
Inflammation	Pain, and swelling redness, and increased heat in an injured or infected tissue produced as a result of the body's healing response.
Infusion	The introduction of a substance, such as a drug or nutrient, into the bloodstream or a body cavity.
Ingestion	Taking something into the body through the mouth.
Ingrown toenail	A painful condition of the big toe in which the nail grows into the skin on either side, causing inflammation and/or infection.
Inheritance	The passing of traits from parent to child through genes.
Injection	The use of a syringe and needle to insert a drug into a vein, muscle, or joint or under the skin.
Insertion	The attachment of a muscle or ligament farthest from the trunk or center of the body.
Insidious	A disease existing, without marked symptoms, but ready to become active upon some slight occasion; a disease not appearing to be as bad as it really is.
Insomnia	Difficulty falling asleep or to sustain sound sleep.
Insulin	A hormone made in the pancreas that stimulates cellular absorption of glucose from the blood.
Insulin resistance	A condition in which the cells of the body become resistant to the effects of insulin.
Insulinoma	A noncancerous tumor of the insulin-producing cells of the pancreas; the tumor releases excess insulin into the blood, causing glucose levels to drop dangerously low.

Intensive care	Close monitoring of a patient who is seriously ill.
Interferon	A protein produced by body cells that fights viral infections and certain cancers.
Interstitial	Lying between body structures or in the interspaces of tissues.
Interstitial radiation therapy	A treatment for cancer in which a radioactive material is inserted into or near a tumor to provide direct radiation.
Intervertebral foramen	The opening between two adjacent vertebrae through which the nerve root exits the spinal canal.
Intestinal bypass	A surgical procedure in which the beginning of the large intestine is joined to its end so that less food is absorbed.
Intestine	A long, tube-shaped organ that extends from the stomach to the anus; absorbs food and water and passes the waste products of digestion as feces.
Intra-aortic balloon pump	A small balloon inserted into the aorta that helps to circulate blood by inflating between heartbeats.
Intractable	Something that does not respond to treatment.
Intraocular pressure	The pressure of the fluids within the eye.
Intrauterine device	A device inserted into the uterus that helps to prevent pregnancy.
Intravenous	Inside of or into a vein.
Intrinsic	A term used to describe something originating from or located in a tissue or organ.
Intrinsic factor	A substance produced by the mucosa of the stomach and intestines that is essential for the absorption of vitamin B12.
Intubation	The passage of a tube into an organ or body structure; commonly used to refer to the passage of a tube down the windpipe for artificial respiration.
Invasive	Describes something that spreads throughout body tissues, such as a tumor or microorganism; also describes a medical procedure in which body tissues are penetrated.
Involuntary	Occurring without a person's control or participation.

Ionizing radiation	Radiation that damages cells or genes; can be used to treat cancer.
Iris	The colored part of the eye.
Iron-deficiency anemia	A type of anemia caused by a loss of iron due to bleeding, a lack of iron in the diet or problems absorbing iron.
Irrigation	The cleansing of a wound by flushing it with water, a medicated solution, or some other fluid.
Irritable bladder	Involuntary contractions of muscles in the bladder, which can cause lack of control of urination.
Ischemia	A condition in which a tissue or organ does not receive a sufficient supply of blood.
Jaundice	Yellowing of the skin and whites of the eyes because of the presence of excess bilirubin in the blood.
Jock itch	A fungal infection in the groin area.
Keloid	A raised, firm, thick scar that forms from excessive stress during healing. Some African descended genes also trigger the formation of keloids.
Keratin	A tough protein found in the eye, skin, nails, and hair.
Keratitis	Inflammation of the cornea.
Keratolytic	Drugs that remove the keratin-containing outer layer of skin.
Keratoplasty	Surgical replacement or reshaping of the cornea.
Keratosis	A growth on the skin that is the result of overproduction of the protein keratin.
Ketoacidosis	The dangerous accumulation of chemicals called ketones in the blood, sometimes occurring as a complication of diabetes mellitus; also called ketosis.
Kidney	One of two organs that are part of the urinary tract, responsible for filtering the blood and removing waste products and water as urine.
Kidney stone	A hard mass composed of calcium and other substances that form in the kidneys.
Killer T cells	White blood cells that are part of the immune system and destroy microorganisms and cancer cells.

Kilocalorie A unit of energy; equal to a nutritional calorie.

Kneading Squeezing, rolling and picking up of body tissues. Also called Petrissage.

Kyphosis The normal curvature of the thoracic and sacral sections of the spine as viewed from the side. Also used to refer to hyperkyphosis.

Labor The interval from onset of contractions to birth of a baby.

Laceration A torn or ragged wound.

Lactation The production of breast milk.

Lactation suppression A decrease in milk production during pregnancy as a result of high levels of estrogen in the blood.

Lactic acid An acid produced when cells have an insufficient supply of oxygen.

Lactose The sugar found in dairy products.

Lactose intolerance Inability to break down and absorb lactose.

Laminectomy A surgical procedure that removes part of a vertebra to relieve pressure on the spinal cord or a nerve branching from the spinal cord.

Laparoscope A viewing instrument used to examine and treat disorders in the abdominal cavity; it consists of a long fiber optic cable that transmits images on to a monitor.

Laparoscopy A procedure done to examine the abdominal cavity using a laparoscope.

Laryngectomy Surgical removal of all or part of the voice box (larynx).

Laryngitis Inflammation of the larynx, possibly caused by an infection.

Larynx The medical term for the voice box, the organ in the throat that produces sounds.

Latent infection An infection that lies dormant in the body for months or years but can reappear.

Lateral The position of a structure is farther away from the midline of the limb, trunk, or head; also pertaining to one side.

LDL	See Low-density lipoprotein.
Leiomyoma	A noncancerous tumor of smooth muscle.
Lesion	Any skin abnormality, wound or condition.
Lethargic	An unusual lack of energy and activity.
Lethargy	A feeling of tiredness, drowsiness, or lack of energy.
Leukocyte	Another name for a white blood cells.
Leukocyte count	The number of white blood cells in the blood, which is used as a measure of health and possible infection.
Lichenification	A skin area with exaggerated skin lines. It is rough and thick.
Ligament	A tough band of tissue that connects bones and supports organs.
Ligation	The process of closing a blood vessel or duct by tying it off.
Lipid-lowering drugs	Drugs taken to lower the levels of specific fats called lipids in the blood in order to reduce the risk of narrowing of the arteries.
Lipids	A group of fats stored in the body and used for energy.
Lipoproteins	Substances containing lipids and proteins, comprising most fats in the blood.
Liposuction	A surgical procedure in which fat is removed from areas of the body using a suction pump.
Lithotripsy	A procedure done to break up stones in the urinary tract using ultrasonic shock waves, so that the fragments can be easily passed from the body.
Lobe	A well-defined part of an organ such as the lung.
Lobectomy	Surgical removal of a lobe.
Local anesthesia	A method of preventing pain by inducing the loss of sensation in a certain area of the body while the patient remains awake.
Locked joint	A joint that cannot be moved because of a disease or a lodged piece of bone or cartilage.
Lockjaw	A spasm of the jaw muscles that prevents the mouth from moving, such as that caused by tetanus.

Lordosis	The normal curve of the lumbar and cervical spine as viewed from the side. It can also be used to refer to an exaggerated curve in the low back.
Low-density lipoprotein	A type of lipoprotein that is the major carrier of cholesterol in the blood. High LDL levels are associated with narrowing of the arteries and heart disease.
Lumbago	Dull, aching pain in the lower back.
Lumbar puncture	A procedure in which a needle is inserted into the lower region of the spinal canal to take out a sample of spinal fluid or to inject a drug.
Lumbar spine	The lower part of the spine between the lowest pair of ribs and the pelvis; made up of five vertebrae. The "low back."
Lumpectomy	Surgical removal of a section of breast containing cancer.
Lung collapse	A condition in which all or part of a lung cannot expand and fill with air.
Lupus erythematosus	A disorder of the immune system that causes inflammation of connective tissue. Also called systemic lupus erythematosus.
Luteinizing hormone	A hormone produced by the pituitary gland that causes the ovaries and testicles to release sex hormones and plays a role in the development of eggs and sperm.
Lymph	A milky fluid containing white blood cells, proteins, and fats; plays an important role in absorbing fats from the intestine and in the functioning of the immune system.
Lymph node	A small gland that is part of the immune system; contains white blood cells and antibodies and helps fight against the spread of infection.
Lymphadenopathy	Swollen lymph nodes.
Lymphangiography	An X-ray procedure that creates images of the lymphatic system.
Lymphangioma	A benign tumor whose cells form lymph vessels.

Lymphatic system	A network of vessels that drain lymph back into the blood.
Lymphocyte	A white blood cell that is an important part of the body's immune system, helping to destroy invading microorganisms.
Lymphocytic leukemia	A disease in which white blood cells called lymphocytes divide uncontrollably.
Lymphogranuloma venereum	A sexually transmitted chlamydial infection.
Lymphoma	A group of cancers of the lymph nodes and spleen that can spread to other parts of the body.
Lymphosarcoma	Another name for a non-Hodgkin's sarcoma; a cancerous tumor in lymphoid tissue.
Lysis	The breakage of the cell wall and subsequent death of the cell.
Lysosome	Lysosomes are the cells' garbage disposal system; they are enzymes that break down cellular components for elimination.
Macrophage	Cells derived from white blood cells that eat antigens, immune complexes, bacteria, & viruses.
Macula	The area of the retina that allows fine details to be observed at the center of vision; also refers to any small, flat spot on the skin.
Macular degeneration	Gradual loss of vision due to deterioration of nerve tissue in the retina.
Macule	A flat, colored area of the skin less than 10 millimeters in diameter. Example: a freckle.
Magnesium	A mineral that is essential for many body functions, including nerve impulse transmission, formation of bones and teeth, and muscle contraction.
Magnetic resonance imaging	A technique that uses magnetic fields and radio waves to create high-quality cross- sectional images of the body without using radiation. Also called an MRI.
Malabsorption	An impaired ability of the lining of the small intestine to absorb nutrients from food.

Malabsorption syndrome	A group of symptoms, including weight loss, weakness, and immune suppression, that result from the body's inability to absorb nutrients from food.
Malaise	Feelings of general discomfort, distress, or uneasiness.
Malaria	A parasitic disease spread by mosquitoes that causes chills and fever; potentially fatal complications in the liver, kidneys, blood, and brain are possible.
Malformation	Abnormal development of an organ or tissue
Malignant	Refers to cancer; a neoplasm or tumor that grows in an uncontrolled manner, invading nearby tissue and spreading (metastasize) to distant sites.
Malignant hyperthermia	A reaction to certain anesthesia gases involving intense muscle contractions and a high fever.
Malignant melanoma	The most serious type of skin cancer, in which a mole changes shape, darkens, becomes painful, and/or bleeds easily.
Mallory-Weiss syndrome	A condition associated with alcoholism in which the lower end of the esophagus tears, causing vomiting of blood.
Mammography	An X-ray procedure done to detect breast cancer.
Mammoplasty	A general term for a cosmetic operation on the breasts; includes breast reduction, enlargement, and reconstruction after a mastectomy.
Mania	A mental disorder characterized by extreme excitement, happiness, overactivity, and agitation; usually refers to the high of the highs and lows experienced in manic-depressive disorder.
Marfan's syndrome	A rare genetic disorder that affects connective tissue, leading to abnormalities of joints, bones, tendons, ligaments, arteries, and/or the heart.
Mast cell	Mast cells play an important role in the body's allergic response. Following subsequent allergen exposure, the mast cells release substances such as histamine into the tissue.
Mastectomy	A surgical procedure in which all or part of the breast is removed to prevent the spread of cancer.

Mastitis	Inflammation of the breast, which is usually caused by a bacterial infection.
Maxilla	One of two bones that form the upper jaw, the roof of the mouth, and the center portion of the face.
Measles	A typically mild illness caused by a viral infection, causing a characteristic rash and a fever, primarily affecting children.
Medial	A term used to describe something situated on or near the midline of the body or a body structure.
Mediastinoscopy	Investigation of the central chest compartment using an endoscope that is inserted through an incision in the neck.
Medulla	The center part of an organ or body structure; sometimes used to refer to the lower part of the brain stem.
Megacolon	A severely swollen large intestine, causing severe constipation and abdominal bloating; may be present at birth or develops later.
Meiosis	The type of cell division that occurs only in the ovaries and testicles, producing cells with half the genes of the original cell; these cells then form eggs and sperm.
Melanin	The pigment that gives skin, hair, and eyes their coloring.
Melanocyte	A type of pigment cell located in the lower epidermis that produces melanin.
Melanocyte-stimulating hormone	A hormone that coordinates pigmentation of the skin, eyes, and hair.
Melanoma	A skin tumor composed of cells called melanocytes
Menarche	The beginning of menstruation.
Meniere's disease	A disorder of the inner ear, causing hearing loss, ringing in the ear, and the sensation that one's surroundings are spinning.
Meninges	The three membranes that surround and protect the spinal cord and brain.

Meningioma	A rare noncancerous tumor developing in the protective membranes covering the brain called the meninges; can cause headaches and problems with vision and mental function.
Meningitis	Inflammation of the meninges; usually caused by infection by a microorganism (meningitis caused by bacteria is life-threatening; viral meningitis is milder).
Meningocele	A protrusion of the meninges through an opening in the skull or spinal cord due to a genetic defect.
Meniscectomy	Surgical removal of all or part of a cartilage disk from a joint.
Meniscus	A crescent-shaped pad of cartilage in the knee and other joints that reduces friction.
Menopause	The period in a woman's life when menstruation stops, resulting in a reduced production of estrogen and cessation of egg production.
Menorrhagia	Excessive loss of blood during menstruation, which can be caused by disorders of the uterus.
Menstrual cycle	The periodic discharge of blood and mucosal tissue from the uterus, occurring from puberty to menopause in a woman who is not pregnant.
Menstruation	The shedding of the lining of the uterus during the menstrual cycle.
Mesenteric infarction	Death of tissue in the intestine due to lack of blood supply to that tissue.
Mesenteric lymphadenitis	Inflammation of lymph nodes in an abdominal membrane.
Mesothelioma	A cancerous tumor occurring in the lining of the lungs and chest cavity, often associated with exposure to asbestos dust.
Mesothelium	A tissue layer that lines the heart, abdomen, chest cavity, and lungs.
Messenger RNA	An RNA molecule that transports the information stored in DNA out of a cell's nucleus in order to make proteins.
Metabolic rate	The speed at which the body uses energy.

Metabolism	A general term for all of the chemical processes that occur in the body.
Metabolite	Any substance that takes part in a chemical reaction in the body.
Metaplasia	A change in the development of a tissue from one type of functional differentiation to another not normally found in that area of the body.
Metastasis	The spreading of a cancerous tumor to another part of the body through lymph, blood, or across a cavity; also sometimes refers to a tumor that has been produced in this way.
Microbe	Another term for a microorganism, especially one that causes disease.
Microbiology	The study of microorganisms.
Microcephaly	An abnormally small head.
Microdiscectomy	Surgical removal of the protruding part of a herniated disc.
Microorganism	Any tiny, single-celled organism (such as a bacterium, virus, or fungus).
Microsurgery	A surgical technique that uses a special binocular microscope to operate on tiny, delicate, or hard-to-reach tissue.
Micturition	The discharge of urine.
Middle ear	The small cavity between the eardrum and inner ear; contains three tiny, linked bones that transmit sound to the inner ear.
Midsagittal	The plane passing through the midplane of the body from the front to the back that divides the body into two equal halves.
Migraine	A severe headache, usually accompanied by vision problems and/or nausea and vomiting, and that typically recurs.
Mineral	A substance that is a necessary part of a healthy diet (such as potassium, calcium, sodium, phosphorus, and magnesium).

Minipill	An oral contraceptive containing only the synthetic hormone progesterone (birth control pills contain estrogen and progesterone).
Miotic	A drug that causes the pupil to constrict.
Miscarriage	Expulsion of a fetus before it has developed sufficiently to survive on its own.
Mitosis	The process by which most cells divide in order to reproduce cells that are genetically identical to each other and to the parent.
Mitral insufficiency	A problem with the ability of the mitral valve in the heart to close, which causes the heart to pump harder and reduces its efficiency.
Mitral stenosis	A condition in which the mitral valve in the heart becomes narrowed, making the heart work harder to pump blood.
Mitral valve	A two leaflet valve between the upper and lower chambers on the left side of the heart (the right atrium and right ventricle). Also called the bicuspid valve.
Mitral valve prolapse	A common condition in which the mitral valve in the heart is deformed, causing blood to leak back across the valve; characterized by a heart murmur and sometimes chest pain and disturbed heart rhythm.
Modified radical mastectomy	A treatment for breast cancer in which the entire breast, a section of the chest muscle, and lymph nodes in the chest and underarm are removed.
Mole	A brown to dark brown spot on the skin that can be flat or raised.
Molecule	The smallest unit of a substance that possesses its characteristics.
Molluscum contagiosum	A viral infection that causes white bumps on the skin; usually clears up in a few months.
Monoclonal antibodies	An antibody that is produced in the laboratory so that it will react with only one specific foreign protein; used to help diagnose certain kinds of cancer.

Mononucleosis	An infection caused by a virus that invades a type of white blood cell called a monocyte, causing fever, sore throat, and swollen lymph nodes.
Monounsaturated fat	A type of fat that is thought to be beneficial in the prevention of coronary heart disease; found in foods such as olive oil and peanut oil.
Morbidity	The state of being ill or having a disease.
Morning sickness	Nausea and vomiting experienced early in a pregnancy, affecting about half of all pregnant women.
Mortality	The death rate, measured as the number of deaths per a certain population; may describe the population as a whole, or a specific group within a population (such as infant mortality).
Motor nerve	A nerve that carries messages to a muscle that cause the muscle to contract. Also called efferent.
Motor neuron disease	Degeneration of the nerves in the spinal cord and brain that are responsible for muscle movement, causing weakness and muscle deterioration.
MRI	See magnetic resonance imaging.
Mucocele	A sac or body cavity that is swollen because of the production of mucus by the cells in its lining.
Mucolytic	A drug that lessens the sticky quality of phlegm and makes it easier to cough up.
Mucous membranes	The soft, pink layer of cells that produce mucus in order to keep body structures lubricated; found in structures such as the eyelids, respiratory tract, and urinary tract.
Mucus	A slippery fluid produced by mucous membranes that lubricates and protects the internal surfaces of the body.
Multiple pregnancy	The presence of more than one fetus in the uterus, such as occurs with twins.
Multiple-gated acquisition scan	A technique for evaluating heart efficiency by measuring blood flow into and out of the heart.
Mumps	A viral infection that causes inflammation of salivary glands; primarily affects children.

Murmur	A characteristic sound (heard through a stethoscope) of blood flowing irregularly through the heart; can be harmless or may be an indication of disease.
Muscle tone	The natural tension in resting muscles.
Muscle wasting	The degeneration of a muscle (loss of bulk), caused by disease or starvation.
Mutagen	Anything that can increase the rate of abnormal change in cells, which can lead to cancer.
Mutation	A change in the genetic information within a cell.
Myalgia	The medical term for muscle pain.
Mycobacterium	A type of slow growing bacterium; resistant to the body's defense mechanisms and are responsible for diseases such as tuberculosis and leprosy.
Mycosis	Any disease caused by a fungus.
Myelin sheath	The fat and protein containing material that surrounds and protects some nerves.
Myelitis	Inflammation of the spinal cord, which can cause headaches, fever, muscle stiffness, pain, weakness, and eventually paralysis.
Myelocele	Protrusion of the spinal cord and its coverings out from the spine; one of the more severe forms of spina bifida.
Myeloma	A cancer affecting cells in the bone marrow; sometimes used as an abbreviation for multiple myeloma.
Myelosclerosis	Buildup of fibrous connective tissue in the bone marrow, affecting the production of blood components.
Myocardial infarction	The death of an area of heart muscle as a result of being deprived of its blood supply; characterized by severe pain in the chest; commonly called a heart attack or **MI**.
Myocarditis	Inflammation of the heart muscle, which can be caused by a virus, certain drugs, or radiation therapy.
Myocardium	The medical term for heart muscle.

Myogram	A test that measures muscle response to nervous stimulation (electrical activity within muscle fibers). Also called electromyography.
Myomectomy	The surgical removal of a noncancerous tumor from muscle.
Myopathy	A muscle disease, usually one that results in the deterioration of muscle.
Myopia	The medical term for nearsightedness.
Myositis	Muscle inflammation, causing pain and weakness.
Myringotomy	A surgical opening in the eardrum that allows for drainage.
Myxoma	A noncancerous tumor made of mucous material and fibrous connective tissue.
Narcolepsy	A disorder that causes excessive sleepiness during the day and frequent and uncontrollable episodes of falling asleep.
Narcosis	A drug (or other chemical) induced drowsiness or stupor.
Nasal septum	The section of the nose that divides the left and right nostrils; made of cartilage and bone and covered by a mucous membrane.
Nasogastric tube	A thin, plastic tube that is inserted through the nose, down the esophagus, and into the stomach; used to drain, wash, or take samples from the stomach, or to feed very sick patients who cannot eat.
Nasopharynx	The passageway connecting the back of the nose to the top of the throat.
Nausea	Feeling the need to vomit.
Nebulizer	An instrument that provides a drug in its misted form through a face mask; used for severe asthma attacks and for children who have asthma but cannot use an inhaler.
Necrosis	The medical term for the death of tissue cells.
Needle aspiration	The use of a thin, hollow needle and syringe to remove body fluid for examination.
Neonate	A term used to describe a newborn infant from birth to 1 month of age.

Neoplasm	Any abnormal, uncontrolled growth of new tissue; a proliferation of cells no longer under control of the hosts' nervous system. These may be benign or malignant.
Nephrectomy	The surgical removal of one or both kidneys.
Nephritis	Inflammation of one or both kidneys because of an infection, an abnormal immune system response, or a disorder of metabolism.
Nephrolithotomy	Surgical removal of a kidney stone.
Nephrons	The tiny filtering units of the kidney.
Nephrosclerosis	The replacement of normal kidney structures with scar tissue.
Nephrostomy	The surgical placement of a tube into the kidney to drain urine.
Nephrotic syndrome	Symptoms that result from damage to the filtering units of the kidney.
Nerve block	The dulling of sensation in an area of the body by injecting a painkiller into or around a nerve leading to that section of the body.
Nerve compression	Pressure on a nerve, which can cause nerve damage and muscle weakness.
Neural tube	The tube located along the back of an embryo that later develops into the spinal cord and brain.
Neural tube defects	Problems in the development of the spinal cord and brain in an embryo, such as the failure of the spine to enclose the spinal cord (spina bifida) and the failure of the brain to develop (anencephaly).
Neuralgia	Pain along the course of a nerve caused by irritation or damage to the nerve.
Neuritis	Inflammation of a nerve, often characterized by pain, numbness or tingling.
Neuroblastoma	A cancerous childhood tumor located in the adrenal glands or the sympathetic nervous system.
Neurofibrillary tangles	Abnormal spiral filaments on nerve cells in the brain; characteristic of Alzheimer disease.
Neurofibromatosis	A condition in which connective tissue tumors occur on nerves in the skin.

Neuroleptic	An antipsychotic drug.
Neuroma	A noncancerous tumor occurring in nerve tissue.
Neuron	Another term for a nerve cell.
Neuropathy	Disease, inflammation, or damage to the nerves connecting the brain and spinal cord to the rest of the body.
Neurosis	Relatively mild emotional disorders (such as mild depression and phobias).
Neurotoxins	Chemicals that attack and damage nerve cells.
Neurotransmitters	Chemicals that transfer messages from one nerve cell to another or from a nerve cell to a muscle cell.
Neutrophil	A type of white blood cell.
Nevus	A marking on the skin; can be present at birth (birthmark) or develop later (such as a mole).
Newborn respiratory distress syndrome	A disorder in which premature babies lack surfactant, a substance that stops the lungs from collapsing.
Night terrors	A form of nightmare causing abrupt awakening in terror; occurs mostly in children.
Nitrates	A group of drugs that widen blood vessels; used to treat insufficient blood supply to the heart (angina pectoris) and reduced pumping efficiency of the heart (heart failure).
Nocturia	Urination or a sleep-disturbing need to urinate during the night.
Nocturnal	Occurring at night.
Node	A small, rounded tissue mass.
Nodule	A solid mass, usually round, that may or may not be elevated.
Nondisjunction	An error that occurs during the division of sex chromosomes, causing either too much or too little genetic information to be placed in an egg or sperm when it is formed.
Non insulin-dependent diabetes	Type 2 diabetes, where the body builds a resistance to insulin and requires ever increasing amounts to entice the cells to accept sugar.

Noninvasive	A term that is used to describe medical procedures that do not enter or penetrate the body; also refers to noncancerous tumors that do not spread to other sections of the body.
Norepinephrine	A hormone that regulates blood pressure by causing blood vessels to narrow and the heart to beat faster when blood pressure drops.
Norwalk virus	A virus that causes acute gastroenteritis.
Nosocomial infection	An infection acquired in a hospital.
Nuclear Magnetic Resonance	A technique that uses magnetic fields and radio waves to create high-quality cross- sectional images of the body without using radiation. Also called NMR. More commonly called magnetic Resonance Imaging; MRI.
Nucleic acids	Substances found in every living organism that provide the instructions for development; includes DNA and RNA.
Nucleotide bases	Molecules that form nucleic acids.
Nucleus	The center or most important point of an object.
Nucleus pulposus	Thich, jellylike material contained in the vertebral discs.
Numbness	The lack of sensation in a part of the body due to interruption of nerve impulses.
Nutrient	Any substance that the body can use to maintain its health.
Nystagmus	Persistent, rapid, involuntary movement of the eyes.
Obesity	A condition in which there is an excess of body fat; used to describe those who weigh at least 20 percent more than the maximum amount considered normal for their age, sex, and height.
Obstructive sleep apnea	The blockage of the airways during sleep which causes breathing to stop for a period of time
Occlusion	The blocking of an opening or passageway in the body.
Occult blood	Blood in the feces that can be detected only by chemical tests.

Occupational disease	A disease that occurs as a result of factors in the workplace.
Occupational therapy	Treatment to relearn physical skills lost as a result of an illness or accident.
Ocular	Describes something related to the eyes.
Oncogenes	Genes that, when altered by environmental factors or viruses, can cause abnormal cell growth.
Oncology	The study of neoplasms and the clinical specialty of managing them.
Oophorectomy	The surgical removal of one or both ovaries; used to treat the growth of ovarian cysts or tumors.
Open heart surgery	Any operation in which the heart is stopped temporarily and a machine is used to take over its function of pumping blood throughout the body.
Ophthalmia	Severe inflammation of the eyes.
Ophthalmoplegia	Partial or total loss of the ability to move the eyes.
Ophthalmoscopy	Examination of the inside of the eye using a lighted viewing instrument.
Opportunistic infection	Infection by organisms that would be harmless to a healthy person, but cause infection in those with a weakened immune system (for example, persons with AIDS or chemotherapy patients).
Optic	Pertaining to the eyes.
Optic neuritis	Inflammation of the optic nerve, often causing a partial loss of vision.
Oral contraceptives	Drugs taken in pill form to prevent pregnancy.
Orbit	The socket in the skull that contains the eyeball, along with its blood vessels, nerves, and muscles.
Organ donation	An agreement to allow one or more organs to be removed and transplanted into someone else.
Origin	The attachment of a muscle or ligament closest to the trunk or center of the body.
Orphan drugs	Drugs used to treat rare diseases; not normally produced because potential sales are small.
Orthopnea	Breathing difficulty experienced while lying flat; can be a symptom of heart failure or asthma.

Orthostatic hypotension	An excessive fall in BP (typically > 20/10 mm Hg) upon assuming the upright posture often resulting in lightheadedness or fainting. Also called postural hypotension.
Orthotic	A device used to correct or control deformed bones, muscles, or joints.
Osmosis	The process of passage of the solvent portion of a lesser-concentrated solution through a semipermeable membrane into a higher-concentrated solution until the two solutions are equal in concentration; plays an important role in water distribution in the body.
Ossification	The formation and maintenance of bone.
Osteitis	Inflammation of bone.
Osteoblast	A cell that forms bone.
Osteochondroma	A noncancerous tumor made up of bone and cartilage
Osteoclast	A cell that breaks down unwanted bone tissue; also refers to a device for fracturing a bone to correct a deformity.
Osteoma	A noncancerous bone tumor.
Osteomyelitis	The inflammation of bones and bone marrow because of an infection, usually caused by bacteria.
Osteopetrosis	A rare hereditary disorder in which bones become harder and more dense, causing them to break more easily.
Osteophyte	An outgrowth of bone near a joint.
Osteosarcoma	A cancerous bone tumor.
Osteosclerosis	An abnormal increase in density and hardness of bone.
Otalgia	The medical term for an earache.
OTC	Over-The-Counter; referring to medicine that does not require a prescription to obtain.
Otitis externa	Inflammation of the outer ear due to an infection; commonly called swimmer's ear.

Otitis media	Inflammation of the middle ear (between the eardrum and inner ear) because of the spread of an infection from the nose, sinuses, and throat.
Otorrhea	A discharge from an inflamed ear.
Otosclerosis	Progressive deafness caused by bone formation around structures in the middle ear.
Ototoxicity	Harmful effect that some drugs have on the organs or nerves in the ears, which can lead to hearing and balance problems.
Outpatient treatment	Medical attention that does not include an overnight stay at a hospital.
Overdose	An excessively large dose of a drug, which can lead to coma and death.
Ovulation	The development and release of the egg from the ovary, which usually occurs halfway through a woman's menstrual cycle.
Ovum	Another term for an egg cell.
Oxidation	A chemical reaction involving active sources of oxygen (called oxygen free radicals) that damage cells.
Oximetry	Determination of the amount of oxygen in the blood by measuring the amount of light transmitted through an area of skin.
Oxygen free radicals	Active forms of oxygen found in pollution, cigarette smoke, and radiation that can damage cells and are believed to play a role in the aging process and cancer.
Oxytocin	A hormone produced in the pituitary gland that causes contraction of the uterus during childbirth and stimulation of milk flow during breast feeding.
Ozone	A poisonous form of oxygen that is present in the earth's upper atmosphere, where it helps to screen the earth from damaging ultraviolet rays.
Pacemaker	A small electronic device that is surgically implanted to stimulate the heart muscle to provide a normal heartbeat.
Palate	The roof of the mouth.

Palliative	Treatment that relieves the symptoms of a disorder without curing it.
Pallor	Abnormally pale skin; usually refers to the skin of the face.
Palpation	The use of the hands to feel parts of the body to check for any abnormalities.
Palpitation	An abnormally rapid and strong heartbeat.
Palsy	Loss of sensation or ability to move.
Pancreatitis	Inflammation of the pancreas, which is often caused by alcohol abuse.
Pandemic	A widespread epidemic.
Pap smear	A test in which cells are scraped off the cervix and examined for abnormalities; used to detect changes that might precede cervical cancer and to diagnose viral infections such as herpes simplex.
Papanicolaou test	A pap smear.
Papilloma	A tumor occurring on the skin or mucous membranes; usually not cancerous.
Papule	This is a solid, elevated skin lesion less than 10 millimeters in diameter.
Paracentesis	The insertion of a needle into a body cavity to relieve pressure, inject a drug, or remove a sample for analysis.
Paralysis	The inability to use a muscle or limb because of injury to or disease of the nerves leading to the tissue.
Paranoia	A disorder in which a person becomes overly suspicious and emotionally sensitive.
Paraplegia	Paralysis of both legs and possibly the lower part of the body.
Parasagittal	A plane passing through the body from the front to the back that divides the body into two unequal halves.
Parasite	An organism that lives on or in other organisms, from which it obtains nutrients.

Parasympathetic nervous system	The part of the autonomic nervous system that is stimulated during times of relaxation
Parathyroid hormone	A hormone released by the parathyroid glands that plays a role in controlling calcium levels in the blood.
Parathyroidectomy	The surgical removal of one or more of the parathyroid glands.
Parenchyma	A bacterial or yeast infection of the skin around the nail.
Parenteral	Administered other than through the digestive system; usually in a vein or under the skin or muscle.
Paresis	Partial paralysis.
Paresthesia	Numbness, tingling or any loss of sensation to the skin; commonly referred to as "pins and needles".
Parotid glands	Salivary glands located in the mouth near the ears.
Paroxysm	A sudden attack or worsening of a disease's symptoms.
Partial mastectomy	A treatment for breast cancer in which a tumor is removed, along with the skin covering it and some of the surrounding tissues and muscles.
Partial seizure	An abnormal electrical discharge in a certain area of the brain, affecting only certain functions.
Partial thromboplastin time	A test that measures clotting time in plasma.
Passive exercise	Exercise of an injured part of the body involving no effort from that injured part.
Patch	A flat, colored area of the skin that is more than 10 millimeters in diameter.
Patent	Not obstructed; open.
Patent ductus arteriosus	A genetic disorder of the heart in which a channel connecting the pulmonary artery and the aorta fails to close.
Pathogen	Any substance capable of causing a disease; usually refers to a disease causing microorganism.

Pathogenesis   The production and development of a disease or disorder.

Pathology   Pathology is the branch of medicine that deals with the nature of disease, especially the structural and functional changes caused by the disease.

Peak flow measurement   The maximum speed that air is exhaled from the lungs; used to diagnose asthma or to determine the effectiveness of asthma medications.

Pedunculated   Hanging from a stalk.

Pepsin   The enzyme found in gastric juice that helps digest protein.

Peptic ulcer   An erosion in the lining of the esophagus, stomach, or small intestine, usually caused in part by the corrosive action of gastric acid.

Percutaneous   A procedure that is performed through the skin, such as an injection.

Perforation   A hole in an organ or body structure caused by disease or injury.

Periarteritis nodosa   Inflammation and weakening of small and medium arteries.

Pericardial effusion   Fluid buildup inside of the pericardium, affecting the performance of the heart.

Pericarditis   Inflammation of the membranous sac that covers the heart, causing chest pain and fever.

Pericardium   The membranous sac that covers the heart and the base of the blood vessels that are attached to the heart.

Perinatal   Occurring just before or just after birth.

Periosteum   The tissue covering bones, except the surfaces in joints

Periostitis   Inflammation of the periosteum.

Peripheral nervous system   The nerves that branch out from the brain and spinal cord to the rest of the body.

Peripheral neuropathy	A disorder of the peripheral nerves, usually involving the feet, hands and sometimes the legs, arms and face. Symptoms include numbness, tingling or burning sensations, pain, abnormal reflexes, weakness and partial paralysis.
Peripheral vascular disease	The narrowing of blood vessels in the legs or arms, causing pain and possibly tissue death (gangrene) as a result of a reduced flow of blood to areas supplied by the narrowed vessels.
Peristalsis	Wavelike movement of smooth muscle-containing tubes, such as the digestive tract.
Peritoneum	The membrane that lines the abdominal cavity and covers the abdominal organs.
Peritonitis	Inflammation of the peritoneum, the membrane that lines the wall of the abdomen and covers the abdominal organs, usually from serious infection or kidney failure.
Pertussis	A bacterial infection of the respiratory tract characterized by short, convulsive coughs that end in a whoop sound when breath is inhaled (commonly called whooping cough); mainly affects children.
PET scan	See Positron emission tomography scanning.
Petit mal	An older term for an absence seizure: an epileptic seizure, usually lasting less than 20 seconds, characterized by a stare and sometimes associated with blinking or brief automatic movements of the mouth or hands.
Petrissage	Squeezing, rolling and picking up of body tissues. (also called kneading)
Peutz-Jeghers syndrome	A genetic disorder in which there are polyps in the small intestine and brown melanin spots on the lips, mouth, fingers, and toes.
pH	Potential of Hydrogen: A measure of the acidic or basic character of a substance.
Phagocyte	An immune system cell that can surround and digest foreign bodies, unwanted cellular material, and microorganisms.
Phantom limb	The sensation of a limb after it has been amputated.

Pharmacology The study of medications, including drug development.

Pharyngitis Inflammation of the throat (the pharynx), causing sore throat, fever, earache, and swollen glands.

Pharynx The throat; the tube connecting the back of the mouth and nose to the esophagus and windpipe.

Phenylketonuria A hereditary disorder in which the enzyme that converts the amino acid phenylalanine into another amino acid is defective, meaning phenylalanine must be kept out of the diet.

Pheochromocytoma A noncancerous tumor of cells that produce epinephrine and norepinephrine, causing higher levels of these hormones in the blood and an increase in blood pressure.

Phlebectomy The surgical removal of varicose veins. A small incision is made and the vein is pulled out through the opening, producing little scarring.

Phlebitis Inflammation of a vein.

Phlebothrombosis Formation of a blood clot in a vein.

Phlegm Mucus and other material produced by the lining of the respiratory tract; also called sputum.

Phobia A persisting fear of and desire to avoid something.

Phosphates Salts containing phosphorus; essential to some body functions such as the bones and teeth.

Phospholipids Fatty substances that make up the membranes surrounding cells.

Phosphorus A mineral that is an important part of structures such as bones, teeth, and membranes in the body; also involved in numerous other chemical reactions.

Photocoagulation Tissue destruction using a focused beam of light.

Photophobia An abnormal sensitivity of the eyes to light.

Photosensitivity An abnormal reaction to sunlight, which usually occurs as a rash.

Phototherapy Treatment with some form of light.

Physiology The study of the body's functions.

Phytochemicals	Chemicals in plants that might help protect against disorders such as cancer.
Pica	A desire to eat materials that are not food.
Pickwickian syndrome	Extreme obesity along with shallow breathing, sleep apnea, excessive sleepiness, and heart failure.
Pigmentation	The coloration of the skin, hair, and eyes by the pigment melanin.
Pimple	A lesion smaller than 5 millimeters in diameter that is filled with serous fluid. See vesicle.
Pinkeye	Inflammation of the membrane that covers the white of the eyes and lines the eyelids, causing redness, discomfort, and a discharge; can be caused by infection or allergies. Also called conjunctivitis.
Pinworm	A small parasite worm that can live in the intestines; commonly affects children.
Pituitary adenoma	A noncancerous tumor of the pituitary gland.
Pityriasis alba	A common childhood or adolescent disorder in which there are pale, scaly patches on the skin of the face.
Pityriasis rosea	A mild skin condition in which flat, scaly spots occur on the trunk and upper arms.
PKU	See Phenylketonuria.
Placebo	A chemically inactive substance given in place of a drug to test how much of a drug's effectiveness can be attributed to a patient's expectations that the drug will have a positive effect.
Placebo effect	The positive or negative response to a drug that is caused by a person's expectations of a drug rather than the drug itself.
Plantar reflex	The normal curling of the toes downward when the sole of the foot is stroked.
Plantar wart	A rough surfaced, hard spot on the sole of the foot that is caused by a virus.
Plaque	This is a solid, elevated skin lesion greater than 10 millimeters in diameter. Also an area of buildup of cholesterol and fat deposits in an artery, causing narrowing of the artery.

Plasma	The liquid part of the blood, containing substances such as nutrients, salts, and proteins.
Plasma cell	A white blood cell that makes antibodies.
Plasmapheresis	A procedure in which autoantibody-filled plasma is filtered from the blood.
Platelet	The smallest particle found in the blood, which plays a major role in forming blood clots.
Pleura	The double layered membrane that lines the lungs and chest cavity and allows for lung movement during breathing.
Pleural effusion	A buildup of fluid between the membranes that line the lungs and chest cavity (the pleura); causes compression of the lungs, which leads to breathing difficulty.
Pleural rub	A rubbing sound produced by inflamed pleural membranes that can be heard when breathing.
Pleurisy	Inflammation of the lining of the lungs and chest cavity, usually caused by a lung infection; characterized by sharp chest pain.
Pleurodynia	Pain in the chest caused by a virus.
Plummer Vinson syndrome	Difficulty swallowing due to an abnormal web of tissue across the upper part of the esophagus.
PMS	See Premenstrual syndrome.
Pneumoconiosis	A respiratory disease caused by dust inhalation.
Pneumocystis pneumonia	An opportunistic infection of the lungs caused by a single celled parasite.
Pneumonectomy	Surgical removal of a lung.
Pneumonia	Inflammation of the lungs due to a bacterial or viral infection, which causes fever, shortness of breath, and the coughing up of phlegm.
Pneumothorax	A condition in which air enters the space between the chest wall and the lungs, causing chest pain and shortness of breath; may occur spontaneously or be the result of a disease or an accident.

Poliomyelitis

A rare viral disease (also called Polio). The resulting skeletal muscle paralysis without sensory nerve dysfunction is called Post-Polio Syndrome.

Polyarthritis

Arthritis occurring in more than one joint.

Polycystic kidney disease

A condition in which there are multiple, slow growing cysts on both kidneys.

Polycythemia

An increased amount of red blood cells in the blood.

Polydactyly

The presence of an excessive number of fingers or toes.

Polydipsia

Excessive thirst.

Polymyalgia rheumatica

A rare disease of the elderly, characterized by muscle stiffness and pain in the hips, thighs, shoulders, and neck.

Polymyositis

An autoimmune disease of connective tissue in which muscles weaken and become inflamed.

Polyp

A growth that occurs on mucous membranes such as those in the nose and intestine; bleeds easily and can become cancerous.

Polysaccharide

A complex carbohydrate composed of three or more simple carbohydrate molecules joined together.

Polyunsaturated fat

A fat or oil that contains well below the maximum number of hydrogen atoms possible; thought to reduce the risk of coronary heart disease.

Polyuria

The excessive production of urine; can be a symptom of various diseases, most notably diabetes mellitus.

Porphyria

A group of genetic disorders in which substances called porphyrins build up in the blood, often causing rashes brought on by exposure to sunlight and reactions to certain drugs.

Portal hypertension

Increased blood pressure in the portal vein.

Portal vein

The vein connecting the stomach, intestines, and spleen to the liver.

Positron emission tomography scanning	An imaging method in which substances emitting positrons (positively charged particles) are introduced into the body, and detectors connected to a computer are used to form images of the tissues. Also called PET scan.
Posterior	Describes something that is located in or relates to the back of the body.
Postmortem examination	Examination of a body after death to determine the cause of death; commonly called an autopsy.
Postmyocardial infarction syndrome	A condition that occurs following a heart attack or heart surgery; characterized by fever, chest pain, pericarditis, and pleurisy.
Postnatal	Describes something that occurs after birth, usually to the baby.
Postpartum	A term that describes something that occurs after childbirth, usually to the mother.
Postural drainage	Drainage of mucus from specific areas of the lungs by placing the body in a specific position.
Postural hypotension	An excessive fall in BP (typically > 20/10 mm Hg) upon assuming the upright posture often resulting in lightheadedness or fainting. Also called Orthostatic hypotension.
Precancerous	Describes a condition from which cancer is likely to develop.
Precordial movement	Movement of the heart that is seen and felt through the chest wall.
Premature labor	Labor that begins before the full term of pregnancy (about 37 weeks).
Premedication	Drugs, usually painkillers, taken 1 to 2 hours before surgery.
Premenopausal	A term that describes the period of a few years in a woman's life just before menopause.
Premenstrual syndrome	Physical and emotional changes that occur in a woman 1 or 2 weeks before menstruation, at or after ovulation; characterized by irritability, tension, depression, and fatigue. Also called PMS.
Prenatal care	Medical care of a pregnant woman and the fetus.

Prenatal diagnosis	Techniques used to diagnose abnormalities in a fetus.
Prenatal testing	Tests performed on a pregnant woman or her fetus to prevent or diagnose abnormalities.
Presbycusis	The loss of hearing that occurs naturally with age.
Presbyopia	The loss of the ability to focus the eyes on near objects that occurs naturally with age, as a result of loss of elasticity of the lens of the eyes.
Pressure point	Specific points on the body where external pressure can be applied to prevent excessive arterial bleeding.
Pressure sore	An ulcer on the skin that is a result of being bedridden; commonly called a bedsore or decubitus ulcer.
Priapism	A painful, persistent erection without sexual arousal, requiring emergency treatment.
Prickly heat	A rash involving small, red, itchy spots and a prickly sensation that usually appears where sweat builds up.
Primary	A disease that began in the affected location.
Proctalgia	Pain in the rectum.
Proctitis	Inflammation of the rectum, which causes soreness and sometimes mucus and/or pus in the stool.
Proctoscopy	Examination of the rectum using a viewing instrument.
Productive cough	A cough that brings up phlegm, which is the body's natural way of clearing blocked airways.
Progeria	An extremely rare condition in which the body ages prematurely.
Progesterone	A female sex hormone that plays many important roles in reproduction, including the thickening of the lining of the uterus during the menstrual cycle; and during pregnancy, the functioning of the placenta, and the initiation of labor.
Prognosis	The predicted outcome of a disease or condition following either treatment or no treatment.
Progressive muscular atrophy	Gradual degeneration and weakening of muscles due to a degenerative spinal cord.

Prolactin A hormone released by the pituitary gland that is responsible for the development of breasts and milk production in females.

Prolapse The displacement of an organ from its normal position to a new one.

Prolapsed disc See herniated disc.

Pronation The foot position that places the smallest toe higher than the big toe.

Prophylactic Anything used to prevent disease.

Proprioception The body's system for determining its position relative to the outside world.

Prostaglandins Naturally occurring body chemicals that induce pain, inflammation and fever.

Prostatectomy The partial or complete surgical removal of the prostate gland.

Prostatitis Inflammation of the prostate gland.

Prosthesis An artificial replacement for a missing part of the body.

Proteins Large molecules made up of amino acids that play many major roles in the body, including forming the basis of body structures such as skin and hair, and important chemicals such as enzymes and hormones.

Protozoan A simple, single celled organism.

Protraction An anterior movement used with movements of the mandible.

Proximal Located nearer to the center of the body.

Pruritus Itchiness; a disagreeable sensation of the skin that provokes the desire to scratch or rub the skin to obtain relief.

Pseudogout A form of arthritis with symptoms similar to gout that results from the depositing of calcium salts in a joint.

Psittacosis A chlamydial infection resembling influenza that is spread to humans by the droppings of infected birds.

Psychogenic Resulting from psychological or emotional disorders.

Psychological	Relating to the mind and the processes of the mind.
Psychosis	A mental disorder in which a serious inability to think, perceive, and judge clearly, causes loss of touch with reality.
Psychosomatic	Describes a physical condition that is influenced by psychological or emotional factors.
Psychotherapy	The treatment of mental and emotional disorders using psychological methods, such as counseling, instead of physical means.
Psychotic	Relating to psychosis.
Psychotropic drug	A drug that has a psychological effect.
Ptosis	The drooping of the upper eyelid.
Puberty	The period during which a child's body becomes sexually mature and develops into adult form.
Pudendal block	A local anesthesia procedure used during childbirth, causing the lower part of the vagina to be insensitive to pain.
Puerperal sepsis	Infection of the female genital tract following childbirth, abortion, or miscarriage.
Puerperium	The time period after childbirth (about 6 weeks) during which a woman's body returns to its normal physical state.
Pulmonary edema	The buildup of fluid in lung tissue, which is usually caused by heart failure.
Pulmonary fibrosis	A condition in which the tissue of the lungs has become thick and scarred, usually because of inflammation caused by lung conditions such as pneumonia or tuberculosis.
Pulmonary heart valve	The heart valve that stops blood pumped to the lungs from leaking back into the heart.
Pulmonary hypertension	Increased blood pressure in the arteries supplying blood to the lungs; caused by increased resistance to blood flow in the lungs, usually a result of a lung disease.

Pulmonary insufficiency	A rare defect in the pulmonary heart valve in which it fails to close properly after each muscle contraction, allowing blood to leak back into the heart; weakens the heart's pumping ability.
Pulmonary stenosis	Obstruction of the flow of blood from the heart to the lungs.
Pulse	The expansion and contraction of a blood vessel due to the blood pumped through it; determined as the number of expansions per minute.
Purines	Components of certain foods that metabolize into uric acid in the body. Foods high in purines include meats, mushrooms, lentils, asparagus and spinach.
Purpuric rash	Areas of purple or reddish brown spots on the skin, which are caused by bleeding from underlying tissues.
Pus	A thick, yellowish or greenish fluid that contains dead white blood cells, tissues, and bacteria; occurs at the site of a bacterial infection.
Pustule	An elevated lesion containing pus.
Pyelolithotomy	Surgical removal of a kidney stone.
Pyelonephritis	Inflammation of the kidney, usually due to a bacterial infection.
Pyloric sphincter	A circular muscle located at the junction of the stomach and small intestine that controls the passage of food into the small intestine.
Pyloric stenosis	Narrowing of the outlet located at the junction of the stomach and small intestine.
Pyloroplasty	Surgical widening of the outlet between the stomach and small intestine.
Pyrexia	A body temperature of above 98.6 F in the mouth or 99.8 F in the rectum.
Pyrogen	Any substance that causes a fever.
Pyuria	The presence of white blood cells in the urine; usually an indication of kidney or urinary tract infection.
Quadriplegic	A person who is paralyzed in both arms and both legs as well as the torso.

Rabies

An infectious viral disease primarily affecting animals; can be transmitted to humans through an infected animal's bite; if untreated, can result in paralysis and death.

Radiation

A variety of types of energy, such as X-rays and ultraviolet.

Radiation therapy

Treatment of a disease, such as cancer, using forms of radioactivity that damage or destroy abnormal cells.

Radical surgery

Treatment of disease by surgically removing all tissue that is or may be affected.

Radiculopathy

Any disease of the nerve roots; can be caused by herniated disc, arthritis, and other problems.

Radioallergosorbent test

A blood test performed to help determine the cause of an allergy by detecting the presence of antibodies to various allergens.

Radiography

The formation of images of the inside of the body using radiation projected through the body and onto film; a radiograph is also called an X-ray.

Radionuclide scanning

An imaging technique in which a radioactive substance is introduced into the body and its emitted radiation is detected; specific organs can be studied according to the amount of the radioactive substance that they absorb.

Radon

A colorless, odorless, tasteless radioactive gas that is produced by materials in soil, rocks, and building materials; suspected of causing cancer.

Rales

Abnormal crackling or bubbling sounds heard in the lungs during breathing.

Rash

An area of inflammation or a group of spots on the skin.

Receptor

A nerve cell that responds to a stimulus and produces a nerve impulse; also refers to the area on the surface of a cell that a chemical must bind to in order to have its effect.

Recessive gene

A gene that does not produce its effect when it occurs with a dominant gene, but produces its effect only when there are two copies of it.

Reconstructive surgery
Surgery to rebuild part of the body that has been damaged or defective from birth.

Rectal prolapse
Bulging of the lining of the rectum through the anus, usually due to straining during a bowel movement.

Red blood cell
A doughnut-shaped blood cell that carries oxygen from the lungs to body tissues.

Referred pain
Pain felt in a part of the body remote from the site where pain originates.

Reflex
An automatic, involuntary response of the nervous system to a stimulus.

Reflexology
Massage technique based around a system of points in the hands and feet thought to correspond, or "reflex," to all areas of the body.

Regurgitation
The backflow of fluid; can refer to food and drink flowing back up from the stomach into the mouth or blood flowing back into the heart through a defective heart valve.

Rehabilitation
Treatment for an injury or illness aimed at restoring physical abilities.

Rehydration
Treatment for dehydration (an abnormally low level of water in the body) in which levels are restored by taking fluids containing water, salt, and glucose by mouth or, if severe, through a vein.

Relapse
The return of a disease or symptom after it had disappeared.

REM sleep
Rapid Eye Movement sleep; the lightest stage of sleep in which most dreams occur.

Remission
The temporary disappearance of a disease or its symptoms, either partially or completely; also refers to the time period in which this occurs.

Renal cell carcinoma
The most common type of kidney cancer

Renal colic
Severe pain on one side of the lower back, usually as a result of a kidney stone.

Renal tubular acidosis
Inability of the kidneys to remove sufficient amounts of acid from the body, making the blood more acidic than normal.

Repetitive strain injury An injury that occurs when the same movement is repeated continuously.

Reproductive system The organs and structures that allow men and women to have sexual intercourse and produce children.

Resection Partial or complete surgical removal of a diseased organ or structure.

Resorption The breakdown and assimilation of bone.

Respiration The process by which oxygen is taken in and used by tissues in the body and carbon dioxide is released.

Respirator Another term for a ventilator.

Respiratory arrest A condition in which a person suddenly stops breathing.

Respiratory distress syndrome A condition experienced after an illness or injury damages the lungs, causing severe breathing difficulty and resulting in a life threatening lack of oxygen in the blood.

Respiratory failure The failure of the body to exchange gases properly, which leads to a buildup of carbon dioxide and a lack of oxygen in the blood.

Respiratory system The organs that carry out the process of respiration.

Resting pulse The pulse rate when a person is not experiencing any physical activity or mental stress.

Reticulocyte An immature red blood cell.

Retina A membrane lining the inside of the back of the eye that contains light sensitive nerve cells that convert focused light into nerve impulses, making vision possible.

Retinal artery occlusion Obstruction of an artery that supplies blood to the retina, resulting in some degree of temporary or permanent blindness.

Retinitis pigmentosa Gradual loss of the field of vision, owing to a degeneration of the light sensitive nerve cells of the retina.

Retinoblastoma A hereditary, cancerous tumor of the retina affecting infants and children.

Retinoid

A substance resembling vitamin A that is used to treat skin conditions such as acne and has been reported to reduce skin wrinkling.

Retinopathy

Any disease or disorder of the retina; usually refers to damage to the retina caused by high blood pressure or diabetes mellitus.

Retinoscopy

A method of determining focusing errors of the eye in which light is shined through the pupil and the reflected beam is measured.

Retraction

A posterior movement of some joints like the jaw and shoulder.

Retrovirus

A group of viruses made up of RNA instead of DNA, including HIV and the virus that causes T-cell leukemia.

Reye's syndrome

A rare disorder mainly affecting those under the age of 15 that is characterized by brain and liver damage following a viral infection such as chickenpox or the flu; may be linked to taking aspirin to treat a viral infection.

Rh blood group

A blood group classifying whether the substances called Rhesus (Rh) factors are present on the surface of red blood cells; the "positive" or "negative" designation in blood classification (e.g., "O negative").

Rh immunoglobulin

A substance used to prevent a woman who is Rh incompatible with her fetus from becoming Rh sensitized.

Rh incompatibility

A condition in which a pregnant woman's Rh factor does not match that of the fetus; can lead to the production of antibodies by the mother that destroy the fetus' red blood cells.

Rh sensitized

A condition in which a woman who has a negative Rh factor develops permanent antibodies against Rh positive blood as a result of exposure to the blood of her fetus; can cause fetal hemolysis in subsequent pregnancies.

Rheumatic fever

A disorder that follows a throat infection by the streptococcus bacteria and causes inflammation in body tissues.

Rheumatoid factors	Antibodies that are present in about 80 percent of people with rheumatoid arthritis; their detection through blood testing can help to diagnose the disorder.
Rhinitis	Inflammation of the mucous membrane lining the nose, which can cause sneezing, runny nose, congestion, and pain; when caused by substances in the air, it is called allergic rhinitis or hay fever.
Rhinophyma	A bulb shaped deformity and redness of the nose as a result of severe rosacea.
Rhinoplasty	Surgery that changes the structure of the nose, either to improve appearance or to correct a deformity or injury.
Riboflavin	A vitamin belonging to the vitamin B complex that is important in many processes in the body and helps to maintain healthy skin.
Righting reflex	An attempt to keep the head upright and eyes horizontal which begins in infancy.
Rigor mortis	General stiffening of muscle after death.
Ringworm	A fungal skin infection that spreads out in an even circle, characterized by ring like, scaly patches of red skin.
Rinne's test	A test that uses a tuning fork to diagnose hearing loss resulting from poor conduction of sound from the outer to the inner ear.
Risk factor	Anything that increases a person's chances of developing a disease, for example, smoking and lung cancer.
RNA	RiboNucleic Acid helps to decode and process the information contained in DNA.
Rocky mountain spotted fever	A rare disease transmitted to humans through the bites of ticks; characterized by small pink spots on the wrists and ankles that spread to other parts of the body, become larger, and bleed.
Rosacea	A skin disorder that is characterized by patches of red skin on the nose and cheeks and acne like bumps; most commonly occurs in middle aged women.

Roseola infantum	A common disease in young children characterized by a sudden fever and rash.
Rostral	Describes a structure on the head that is closer to the nose.
Roundworm	A group of worms that includes many of the major human parasites.
Rubella	A mild viral infection (also known as German measles) that produces a rash and fever; dangerous when it infects a woman during the early stages of pregnancy, when it can spread causing birth defects in the fetus.
Rubeola	Another term for measles.
Rupture	A tear or break in an organ or tissue.
Saccharides	A group of carbohydrates, including sugars and starches.
Sagittal	Any plane passing through the body from the front to the back dividing the body into two halves.
Saline	A salt solution or any substance that contains salt.
Salivary glands	A group of glands that secrete saliva into the mouth.
Salmonella	A group of bacteria; includes a species that causes food poisoning and another responsible for typhoid fever.
Salmonellosis	Infection by salmonella bacteria.
Salpingectomy	Surgical removal of one or both fallopian tubes.
Salpingitis	Inflammation of a fallopian tube.
Salpingography	X-ray examination of the fallopian tubes.
Salpingolysis	Removal of abnormal scar tissue between a fallopian tube and nearby tissue.
Salpingo-oophorectomy	The surgical removal of one or both of the fallopian tubes and one or both of the ovaries.
Salpingostomy	Surgical opening of a fallopian tube for drainage or removal of an obstruction.
Sarcoidosis	A rare disease with no known cause that leads to inflammation in tissues throughout the body, including the lymph nodes, lungs, liver, skin, and eyes.

Sarcoma	A cancer in connective tissue, fibrous tissue, or blood vessels.
Saturated fat	Fats that contain the maximum amount of hydrogen possible, such as those found in meats and dairy products; can contribute to coronary heart disease and the development of some cancers.
Scabies	A highly contagious skin disorder caused by a mite that burrows into the skin and produces an intense, itchy rash.
Scales	These are heaped up particles of keratin in the surface epithelium of the body. They are loose and hardened.
Scar	Fibrous tissue where a skin lesion has healed.
Scarlet fever	An infectious fever of children from a strain of Streptococcus pyogenes; symptoms include a sore throat and a scarlet rash.
Schistosomiasis	Infestation by a parasitic blood worm that can damage the liver, bladder, and intestines.
Schizophrenia	A group of mental disorders characterized by abnormal thoughts, moods, and actions; sufferers have a distorted sense of reality and thoughts that do not logically fit together.
Sclera	The tough, white coating that covers and protects the inner structures of the eye.
Sclerosis	A hardening of tissue.
Sclerotherapy	Treatment of varicose veins by injection of a solution that destroys them.
Scoliosis	Lateral abnormal curvature of the spine beginning early in puberty, resulting in postural deformity and possibly organ dysfunction due to internal pressure.
Screening	The testing of an otherwise healthy person in order to diagnose disorders at an early stage.
Scurvy	A disease caused by a lack of vitamin C, characterized by weakness, bleeding and pain in joints and muscles, bleeding gums, and abnormal bone and tooth growth.

Sebaceous cyst

A swelling that occurs under the skin, most commonly on the scalp, face, ears, and genitals; although usually harmless, can grow very large and become painful if infected.

Sebaceous gland

A small subcutaneous gland, usually connected with hair follicles, that secretes sebum.

Seborrhea

Excessive oiliness of the face and scalp.

Sebum

The oily, lubricating substance that is secreted by sebaceous glands in the skin.

Secondary

Describes a disease or disorder that follows, or is caused by, another one.

Sedative

A group of drugs that have a calming effect; used to treat anxiety and pain, bring on sleep, and help relax a person before surgery.

Seizure

Sudden uncontrolled waves of electrical activity in the brain, causing involuntary movement or loss of consciousness.

Sensory nerve

Nerves that carry information about the body's senses toward the brain. Also called an afferent nerve.

Sensory organ

An organ that receives and relays information about the body's senses to the brain.

Sepsis

A life-threatening illness caused by an overwhelming bacteria infection of the bloodstream. Also called systemic inflammatory response syndrome.

Septal defect

A birth defect in which a hole is present in the wall that separates the left and right sides of the heart.

Septic shock

A life threatening condition in which tissues become damaged and blood pressure drops due to bacteria multiplying and producing poisons in the blood.

Serotonin

A chemical that transmits nerve impulses in the brain, causes blood vessels to constrict (narrow) at sites of bleeding, and stimulates smooth muscle movement in the intestines.

Serum

The clear, watery fluid that separates from clotted blood.

Sex chromosomes	The X and Y chromosomes that determine a person's gender; women normally have two X chromosomes and men normally have one X and one Y.
Sex hormones	Hormones responsible for producing sex characteristics and controlling sexual functions.
Shigellosis	A bacterial infection of the intestines, causing abdominal pain and diarrhea.
Shock	A dangerous combination of lowered blood pressure and depressed metabolism causing a decreased core temperature. Shock can be life threatening without prompt treatment.
Shunt	An artificially constructed drainage system.
Sick sinus syndrome	Abnormal functioning of the structure that regulates the heartbeat, causing episodes of abnormal heart rhythm.
Sigmoidoscopy	An examination of the rectum and the lowest part of the large intestine using a flexible viewing tube inserted through the anus.
Sign	Some characteristic that can be observed or recognized by someone other than the client.
Silicone	A group of compounds of silicon and oxygen; commonly used as implants in cosmetic surgery because they resist body fluids and are not rejected by the body.
Silicosis	A respiratory disease caused by inhalation of dust containing the mineral silica.
Single photon emission computed tomography	An imaging technique in which a radioactive substance is introduced into the body and the radiation emitted by the substance is detected by a camera and is transformed into cross-sectional images by a computer. Also called SPECT.
Sinoatrial node	The structure that regulates the heartbeat; a natural "pacemaker".
Sinus	A cavity within bone or a channel that contains blood; also refers to an abnormal tract in the body.
Sinus bradycardia	A regular heart rate of less than 60 beats per minute.

Sinus rhythm	Normal heart rhythm.
Sinus tachycardia	A regular heart rate of over 100 beats per minute.
Sinusitis	Inflammation of the lining of the cavities in the bone surrounding the nose (the sinuses), usually as a result of a bacterial infection spreading from the nose.
Skin graft	A method of treating damaged or lost skin in which a piece of skin is taken from another area of the body and transplanted in a damaged or missing section.
Skin patch	A sticky patch attached to the surface of the skin that releases drugs into the bloodstream.
Skin patch test	A diagnostic test in which different allergens are taped to the skin to determine which causes an allergic reaction.
Skin prick test	A test performed to determine a person's sensitivity to a certain allergen by applying it to a small needle and using that needle to pierce the skin.
Sleep apnea	A condition in which breathing stops for very short periods of time during sleep.
Slipped disc	The obsolete term for herniated disc.
Small cell carcinoma	The most serious form of lung cancer.
Smallpox	A highly contagious and often fatal viral infection that has been completely eradicated by immunization.
Smear	A sample of cells spread across a glass slide to be examined through a microscope.
Solar plexus	The largest network of nerves in the body, located behind the stomach.
Somatic	Pertaining to the body.
Spasm	An involuntary muscle contraction; can sometimes be powerful and painful.
Spastic paralysis	Spasticity involving partial paralysis where muscle tissues are hypertonic.
Spasticity	Muscle stiffness caused by an increase in contractions of the muscle fibers.

SPECT	Single Photon Emission Computed Tomography: An imaging technique in which a radioactive substance is introduced into the body and the radiation emitted by the substance is detected by a camera and is transformed into cross-sectional images by a computer.
Sphincter	A ring of muscle fibers located around a naturally occurring passage or opening in the body that opens and closes to regulate passage of substances.
Sphygmomanometer	An instrument used to measure blood pressure.
Spider nevus	A collection of dilated (widened) capillaries on the skin that creates a patch resembling a spider.
Spider vein	Small, superficial blood vessels that have dilated. They are visible as clusters of red, blue or purple lines. Also called telangiectasia.
Spina bifida occulta	The least dangerous form of spina bifida, in which bones in the spine fail to close but there is no protrusion of the spinal cord or its fluid cushion out of the body.
Spinal fusion	The surgical joining of two or more adjacent vertebrae using bone fragments; used to help severe back pain or prevent damage to the spinal cord.
Spinal tap	Another term for a lumbar puncture.
Spirometry	A test of lung condition; a person breathes into a machine called a spirometer that measures the volume of air exhaled.
Splenectomy	Surgical removal of the spleen.
Splint	A device that is used to immobilize a part of the body.
Splinter hemorrhage	A splinter shaped area of bleeding under a fingernail or toenail.
Splinting	A reflexive immune response to underlying instability or trauma where the muscles remain tense and inflexible; muscle splinting acts to immobilize the joint(s).
Spondylitis	Inflammation of the joints in the spine.

Sprue	A digestive disorder in which nutrients cannot be properly absorbed from food, causing weakness and loss of weight.
Sputum	Mucus and other material produced by the lining of the respiratory tract; also called phlegm.
Staging	Classifying tumor cells on the basis of their abnormality, invasiveness, and metastasis.
Stapedectomy	Surgical removal of a stapes (a sound conducting bone in the middle ear) that cannot move to transmit sound; performed to treat hearing loss caused by otosclerosis.
Staphylococci	Common bacteria that cause skin infections and a number of other disorders.
Status asthmaticus	A life threatening asthma attack requiring immediate treatment.
Status epilepticus	A life threatening succession of epileptic seizures.
Stem cells	Cells that give rise to the different types of blood cells.
Stenosis	Narrowing of a body passageway.
Stent	A device used to hold tissues open or in place, such as to support a skin graft or hold an artery open.
Stereotaxic surgery	Brain surgery done through a small opening in the skull and guided by X-rays or computer-aided imaging techniques.
Sterilization	A surgery performed to make a person incapable of reproducing; also refers to the process of killing microorganisms on objects such as surgical instruments.
Steroids	A group of drugs that includes corticosteroids, which resemble hormones produced by the adrenal glands, and anabolic steroids, which are similar to the hormones produced by the male sex organs.
Stoma	A surgically formed opening on a body surface.
Stomach bypass	A surgical procedure to treat an obstructed stomach or severe obesity in which the passage of food is diverted around the stomach and directly into the small intestine.

Stomach stapling	A dangerous procedure in which the stomach is made smaller by partitioning it off using metal staples; used as an extreme treatment of severe obesity.
Stool	Another term for feces.
Strabismus	A condition in which the eyes are not aligned correctly.
Strawberry nevus	A bright red, raised birthmark that usually disappears without treatment.
Strep throat	A throat infection caused by streptococcus bacteria; characterized by a sore throat, fever, and enlarged lymph nodes in the neck.
Streptococci	Bacteria that cause a variety of diseases, including pneumonia and strep throat.
Stye	A pus filled abscess in the follicle of an eyelash; caused by a bacterial infection.
Subacute	A state between acute and chronic when symptoms have lessened in severity or duration.
Subcutaneous	A medical term meaning "beneath the skin"
Subluxation	A loss of normal joint mobility coupled with a nervous system deficit.
Submucosa	The layer of connective tissue under a mucous membrane.
Suction lipectomy	See Liposuction.
Superficial	The structure near the surface of the body.
Superior	Anatomically above another structure or toward the top.
Supination	A foot position in which the big toe is higher than the smallest toe.
Suppository	A solid cone or bullet-shaped object made up of a chemically inactive substance and a drug that is inserted into the rectum or vagina; used to administer a drug.
Suppuration	The production of pus.

Surfactant A mixture of substances secreted by the air sacs of the lungs that prevents the air sacs from collapsing during exhalation.

Suture A surgical stitch that helps close an incision or wound so that it can heal properly.

Sweat test A measure of the saltiness of sweat to help diagnose cystic fibrosis.

Swimmer's ear See Otitis externa.

Sycosis barbae A bacterial infection of the hair follicles in the beard area.

Sympathetic nervous system The part of the autonomic nervous system that raises blood pressure and heart rate in response to stress.

Symptom Any sensation or change in bodily function that is experienced by a patient

Syncope A sudden brief loss of consciousness, with loss of postural tone. Commonly called fainting.

Syndactyly A condition in which fingers or toes are fused together.

Syndrome A group of symptoms that indicate a certain disorder when they occur together.

Synovectomy Surgical removal of the synovial membrane.

Synovial fluid A lubricating joint fluid secreted by the synovial membrane.

Synovial membrane The thin membrane that lines the inside of a joint capsule.

Synovitis Inflammation of the joint capsule as a result of injury or infection.

System The combination of various organs that have similar or related functions

Systemic Affecting the whole body.

Systemic inflammatory response syndrome A life-threatening illness caused by an overwhelming bacteria infection of the bloodstream. Also called sepsis.

Systolic pressure The blood pressure measured while the heart is contracting.

T cell	See T lymphocyte.
T cell leukemia	A type of leukemia caused by a virus in which T lymphocytes divide uncontrollably.
T lymphocyte	A type of white blood cell that fights infections and destroys abnormal cells directly; as compared with releasing antibodies to fight infection.
T lymphocyte killer cell	A type of T lymphocyte white blood cell that attaches to abnormal cells and releases chemicals that destroy them.
Tachycardia	A rapid heart rate (over 100 beats per minute).
Tapeworm	A parasitic worm that lives in the intestines; causes diarrhea and abdominal discomfort.
Tapotement	Short, alternating taps to the client, executed with cupped hands, fingers or the edge of the hand.
Tear duct	A tiny passageway that drains lubricating tears from the surface of the eye to the back of the nose.
Telangiectasia	Small, superficial blood vessels that have dilated. They are visible as clusters of red, blue or purple lines. Also called spider veins or sunburst varicosities.
Temporal arteritis	Inflammation and narrowing of arteries in the head and neck, including those in the scalp near the temple, which can cause blindness if untreated.
Tendinitis	Inflammation of a tendon, usually caused by injury, characterized by pain, tenderness, and sometimes limited movement in the attached muscle.
Tendon	Strong connective tissue cords that attach muscle to bone or muscle to muscle.
Tendon transfer	Surgical cutting and repositioning of a tendon so that the muscle attached to it has a new function.
Tennis elbow	A form of tendinitis that causes pain and tenderness in the elbow and forearm.
Tenosynovitis	Inflammation of the inner lining of the sheath that covers a tendon.
Tenovaginitis	Inflammation of the fibrous wall of the sheath that covers a tendon.

TENS	Transcutaneous Electrical Nerve Stimulation: A therapy that applies specific electrical pulses across the upper layer of skin to "crowd out" pain signals. Also called TENS therapy.
Teratoma	A tumor composed of cells not normally found in the part of the body when the tumor occurred.
Testosterone	The sex hormone that stimulates development of male sex characteristics and bone and muscle growth; produced by the testicles and in small amounts by the ovaries.
Tetanus	A sometimes fatal disease affecting the brain and spinal cord; caused by infection with bacterium present in soil and manure. Also called lockjaw.
Tetralogy of Fallot	A genetic heart disease involving four structural defects in the heart, which result in insufficient levels of oxygen in the blood.
Tetraplegic	A person who is paralyzed in both arms and both legs (also called quadriplegic).
Thalamus	A structure in the brain that relays and processes incoming sensory information from the eyes and ears and from pressure and pain receptors.
Thalassemia	A group of genetic blood disorders characterized by a defect in the ability to produce hemoglobin, leading to the rupturing of red blood cells (called hemolytic anemia).
Thallium scan	A method of examining the heart to obtain information about the blood supply to the heart muscle.
Therapeutic range	The range of doses of a drug that will produce beneficial results without side effects.
Thoracoscopy	Examination of the membranes covering the lungs using an endoscope.
Thoracotomy	A procedure in which the chest is surgically opened to operate on an organ in the chest cavity.
Thorax	The chest.
Thrombectomy	Removal of a blood clot.
Thrombi	Plural of thrombus.

Thromboembolism	Blockage of a blood vessel by a blood clot fragment that has broken off and traveled from another area of the body.
Thrombophlebitis	Inflammation of a vein, along with clot formation in the affected area.
Thrombosis	A condition in which an attached blood clot (thrombus) has formed inside a blood vessel.
Thrombus	An attached blood clot in a blood vessel.
Thrush	A yeast infection of the mouth, throat and esophagus that may be a result of a candida infection.
Thymus gland	An immune system gland located in the upper part of the chest that plays an important role in the production of T lymphocytes.
Thyroglossal cyst	A swelling at the front of the neck; forms from a duct that fails to disappear during embryonic development.
Thyroid gland	A gland located in the front of the neck below the voice box that plays an important role in metabolism (the chemical processes in the body) and growth; the gland produces thyroid hormone.
Thyroiditis	Inflammation of the thyroid gland.
Thyrotoxicosis	A toxic condition resulting from overactivity of the thyroid gland.
Thyroxin	A hormone produced by the thyroid gland that helps regulate energy production in the body.
Tic	An involuntary, repetitive movement such as a twitch.
Ticks	Small, eight legged animals that can attach to humans and animals and feed on blood; sometimes spread infectious organisms via their bites.
Tietze's syndrome	Inflammation of the cartilage that joins ribs to the breastbone, causing chest pain.
Tinea	A group of common infections occurring on the skin, hair, and nails that are caused by a fungus; commonly referred to as ringworm.
Tinnitus	A persistent ringing or buzzing sound in the ear.

Tissue	Tissues are layers of cells that perform specific functions. An example of a tissue is a muscle.
Tissue typing	Tests used to determine the compatibility of tissues used in grafts and transplants.
TMJ syndrome	Headache, facial pain, and jaw tenderness caused by irregularities in the way the joints, muscles, and ligaments in the jaw work together. Also called temporomandibular joint syndrome.
Tolerance	Decreased sensitivity of the body to a certain drug, usually either because the liver becomes more efficient at breaking down the drug or the body's tissues become less sensitive to it; increased tolerance creates a need for a higher dose of the drug in order to have the same effects.
Tonometry	The procedure used to measure the pressure within the eye; is useful in detecting glaucoma.
Tonsillectomy	Surgical removal of the tonsils, usually to treat tonsillitis.
Tonsillitis	Infection and inflammation of the tonsils.
Tonsils	Masses of lymphoid tissue located at either side of the back of the throat.
Tourette's syndrome	A movement disorder characterized by involuntary tics and noises, and in some cases uncontrollable shouting of obscenities.
Tourniquet	A device placed tightly around an arm or leg in order to stop blood flow; can be used to locate veins in order to take a blood sample or to control blood flow during some operations.
Toxemia	The presence of bacterial toxins in the blood.
Toxic epidermal necrolysis	A severe rash in which the outer layers of skin blister and peel off.
Toxic shock syndrome	A life threatening infection caused by staphylococcus bacteria.
Toxicity	The extent to which a substance is poisonous.
Toxin	A poisonous substance.

Toxoplasmosis	A common protozoan infection that is usually only dangerous to a fetus in early pregnancy or a person who is immunocompromised.
Tracheitis	Inflammation of the trachea.
Tracheotomy	Insertion of a tube through a surgical opening in the trachea to maintain an open airway.
Trachoma	A persistent, contagious form of conjunctivitis that can lead to complications such as blindness if untreated.
Traction	The use of tension to hold a body part in place or to correct or prevent an alignment problem.
Transcutaneous	Through the skin.
Transcutaneous Electrical Nerve Stimulation	A therapy that applies specific electrical pulses across the upper layer of skin to "crowd out" pain signals. Also called TENS.
Transferrin	A substance in the blood that transports iron throughout the body.
Transmissible	Able to be passed from one organism to another.
Transplant	Transferring a healthy tissue or organ to replace a damaged tissue or organ; also refers to the tissue or organ transplanted.
Transurethral Prostatectomy	Removal of cancerous tissue from the prostate gland using a resectoscope (a long, narrow instrument passed up the urethra), which allows the surgeon to simultaneously view the prostate and cut away the cancerous tissue.
Transverse	A plane that divides the body into upper and lower portions. It is perpendicular to the longitudinal axis of the mid sagittal section.
Trauma	Physical injury or emotional shock.
Treatment	The procedures, medications and modalities used by a physician in an attempt to cure the diagnosed disease.
Tremor	An involuntary, rhythmic, shaking movement caused by alternating contraction and relaxation of muscles; can be the normal result of age or the abnormal effect of a disorder.

Triage

A system used to classify sick or injured people according to the severity of their conditions.

Tricuspid valve

A three leaflet valve between the upper and lower chambers on the right side of the heart (the right atrium and right ventricle).

Trigger point therapy

Concentrated finger pressure applied to "trigger points" (painful irritated areas in muscles) to break cycles of spasm and pain.

Triglyceride

The main form of fat in the blood; determining levels of triglyceride is useful in diagnosing and treating diabetes, high blood pressure, and heart disease.

Trimester

One of three time periods lasting about three months each into which pregnancy term is divided.

Trisomy

The presence of three copies of a certain chromosome instead of the normal two copies.

Trisomy 21

See Down syndrome.

Tubal ligation

A procedure in which the fallopian tubes are cut and tied off; usually a permanent form of sterilization.

Tuberculin test

Skin tests performed to determine previous infection with tuberculosis; can help rule out the possibility of being currently infected with tuberculosis.

Tuboplasty

Surgical repair of a damaged fallopian tube to treat infertility.

Tumor

An abnormal mass that occurs when cells in a certain area reproduce unchecked; can be cancerous (malignant) or noncancerous (benign).

Tunnel vision

Loss of peripheral vision so that only objects directly ahead can be seen.

Tympanic membrane

The medical term for the eardrum.

Tympanoplasty

A surgical procedure used to treat hearing loss in which the eardrum or structures in the middle ear are repaired.

Typhoid fever

An acute bacterial infection causing fever, headache, abdominal discomfort, and enlargement of the liver and spleen.

Typhus

A group of diseases caused by the microorganism rickettsia, spread by the bites of fleas, mites, or ticks; symptoms include headache, fever, rash, and a series of complications if untreated.

Ulcer

An open lesion of any portion of the skin that destroys the epidermis and disrupts the basement membrane making the body vulnerable to infection.

Ultrasound scanning

An imaging procedure used to examine internal organs in which high-frequency sound waves are passed into the body, reflected back, and used to build an image; also sometimes called sonography.

Ultraviolet light

A form of invisible light in sunlight that is responsible for the tanning and burning of skin and can cause cataracts and skin cancer.

Unconsciousness

A temporary or prolonged loss of awareness of self and of surroundings.

Unsaturated fat

A fat or oil found mainly in vegetables; thought to reduce the risk of coronary heart disease.

Urea

A waste product of the metabolism of proteins that is formed by the liver and secreted by the kidneys.

Uremia

Abnormally high levels of waste products such as urea in the blood.

Urethritis

Inflammation of the urethra.

Urethrocystitis

Inflammation of the urethra and the bladder.

Urinalysis

A group of physical and chemical tests done on a sample of urine to check for various disorders, including those of the kidneys and urinary tract.

Urinary diversion

An operation to allow urine passage when the bladder or urethra has become blocked or been removed.

Urinary incontinence

The involuntary release of urine because of the inability to control bladder muscles; may occur as a natural part of the aging process or be caused by an injury or disorder.

Urinary tract

The structures in the body that are responsible for the production and release of urine, including the kidneys, ureters, bladder, and urethra.

Urticaria	An allergic reaction in which itchy white lumps surrounded by areas of inflammation appear on the skin; commonly called "hives".
Vaccination	A form of immunization in which killed or weakened microorganisms are placed into the body, where antibodies against them are developed; if the same types of microorganisms enter the body again, they will be destroyed by the antibodies.
Vaccine	A preparation of weakened microorganisms given to create resistance to a certain disease.
Vacuum aspiration	Removal of the contents of the uterus using a suction device.
Valve	A structure that allows fluid flow in only one direction.
Valvotomy	Surgical correction of a narrowed heart valve.
Valvular heart disease	A heart valve defect.
Valvuloplasty	Reconstruction or repair of a narrowed heart valve.
Varicella	The medical term for chickenpox.
Varices	Enlarged, fragile blood or lymph vessels.
Varicose veins	Enlarged, twisted veins just below the surface of the skin, caused by defective valves in the veins.
Variola	Another term for smallpox.
Vascular	Pertaining to blood vessels.
Vasculitis	Inflammation of blood vessels.
Vasoconstriction	Narrowing of blood vessels.
Vasodilation	Widening of blood vessels.
Vasovagal attack	A sudden slowing of the heart, causing fainting.
Vein	A blood vessel that carries blood toward the heart.
Venipuncture	Piercing of a vein with a hollow needle to inject fluid or withdraw blood.
Venography	An X-ray procedure for viewing veins.

Ventilation

The process through which oxygen and carbon dioxide are exchanged between the lungs and the air; also refers to the use of a machine to carry out this process in someone who cannot breathe on his or her own.

Ventilator

A machine used to take over breathing when a person cannot breathe on his or her own.

Ventral

Toward anterior portion of the body.

Ventricle

A small cavity or chamber; there are four ventricles in the brain that circulate cerebrospinal fluid through it, and two in the heart that pump blood throughout the body.

Ventricular fibrillation

Ventricular fibrillation is a condition in which the heart's lower (pumping) chambers contract in a rapid, unsynchronized way, pumping little or no blood. Collapse and sudden cardiac death will follow in minutes unless medical help is provided immediately. This is what a defibrillator is used for.

Ventricular septal defect

A hole in the wall that separates the two lower chambers of the heart (called the ventricles).

Vertebra

One of twenty-four moveable bones of the spinal column.

Vertebrae

Plural form of vertebra.

Vertebral arteries

A pair of arteries running up the neck to supply the brain with blood.

Vertebrobasilar insufficiency

Episodes of dizziness and weakness caused by insufficient blood flow to the brain.

Vertigo

The feeling that one or one's surroundings are spinning.

Very low density lipoprotein

Large lipoproteins rich in triglycerides that circulate through the blood giving up their triglycerides to fat and muscle tissue until they are converted into LDLs. Also called VLDLs.

Vesicle

A lesion smaller than 5 millimeters in diameter that is filled with clear, serous fluid. Commonly called a pimple.

Villi
The millions of fingerlike projections on the lining of the small intestine that aid in the absorption of food.

Viral
A term describing something related to or caused by a virus.

Viremia
The presence of a virus in the blood.

Virilization
The process by which a woman develops male characteristics; caused by overproduction of male sex hormones.

Virulence
The relative ability of an organism to cause disease.

Virus
The smallest known disease-causing microorganism; viruses are very simple in structure and can only multiply when they are inside the cell of another organism.

Visual field
The area on both sides that can be seen while looking straight ahead.

Vital sign
Any sign, such as a pulse, that indicates that a person is alive.

Vitamin
Complex molecular substances necessary to ensure proper body development and maintenance.

Vitiligo
A condition in which patches of skin on the body lose their color; thought to be caused by the immune system attacking the skin tissues, causing the absence of melanin.

Vitreous humor
The clear, watery fluid that fills the cavity of the eye behind the lens.

VLDL
Very Low Density Lipoprotein: large lipoproteins rich in triglycerides that circulate through the blood giving up their triglycerides to fat and muscle tissue until they are converted into LDLs.

Volvulus
Twisting and obstruction of an area of intestine.

Wart
A contagious, harmless growth caused by a virus that occurs on the skin or a mucous membrane.

WBC count
The number of white blood cells present in a blood sample; useful in diagnosing and evaluating various diseases and infections.

Wegener's granulomatosis	A disorder in which nodules associated with inflammation of blood vessels develop in the lungs, kidneys, and nasal passageways.
Weight bearing exercise	Exercise that puts gravitational stress on bones of the leg and pelvis, such as walking,
Wheal	A small, solid elevation on the skin that may itch or burn, often characteristic of an allergic reaction. A group of wheals is called hives.
Wheeze	A high pitched sound produced during breathing because of narrowing of the airways; common sign of asthma.
Whipple's disease	A rare disorder that has widespread effects on the body, including impaired absorption of nutrients, weight loss, joint pain, and anemia.
Whipworm	A small, parasitic worm that can live in the intestines of a human and may cause diarrhea, abdominal pain, and anemia.
White blood cell	A group of colorless blood cells that are part of the immune system, helping prevent and fight infection.
Whooping cough	See Pertussis.
Wilm's tumor	A type of kidney cancer that usually affects children under the age of 5.
Wilson's disease	A rare genetic disorder in which copper builds up in the liver and is released into other parts of the body, eventually causing damage to the liver and brain.
X chromosome	The sex chromosome that is paired (XX) in female cells and single (XY) in male cells.
X linked disorder	A genetic disorder in which the abnormal gene is located on the X chromosome; those affected are always male.
Xanthelasma	Fatty deposits around the eyes that are common in elderly people and are associated with high levels of cholesterol in the blood.
Xanthomatosis	A condition in which fatty deposits occur in various parts of the body, possibly leading to atherosclerosis.

Xeroderma pigmentosum	A genetic disorder in which the skin is extremely sensitive to sunlight, causing it to age prematurely and leaving the individual particularly susceptible to skin cancer.
Xerophthalmia	Excessive dryness of the cornea and conjunctiva due to a lack of vitamin A.
X-ray	See Radiography.
XYY syndrome	A disorder in which a man has an extra Y chromosome, causing him to be unusually tall and to have behavioral disorders.
Y chromosome	One of the two sex chromosomes; determines male sex characteristics.
Yeast infection	A term usually referring to a candidiasis infection.
Yellow fever	A life threatening viral infection transmitted by mosquitoes that causes jaundice, fever, headache, and vomiting.

Bibliography

Text References

American Joint Committee on Cancer, *AJCC Cancer Staging Manual,* 5ᵗʰ Ed, Lippincott-Raven Publishers, 1997

Newton, Donald, *Clinical Pathology For The Professional Bodyworker*, Simran Publications, 1998

Griffith, H. Winter, *Complete Guide to Prescription and Nonprescription Drugs, Edition 2003*, The Berkley Publishing Group, 2002

Yochum TR, Rowe LJ: *Essentials of Skeletal Radiology*. Lippincott, Williams and Wilkins, 1987

Chaitow, Leon, *Fibromyalgia Syndrome: A Practitioner's Guide to Treatment*, Churchill Livingstone Publishers, New York, NY, 1999

Saunders, Jeraldine, and Ross, Harvey M., *Hypoglycemia: The Classic Healthcare Handbook*, Kensington Publishing Corporation, 2002

Lawrence D.J., Cox J.M., *Low Back Pain Mechanism, Diagnosis and Treatment, (5ᵗʰ ed)*, Lippincott, Williams & Wilkins, 1990

Premkumar, Kalyani, *The Massage Connection, Anatomy and Physiology*, 2ⁿᵈ Ed, Lippincott, Williams and Wilkins, 2004

Werner, Ruth, *A Massage Therapist's Guide To Pathology, 2nd Ed,* Lippincott, Williams and Wilkins, Philadelphia, PA, 2002

Rattray, Fiona, *Massage Therapy: An Approach To Treatments*, Massage Therapy Texts and Maverick Consultants, 1997

Curties, Debra, *Massage Therapy and Cancer*, Curties-Overzet Publications, 1999

Persad, Randall, *Massage Therapy and Medications.*: Curties-Overzet Publications Inc, 2001

MacDonald, Gayle, *Medicine Hands: Massage Therapy for People with Cancer*. Findhorn Press, 1999. 877 390 4425.

Fritz, Sandy, *Mosby's Fundamentals Of Therapeutic Massage, 3ʳᵈ Ed.*, C.V. Mosby, 2004

Premkumar, Kalyani, *Pathology A To Z: A Handbook For Massage Therapists, 2ⁿᵈ Ed*, Meducational Skills, Tools & Technology, Inc., 2001

Wible, Jean, *Pharmacology for Massage Therapy*, Lippincott, Williams and Wilkins, 2005

Mandell G.L., Bennett J.E., and Dolin R., *Principles and Practices of Infectious Diseases, 5th ed.,* Churchill Livingstone Publishers, 2000

Robins, LN, Regier, DA, *Psychiatric Disorders in America, The Epidemiologic Catchment Area Study*, New York: The Free Press. 1990

Burch, Sharon, *Recognizing Health And Illness: Pathology For Massage Therapists And Bodyworker*, Health Positive Publishing, 1997

Sanders, R.J., M.D.,. Haug, C.E., M.D., *Thoracic Outlet Syndrome: A Common Sequela Of Neck Injuries.*, J.B. Lippincott Co., 1991.

Journal and Website References

Association of Bodywork and Massage Professionals Website, Technique Listing, *Website Content, 2004,* www.massagetherapy.com/glossary/index.php

NDC Health, *Website Content, 2004,* www.ndchealth.com/

AllRefer Health, *Website Content, 2004,* www.health.allrefer.com/

U.S. Food and Drug Administration, *Website Content, 2004,* www.fda.gov

Centers for Disease Control U.S. Department of Health and Human Services, *Website Content, 2004,* www.cdc.gov

Emedicine Online Resource Center, *Website Content, 2004,* www.emedicine.com

Agency for Healthcare Research and Quality (AHRQ), U.S. Department of Health and Human Services, *Website Content, 2004,* www.guideline.gov/

National Institutes of Health National Library of Medicine, *Website Content, 2004,* www.ncbi.nlm.nih.gov

National Cancer Institute, *Website Content, 2004,* www.cancer.gov

American Cancer Society, *Website Content, 2004,* www.cancer.org/docroot/stt/stt_0.asp

U.S. Board Certified Physicians and Allied Health Professionals, *Website Content, 2004,* www.medicinenet.com/script/main/hp.asp

Web M.D. Health, *Website Content, 2004,* http://my.webmd.com/webmd_today/home/default

Currently Approved Drugs for HIV: A Comparative Chart, Article, Aids Meds.com, *Website Content, 2004,* http://www.aidsmeds.com/lessons/DrugChart.htm

Physicians' Desk Reference, Cerner Multum and Thomson Micromedex Databases, *Website Content, 2004,* www.Drugs.com

National Institute of Neurological Disorders and Strokes, *Website Content, 2004,* www.ninds.nih.gov/index.htm

National Digestive Diseases Information Clearinghouse (NDDIC), *Website Content, 2004,* www.digestive.niddk.nih.gov/index.htm

American Academy of Family Physicians, *Website Content, 2004,* http://familydoctor.org/

Drug Digest Online, *Website Content, 2004,* www.drugdigest.org/DD/Home/

Access Health Information Library, *Website Content, 2004,* www.ehendrick.org/healthy/

PDR Health, *Website Content, 2004,* www.pdrhealth.com/drug_info/index.html

Healthwise Inc, *Website Content, 2004,* www.peacehealth.org/kbase/support/multdisc.htm

Pharmaceutical and Drug Manufacturers, *Website Content, 2004,* www.pharmaceutical-drug-manufacturers.com/index.html

Rx List internet drug index *Website Content, 2004,* www.rxlist.com/cgi/generic/asa_ids.htm

Foley D., Nechas E., Perry S.K., Salmon D.K., *The Doctors Book of Home Remedies for Children,* Bantam Publishers, New York, NY, 1995

Smith, Vickie, Filmmaker Becomes 'Super Size' Crusader for Health, Associated Press, *Website Content, 2004,* www.chron.com/cs/CDA/ssistory.mpl/ae/movies/jump/2570221

Shaw, T.W. Chiropractic rehabilitation of the re-traumatized post-surgical lumbar spine with radiculopathy. *Chiropractic* 1994; 9(4):108–111

Wolff, J. *Das Gesetz der Transformation der Knochen*, Hirschwald, Berlin, 1892, *Website Content, 2004,* http://moon.ouhsc.edu/dthompso/pk/physiol/wolfslaw.htm

Management of Soft Tissue Injury with PRICE, National Electronic Library for Health, *Website Content, 2004* www.nelh.nhs.uk/guidelinesdb/html/fulltext-references/SoftTissueInjury.html

Laurence Rosenberg, MD, Wound Healing, Growth Factors, *Website Content, 2004,* www.emedicine.com/plastic/topic457.htm

Achilles Tendon Strain Article, Running Planet.com *Website Content, 2004,* www.runningplanet.com/articles/article_detail.asp?article_id=734

White and yellow ligaments, Article, Project Skeletal, Website Content, 2004, www.members.tripod.com/projectskeletal/Components.htm

Tishya A. L. Wren, PhD; Gary S. Beaupré, PhD; Dennis R. Carter, Tendon and Ligament Adaptation To Exercise, Immobilization, And Remobilization; *Journal of Rehabilitation Research and Development* Vol. 37 No. 2, March/April 2000

Wren TAL, Carter DR. A microstructural model for the tensile constitutive and failure behavior of soft skeletal connective tissues. *Journal of Biomechanical Engineering*, 1998;120:55 61

HONG, J. Ankle Sprain, Article, *Website Content, 2004,* http://www.cecats.com/topics/anklesprain.html

Lee JM, Warren MP, Mason SM., Effects of Ice on Nerve Conduction Velocity, *Physiotherapy* (1978) 64, 1:2-6

Hot Stone Massage Technique Article, Therapy Stones.com, *Website Content, 2004,* www.selfgrowth.com/articles/TherapyStones1.html

Bynum, D. Petri, V., et. al.; Domestic Hot Water Scald Burn Lawsuits - The Who, What, When, Why, Where How; *Website Content, 2004,* www.tap-water-burn.com/

Hot Tubs - Health And Safety Tips, Ministry of Health Services, November 1993 *Website Content, 2004,* www.bchealthguide.org/healthfiles/hfile27a.stm#E46E243

Baths during Pregnancy, *Website Content, 2004,* www.engenderhealth.org/wh/mch/ppreact.html

Benjamin, B. Neurological Conditions: Polio, Post-Polio and Multiple Sclerosis, *Journal of the American Massage Therapy Association, Website Content, 2004,* www.amtamassage.org/journal/ben2_fall01.html

Tramer MR, Moore RA, Reynolds DJM, McQuay HJ. Quantitative Estimation of Rare Adverse Events Which Follow A Biological Progression: A New Model Applied to Chronic NSAID Use. *Pain* 2000;85:169-182.

James, J: Brochure: Aspirin: Upside/Downside, Do It Now Foundation, 1999, *Website Content, 2004* www.doitnow.org/pages/138.html

Food and Drug Administration, Internal Analgesic, Antipyretic, and Antirheumatic Drug Products for Over The Counter Human Use; Final Rule for Professional Labeling of Aspirin, Buffered Aspirin, and Aspirin in Combination with Antacid Drug Products. *Federal Register.* October 23, 1998; 63:56802-56819.

Introduction to Sports Injuries, Merck Online, *Website Content, 2004,* www.merck.com/mmhe/sec05/ch075/ch075a.html

Behrens, F., Shephard, N., Mitchell, N. Alteration of Rabbit Articular Cartilage By Intra-articular Injection of Glucocorticoids. *Journal of Bone & Joint Surgery*, 1975: 57A:70.

Melmed, E.P. Spontaneous Bilateral Rupture of the Calcaneal Tendon During Steroid Therapy. *Journal of Bone & Joint Surgery* 1965; 47B:104.

Introduction to Sports Injuries, Merck Online, *Website Content, 2004,* www.merck.com/mmhe/sec05/ch075/ch075a.html

Nakajima H. Nippon Yakurigaku Zasshi, 2001 Aug;118(2):117-22, A Pharmacological Profile of Clobazam, A New Antiepileptic Drug, *Website Content, 2004,* www.biopsychiatry.com/clobazam.html

The Leukemia and Lymphoma Society, *Website Content, 2004,* www.leukemia-lymphoma.org

CancerBACUP online, *Website Content, 2004,* www.cancerbacup.org.uk/Cancertype/Lymphomanon-Hodgkins/General/WhatareNHLs

International Union Against Cancer, TNM Prognostic Factors, *Website Content, 2004,* www.uicc.org/tnm/index.shtml

University of Pittsburg Medical Center, *Website Content, 2004,* www.upmccancercenters.com/cancer/prostate/TNMsystem.html

Walton, T.H., Contraindications to Massage Part IV: Clinical Thinking and Cancer, *Massage Therapy Journal* 39(3):66-83, Fall 2000. *Website Content, 2004,* http://www.amtamassage.org/journal/fa_00_journal/cancer_and_massage_1.html

Rosenberg, Laurence MD, Wound Healing Growth Factors Article, *Website Content, 2004,* www.emedicine.com/plastic/topic457.htm

Osteopenia Article, MedicineNet.com, *Website Content, 2004,* www.medterms.com/script/main/art.asp?ArticleKey=8048

Paget's Disease of Bone, Article, CNN.com Health Library, *Website Content, 2004* www.cnn.com/HEALTH/library/DS/00485.html

Degenerative Arthritis, Article, MedicineNet.com, 2004, *Website Content, 2004* www.medicinenet.com/Osteoarthritis/article.htm

Lyme Disease, Article, Pediatric Health Center Online, *Website Content, 2004,* http://ww4.americanbaby.com/ab/pediatrichealth/printIllness.jhtml?illnessid=/templatedata/ab/illness/data/10918.xml

Howard, James F. Jr., M.D., Myasthenia Gravis - A Summary, Myasthenia Gravis Organization, *Website Content, 2004,* www.myasthenia.org/information/summary.htm

Myasthenia Gravis, Article, National Institute of Neurological Disorders and Stroke, *Website Content, 2004* http://www.ninds.nih.gov/health_and_medical/disorders/myasthenia_gravis.htm

Facts About Plasmapheresis, Muscular Dystrophy Association, *Website Content, 2004,* www.mdausa.org/publications/fa-plasmaph.html?NS-search-set=/371cc/aaaa005J41ccc8e&NS-doc-offset=7&

Sharpless, S.K., Goldstein M.: Susceptibility of Spinal Roots to Compression Block, *The Research Status of Spinal Manipulative Therapy*, Monograph #15, Bethesda, MD, 1975, NIH/NINCDS, U.S. Department of Health, Education & Welfare

Ruch W.J., Masarsky C.S., Todres-Masarsky M., *Autonomic Neuroanatomy of the Vertebral Subluxation Complex.* Somatovisceral Aspects of Chiropractic: An Evidence-Based Approach, Churchill Livingstone, New York, 2001

Cole, C., Does Acupuncture or Massage Work in People with Persistent Back Pain? *Journal of Family Practice,* Sept, 2001

Newman PH, Stone KH, The Etiology of Spondylolisthesis. *Journal of Bone and Joint Surgery* 45:39, 1963

Rossi F, Spondylolysis, Spondylolisthesis and Sports. *American Journal of Sports Medicine* 18:317, 1978

Toto, BJ. Chiropractic Correction of Congenital Muscular Torticollis., *Journal of Manipulative and Physiological Therapeutics,* 1993 Oct;16(8):556-9.

Bazner, Hubner, Konig, Selective Peripheral Denervation, Article, *Website Content, 2004* http://www.uni-ulm.de/klinik/neurochirurgie/themend/Torticollis/torticollis.html

NINDS Thoracic Outlet Syndrome Information Page, *Website Content, 2004* www.ninds.nih.gov/health_and_medical/disorders/thoracic_doc.htm

Rayan G.M., Lower Trunk Brachial Plexus Compression Neuropathy Due to Cervical Rib in Young Athletes. *American Journal of Sports Medicine* 16,1988:77-79.

What is Thoracic Outlet Syndrome, Article, S-Healthy Roads Website, *Website Content, 2004* www.healthyroads.com/mylibrary/data/ash_ref/htm/art_whatisthoracicoutletsyndrome.asp

Miller M.D., Wirth M.A., Rockwood C.A. Jr., Thawing the Frozen Shoulder, *Orthopedics,* 1996;19:849-53.

Shin Splints Treatment Exercises, Article, Sports Injury Bulletin, *Website Content, 2004,* www.sportsinjurybulletin.com/archive/1079-shin-splints.htm

Anterior Compartment Syndrome, Article, Sports Injury Clinic.net, *Website Content, 2004,* http://www.sportsinjuryclinic.net/cybertherapist/front/lowerleg/anteriorcompart.htm

Cluett, J., M.D., Growing Pains, Article, *Website Content, 2004,* http://orthopedics.about.com/cs/pediatricsurgery/g/growingpains.htm

Extremity Compartment Syndrome, Article, Richard Paula, MD, Director of Research, Emergency Medicine Residency Program, Tampa General Hospital, *Website Content, 2004,* www.emedicine.com/EMERG/topic739.htm

Nochimson G., MD, Legg-Calve-Perthes Disease, Article, *Website Content, 2004,* www.emedicine.com/emerg/topic294.htm

Joshi, A. MD, Osgood-Schlatter's Disease, Article, *Website Content, 2004,* www.emedicine.com/radio/topic491.htm

Baker's Cyst, Article, Arthritis Victoria, *Website Content, 2004,* http://www.betterhealth.vic.gov.au/bhcv2/bhcarticles.nsf/pages/Baker's_cyst?OpenDocument

Cluett, Jonathan, M.D., Meniscus Tear, *Website Content, 2004,* www.orthopedics.about.com/cs/meniscusinjuries1/a/meniscus.htm

Types of Knee Pain, article by Elizabeth Quinn, *Website Content, 2004* http://sportsmedicine.about.com/cs/knee_injuries/a/aa101000b.htm

Continuous Passive Motion Helps After Knee Repair, Reuters, November 19, 2004, *Website Content, 2004,* www.nlm.nih.gov/medlineplus/news/fullstory_21380.html

Muscular Dystrophy, Article, Integrative Medicine Online, *Website Content, 2004*
www.healthandage.com/html/res/com/ConsConditions/MuscularDystrophycc.html

Muscular Dystrophy, Article, Muscular Dystrophy Association, *Website Content, 2004*,
www.mdausa.org/publications/fa-myosi.html

Polymyositis, Article, The National Institute of Neurological Disorders and Stroke, National Institutes of
Health, *Website Content, 2004*, www.ninds.nih.gov/health_and_medical/disorders/polymyos_doc.htm

Pattekar M.A., MD, MS, Myositis Ossificans, *Website Content*, 2003,
www.emedicine.com/ped/topic1538.htm

Folic Acid, Article, Web MD Health *Website Content, 2004*,
www.my.webmd.com/hw/health_guide_atoz/stf15552.asp?navbar=hw152339

Vitamin B12, Article, Vegetarian Society, *Website Content, 2004*, www.vegsoc.org/info/b12.html

Feied C., MD, Pulmonary Embolism, *Website Content, 2004*,
www.emedicine.com/EMERG/topic490.htm

Deep Vein Thrombosis, Article, MedicineNet Online, *Website Content, 2004*,
www.medicinenet.com/deep_vein_thrombosis/page4.htm

Varicose Veins, Article, National Women's Health Information Center, *Website Content, 2004*,
www.4woman.gov/faq/varicose.htm

High Blood Pressure, Article, American Heart Association, *Website Content, 2004*,
www.americanheart.org/presenter.jhtml?identifier=2112

Heart Disease and Stroke Statistics, 2004 Update, American Heart Association, *Website Content, 2004*
http://www.americanheart.org/downloadable/heart/1079736729696HDSStats2004UpdateREV3-19-
04.pdf

American Stroke Association Statistics, 2004 Update, *Website Content, 2004*
http://www.americanheart.org/downloadable/heart/1079736729696HDSStats2004UpdateREV3-19-
04.pdf

Hurst W., The Heart, Arteries and Veins. 10th ed. New York, NY: McGraw-Hill; 2002, *Website Content,
2004*, http://www.americanheart.org/downloadable/heart/1079736729696HDSStats2004UpdateREV3-
19-04.pdf, page 16

Angiotensin Converting Enzyme Inhibitors, Article, Drug Digest Online, *Website Content, 2004*,
http://www.drugdigest.org/DD/HC/HCDrugClass/0,4055,1-9,00.html

Goldberg D., Fibromyalgia Syndrome: An Emerging but Controversial Condition. *Journal of the
American Medical Association.* 257(20):2782-2787, 1987.

Oster H., MD Can You Have Mono More Than Once, Ivillage Health Online, Website Content, 2004,
http://www.ivillagehealth.com/experts/infectious/qas/0,,229709_175994,00.html

Cates L., M.D., F.A.A.P, What to Expect with Mono, *Website Content, 2004*,
http://www.drspock.com/article/0,1510,6112,00.html

Center for Disease Control, National Center for Infectious Diseases, *Website Content, 2004*,
http://www.cdc.gov/ncidod/diseases/ebv.htm

Cates, Lynn, M.D., F.A.A.P, What to Expect with Mono, *Website Content, 2004*
http://www.drspock.com/article/0,1510,6112,00.html

U.S. Department of Health and Human Services, AIDS Info, *Website Content, 2004*,
http://aidsinfo.nih.gov/other/cbrochure/english/01_en.html

National Institute of Allergy and Infectious Diseases, National Institutes of Health, *Website Content, 2004* http://www.niaid.nih.gov/factsheets/hivinf.htm

Mayo Foundation for Medical Education and Research, *Website Content, 2004* http://www.mayoclinic.com/invoke.cfm?objectid=32278E96-F109-4807-8738841CD620091B&dsection=6

Center for Disease Control: Universal Precautions for Prevention of Transmission of HIV and Other Bloodborne Infections, Published 1987, *Website Content, 2004*, http://www.cdc.gov/ncidod/hip/blood/universa.htm

American Academy of Dermatology, *Website Content, 2004*, http://www.aad.org/pamphlets/Scabies.html

Lice, Article, Martin Memorial Health Systems Health Library Online, *Website Content, 2004* http://www.mmhs.com/clinical/peds/english/derm/lice.htm

Whitley, R.J., Kimberlin, D.W., Roizman B., Herpes Simplex Viruses, *Journal of Clinical Infectious Diseases*, 1998;26:541-55.

What are Plantar Warts, Article, American Podiatric Medical Association, *Website Content, 2004*, http://www.apma.org/topics/Warts.htm

Conjunctivitis, Article, All About Vision Online, *Website Content, 2004*, http://www.allaboutvision.com/conditions/conjunctivitis.htm

Dermatitis, Article, Mayo Foundation for Medical Education and Research, *Website Content, 2004* http://www.mayoclinic.com/invoke.cfm?objectid=24EEAE39-2697-4971-95705ABC4DBBE485&slide=6&isagg=0

Psoriasis Facts, Article, The National Psoriasis Foundation, *Website Content, 2004*, http://www.psoriasis.org/facts/psoriasis/

Scleroderma, Article, The International Scleroderma Network, *Website Content, 2004*, http://www.sclero.org/medical/about-sd/a-to-z.html

Burn Types, Article, Burn Survivor Resource Center, *Website Content, 2004*, http://www.burnsurvivor.com/burn_types.html

Birthmarks, Article, University of Florida Shands Healthcare, *Website Content, 2004*, http://www.shands.org/health/information/article/001440.htm

Bacteria, Article, American Museum of Natural History, *Website Content, 2004*, http://www.amnh.org/nationalcenter/youngnaturalistawards/1998/bacteria.html

Chamberlain N.R., Ph.D., Medical Microbiology, *Website Content, 2004*, http://www.kcom.edu/faculty/chamberlain/Website/studio.htm

Wilson S., Chicken: Is It A Healthier Meat, Article, *Website Content, 2004*, http://www.selene.com/healthlink/chicken.html

Burros, M., Poultry Industry Quietly Cuts Back on Antibiotic Use, New York Times, February 10, 2002, *Website Content, 2004*, http://www.mercola.com/2002/feb/27/antibiotic_poultry.htm

Complex Regional Pain Syndrome Fact Sheet, National Institute of Neurological Disorders and Stroke, *Website Content, 2004*, http://www.ninds.nih.gov/health_and_medical/pubs/rsds_fact_sheet.htm

Cluster Headaches, Article, Drug Digest Online, *Website Content, 2004*, http://www.drugdigest.org/DD/HC/AdditionalContent/0,4054,550114,00.html

Oxygen Therapy For Headaches, Sands, Article, G.H., MD, National Headache Foundation, *Website Content, 2004*, http://www.headaches.org/consumer/topicsheets/oxygen.html

Robert T., Sinus Headache May Be Migraine, American Academy of Neurology Study, *Website Content, 2004*, http://headaches.about.com/cs/diagnosis/a/sinus_migr.htm

Trigeminal Neuralgia, Article, National Institute of Neurological Disorders and Stroke, *Website Content, 2004* http://www.ninds.nih.gov/health_and_medical/disorders/trigemin_doc.htm

Huff J.S., MD, Trigeminal Neuralgia, *Website Content* 2001, http://www.emedicine.com/emerg/topic617.htm

Bell's Palsy, Article, National Institute of Neurological Disorders and Stroke, *Website Content, 2004* http://www.ninds.nih.gov/health_and_medical/disorders/bells_doc.htm

Depression Treatments, Article, Drug Digest Online, http://www.drugdigest.org/DD/HC/Treatment/0,4047,11,00.html

Anxiety Disorders, Article, The National Institute of Mental Health, *Website Content, 2004*, http://www.nimh.nih.gov/publicat/anxiety.cfm#anx7

Obsessive-Compulsive Disorder, Article, Obsessive-Compulsive Foundation, *Website Content, 2004*, http://www.ocfoundation.org/ocf1010a.htm

OCD Defined, Article, OCD Online, *Website Content, 2004*, http://www.ocdonline.com/defineocd.htm

New Fronts in Alzheimer's Research, Article, National Institutes of Health, *Website Content, 2004* http://www.nih.gov/news/WordonHealth/apr2004/alzheimers.htm

Parkinson's Disease, Article, National Parkinson Foundation, *Website Content, 2004*, http://www.parkinson.org/site/pp.asp?c=9dJFJLPwB&b=71117

Amyotrophic Lateral Sclerosis, Article, The ALS Association, *Website Content, 2004*, http://www.alsa.org/als/what.cfm?CFID=217957&CFTOKEN=93621910

Benjamin, B. Neurological Conditions: Polio, Post-Polio and Multiple Sclerosis. *Website Content, 2004*, http://www.amtamassage.org/journal/ben2_fall01.html

Teaching MS Patients to Save Energy Curbs Fatigue, Article, *Reuters Health*, October 6, 2004, *Website Content, 2004*, http://www.nlm.nih.gov/medlineplus/news/fullstory_20524.html

Guillain-Barré Syndrome, Article, Guillain-Barré Syndrome Foundation International, *Website Content, 2004,* http://www.guillain-barre.com/overview.html

Guillain-Barré Syndrome, Article, National Institute of Neurological Disorders and Stroke, *Website Content, 2004*, http://www.ninds.nih.gov/health_and_medical/pubs/guillain_barre.htm

Facts About Plasmapheresis, Article, Muscular Dystrophy Association, *Website Content, 2004*, http://www.mdausa.org/publications/fa-plasmaph.html?NS-search-set=/371cc/aaaa005J41ccc8e&NS-doc-offset=7&

Encephalitis and Meningitis, Article, National Institute of Neurological Disorders and Stroke, *Website Content, 2004*, http://www.ninds.nih.gov/health_and_medical/disorders/encmenin_doc.htm

Gutierrez K.M., MD; Prober C.G., MD, Encephalitis, Postgraduate Medicine Online, *Website Content, 2004*, http://www.postgradmed.com/issues/1998/03_98/guti.htm

Glaucoma, Article, Glaucoma Research Foundation, *Website Content, 2004*, http://www.glaucoma.org/learn/index.html

Influenza Fact Sheet, National Institute of Allergy and Infectious Diseases, National Institutes of Health, *Website Content, 2004* http://www.niaid.nih.gov/factsheets/flu.htm

Tenpenny, S.J., D.O, Risks of FluMist Vaccine, *Website Content,* 2004, http://www.mercola.com/2003/oct/4/flumist_vaccine.htm

Mercola, J., D.O., Flu Shot Demand Rises Sharply But Don't Be Fooled, *Website Content, 2004,* http://www.mercola.com/2003/dec/6/flumist.htm

American Lung Association, *Website Content, 2004,* http://www.lungusa.org/site/pp.asp?c=dvLUK9O0E&b=35873

Sinusitis Article, MedicineNet Online, *Website Content, 2004,* http://www.medicinenet.com/sinusitis/page1.htm

Chronic Obstructive Pulmonary Disease, Article, National Institutes of Health COPD Online, *Website Content, 2004* http://www.nlm.nih.gov/medlineplus/copdchronicobstructivepulmonarydisease.html

COPD Fact Sheet, American Lung Association, *Website Content, 2004,* http://www.lungusa.org/site/pp.asp?c=dvLUK9O0E&b=35020

Asthma and Allergy Fact Sheet, American Academy of Allergy, Asthma and Immunology, *Website Content, 2004* http://www.aaaai.org/patients/resources/fastfacts/allergies.stm

American Lung Association, *Website Content, 2004,* http://www.lungusa.org/site/pp.asp?c=dvLUK9O0E&b=35691

Tuberculosis, Article, National Institutes of Health, Department of Health & Human Services, *Website Content, 2004,* http://www.nlm.nih.gov/medlineplus/tuberculosis.html

Tuberculosis, Article, American Lung Association, *Website Content, 2004,* http://www.lungusa.org/site/pp.asp?c=dvLUK9O0E&b=35778

Feied C., MD, Pulmonary Embolism, *Website Content, 2004,* http://www.emedicine.com/EMERG/topic490.htm

Crude and Age-Adjusted Prevalence of Diagnosed Diabetes per 100 Population, United States, 1980-2002, United States Centers for Disease Control and Prevention, *Website Content, 2004,* http://www.cdc.gov/diabetes/statistics/prev/national/figage.htm

National Diabetes Education Program, U.S. National Institutes of Health, *Website Content, 2004* http://www.ndep.nih.gov/diabetes/youth/youth_FS.htm

Diabetic Coma: When Blood Sugar Extremes Aren't Treated, Article, Mayo Clinic Online Diabetes Center, *Website Content, 2004,* http://www.mayoclinic.com/invoke.cfm?id=DA00022

Mathur R., M.D., Hypoglycemia, Low Blood Sugar & Diabetes: How Low Can You Go, *Website Content, 2004* http://www.medicinenet.com/script/main/art.asp?articlekey=19679

Williams D., MD, Hypoglycemia: The Deadly Roller Coaster, *Website Content, 2004,* http://www.hypoglycemia.org/hypo.asp

Hyperthyroidism and Graves' Disease, Article, MedicineNet Online, *Website Content, 2004,* http://www.medicinenet.com/hyperthyroidism/article.htm

Graves' Disease, National Graves' Disease Foundation, *Website Content, 2004,* http://www.ngdf.org/faq.htm

Manifold C.A., DO, Hyperthyroidism, Thyroid Storm, and Graves' Disease, *Website Content,* 2002 http://www.emedicine.com/emerg/topic269.htm

Orlander P.R., MD, Hypothyroidism, *Website Content, 2004,* http://www.emedicine.com/MED/topic1145.htm

Myxedema, Article, EcureMe.com, *Website Content, 2004*,
  http://www.ecureme.com/emyhealth/data/Myxedema.asp

Rowland D.L., Burnett A.L., Pharmacotherapy in the Treatment of Male Sexual Dysfunction. *Journal of Sex Research*, 2000; 37(3):226-230

Clark A.D, MD, Dysmenorrhea, *Website Content, 2004* http://www.emedicine.com/emerg/topic156.htm

Dysmenorrhea, Article, Mayo Foundation for Medical Education and Research, *Website Content, 2004*
  http://www.mayoclinic.com/invoke.cfm?id=DS00506

Abbuhl S., MD, Pelvic Inflammatory Disease, *Website Content, 2004*
  http://www.emedicine.com/EMERG/topic410.htm

Endometriosis, Article, The Endometriosis Association, *Website Content, 2004*,
  http://www.endometriosisassn.org/endo.html

Endometriosis, Article, the Mayo Clinic Online, *Website Content, 2004*,
  http://www.mayoclinic.com/invoke.cfm?id=DS00289

Golladay E.S., MD, Abdominal Hernias, *Website Content, 2004*,
  http://www.emedicine.com/med/topic2703.htm

Inguinal Hernia Repair, article, British United Provident Association, *Website Content, 2004*,
  http://hcd2.bupa.co.uk/fact_sheets/mosby_factsheets/inguinal_hernia.html

Umbilical Hernia, Article, EcureMe Online, *Website Content, 2004*
  http://www.ecureme.com/emyhealth/Pediatrics/Umbilical_Hernia.asp

Gastroesophageal Reflux After Distal Gastrectomy: Possible Significance of the Angle of His, *American Journal of Gastroenterology*. 1998 Jan;93(1):11-5.

Prostate Enlargement: Benign Prostatic Hyperplasia, Article, National Kidney and Urologic Diseases Information Clearinghouse, *Website Content, 2004*,
  http://kidney.niddk.nih.gov/kudiseases/pubs/prostateenlargement

Gastroesophageal Reflux Disease, Article, GERD Information Resource Center, *Website Content, 2004*,
  http://www.gerd.com/

Shayne P., MD, Gastritis and Peptic Ulcer Disease, *Website Content, 2004*,
  http://www.emedicine.com/EMERG/topic820.htm

Helicobacter Pylori and Peptic Ulcer Disease, Article, Centers for Disease Control and Prevention, *Website Content, 2004* http://www.cdc.gov/ulcer/

Peptic Ulcer Disease, Article, MedicineNet.com, *Website Content, 2004*,
  http://www.medicinenet.com/peptic_ulcer/article.htm

Crohn's Disease Article Lori Kam, M.D., MedicineNet.com, *Website Content, 2004*
  http://www.medicinenet.com/crohns_disease/article.htm

Celiac Sprue Association, *Website Content, 2004*, http://www.csaceliacs.org/celiac_defined.php

Ulcerative Colitis, Article, National Institute of Diabetes and Digestive and Kidney Diseases, National Institutes of Health, *Website Content, 2004*, http://digestive.niddk.nih.gov/ddiseases/pubs/colitis/

Kazzi A.A., MD, Diverticular Disease, *Website Content, 2004*,
  http://www.emedicine.com/EMERG/topic152.htm

Diverticulosis and Diverticulitis, Article, National Institute of Diabetes and Digestive and Kidney Diseases, National Institutes of Health, *Website Content, 2004*, http://digestive.niddk.nih.gov/ddiseases/pubs/diverticulosis/#2

Appendicitis and Appendectomy, Article, MedicineNet.com, *Website Content, 2004*, http://www.medicinenet.com/appendicitis/article.htm

Cates L., M.D., F.A.A.P., What To Expect With Mono, *Website Content, 2004*, http://www.drspock.com/article/0,1510,6112,00.html

Viral Hepatitis, Article, National Institute of Diabetes and Digestive and Kidney Diseases, National Institutes of Health, *Website Content, 2004* http://digestive.niddk.nih.gov/ddiseases/pubs/viralhepatitis/index.htm#hepa

The ABC's of Hepatitis, Hepatitis Foundation International, *Website Content, 2004*, http://www.hepfi.org/living/liv_abc.html

Santen S., MD, Cholelithiasis, *Website Content, 2004*, http://www.emedicine.com/EMERG/topic97.htm

Cirrhosis, Article, National Institute of Diabetes and Digestive and Kidney Diseases, National Institutes of Health, *Website Content, 2004*, http://digestive.niddk.nih.gov/ddiseases/pubs/cirrhosis/

Kidney Stones, Article, National Institute of Diabetes and Digestive and Kidney Diseases, National Institutes of Health, *Website Content, 2004* http://kidney.niddk.nih.gov/kudiseases/pubs/stonesadults/

Terris, MK, Issa, MM, Tacker JR., Dietary Supplementation With Cranberry Concentrate Tablets May Increase The Risk Of Nephrolithiasis., *Urology*. 2001 Jan;57(1):26-9

McHarg, T., Rodgers, A. & Charlton, K., Influence of Cranberry Juice on the Urinary Risk Factors for Calcium Oxalate Kidney Stone Formation. *British Journal of Urology International* 2003 92 (7), 765

Pyelonephritis in Adults, Article, National Institute of Diabetes and Digestive and Kidney Diseases, National Institutes of Health, *Website Content, 2004*, http://kidney.niddk.nih.gov/kudiseases/pubs/pyelonephritis/

Urinary System Review, Article, National Institute of Diabetes and Digestive and Kidney Diseases, National Institutes of Health, *Website Content, 2004*, http://kidney.niddk.nih.gov/kudiseases/pubs/yoururinary/#4

Interstitial Cystitis, Article, *Website Content, 2004*, http://www.urologychannel.com/interstitialcystitis/index.shtml

Kidney Failure, Article, Mayo Foundation for Medical Education and Research, *Website Content, 2004* http://www.mayoclinic.com/invoke.cfm?objectid=9E510C36-F9F7-4E3B-A7054C1D1F942043&dsection=1

Kidney Failure, Article, MedicineNet.com, *Website Content, 2004*, www.medicinenet.com/kidney_failure/article.htm

Morbidity and Mortality Weekly Report, News release, CDC., Oct. 8, 2004; vol 53: pp 918-920. *Website Content, 2004* http://my.webmd.com/content/article/95/103177.htm

Index

Botox, 115, 383, 405
Botulinum Toxin Type A, 115
Botulism, 405
BOW, 383
Bowel, 405
Bowen Technique, 17
BP, 383
BPH, 331–32
BPM, 383
BPP, 383
BR, 383
brach., 383
Bradycardia, 405
bradykinesia, 261, 405
Brain Cancer, 60
Brain damage, 406
Brain death, 406
Bravelle, 337
Breaking your back, 89
Breast Cancer, 60
Breema Bodywork, 18
Brethaire, 306
Brevibloc, 176
Bricanyl, 306
brimonidine, 288
brinzolamide, 286
Brittle Bone Disease, 84
Brodspec, 233
bromazepam, 56
bromocriptine, 284
bromodiphenhydramine, 304
brompheniramine, 304
Bronchiolitis, 406
Bronchitis, 406
bronchitis, acute, 293
bronchitis, chronic, 294–95
Bronchoconstrictor, 406
Bronchodilator, 406
bronchogenic cancer, 61
Bronchospasm, 406
Brondelate, 310
Bronkodyl, 310
BroveX, 304
BRP, 383
Brufen, 39
Bruise, 218, 406
Bruxism, 406
BS, 383
BSA, 383
BsL, 383
BT, 384

BTE, 384
BTU, 384
BTW, 384
Buc, 384
budesonide, 43, 308
BUE, 384
Bufferin, 41
bulging disc, 108
Bulimia, 406
bull's eye rash, 95
Bulla, 406
bumetanide, 181
Bumex, 181
Bunion, 406
bupivacaine, 46
Buprenex, 49
buprenorphine, 49
bupropion, 275
BUQ, 384
Burn, First-Degree, 217
Burn, Second-Degree, 217
Burn, Third-Degree, 217
Burns, 217
Bursa, 406
Bursitis, 124, 406
Buscopan, 76, 281
BuSpar, 274
buspirone, 274
busulfan, 73
busulphan, 74
butabarbital, 48
Butace, 49
Butacote, 39
Butalan, 48
butalbital, 49
Butazone, 39
Butisol, 48
butorphanol, 49
butterfly rash, 99–100
BV, 384
BW, 384
Bx., 384
Bypass, 406
c, 384
C, 384
C & S, 384
C., 384
c.m., 384
c.v., 384
c/o, 384
C/O, 384
C1 - C7, 384
Ca, 384

CA, 384
cabergoline, 341
CABG, 384
Cachexia, 406
CAD, 113–14, 151, 384
CADASIL, 259
Caelyx, 78
Caf., 384
Cafatine, 53
Cafergot, 53
Cafetrate, 53
caffeine, 310
Cal, 384
Calan, 177
Calcaneal Periostitis, 139–40
Calcification, 407
Calcimar, 342
calcinosis, 215
calcipotriene, 198
calcitonin, 342, 407
calcium bilirubinate, 362
calcium carbonate, 365
calcium channel blockers, 176–77
Caldecort, 45
Calel-D, 365
callous, 87
Callous formation, 407
callus, 209, 407
Calm-X, 76
Calmydone, 304
Calmylin, 304
Calorie, 407
Caltrate, 365
Campath, 74
Campto, 74
Camptosar, 74
Canadian Deep Muscle Massage, 16
Canal, 407
Canasa, 50
Cancer, 57, 407
Cancer Staging and Grading, 62
Cancer, Causes of, 58
Cancer, Skin, 224–26
candesartan, 172
Candida, 407
Candidiasis, 407
Canker sore, 407
Cantil, 281
Cap, 384
capecitabine, 74

NOTES

NOTES

NOTES

NOTES

NOTES

Quick Order Form

There are a number of convenient ways to order additional copies of *The Essential Massage Companion*. Visit our website at www.theEssentialMassageCompanion.com for an online order form, or Email the information below to order@ConceptsBorn.com. Just dial (248) 891-9116 to be connected with a real, live, friendly person who would be happy to take your order by phone.

You can mail this form to: Concepts Born, llc
                              Attn: Order Department
                              PO Box 721335-701
                              Berkley, MI 48076-0335
                              USA

Please send _____ copies of *The Essential Massage Companion*,
ISBN: 0-9749258-0-2

(We respect your privacy and will never sell, rent or share this information.)

Name: _____

Address: _____ Apt # _____

City: _____ State/Province: _____

Zip/Postal Code: _____ Country: _____

Telephone: _____

Email Address: _____

Sales Tax: We must add 6% for products shipped to Michigan addresses.

Payment: (circle one)   Visa   MasterCard   American Express   Personal Check

Card Number: _____ Exp. Date: _____

Name on card: _____

For current prices and shipping charges, please call us at (248) 891-9116 and we will be happy to help you, or visit our website at www.theEssentialMassageCompanion.com.

Free Stuff Online!

Did you notice how few internet links were inside the book? That's because they're all free and constantly updated at **www.theEssentialMassageCompanion.com**

- ✓ Take the online Quiz (Hint: It's an Open-Book test!)

- ✓ Link to The Essential Internet Reference Guide for dozens of internet reference sites.

- ✓ Read about others like you in our Success Story section.

- ✓ Sign our Guestbook – tell us what you like best, what you like least, or maybe what you think the next edition should include. Tell us your story!

- ✓ Write the Author! DrBryan@ConceptsBorn.com

Visit **theEssentialMassageCompanion.com** today.